Keto Diet
Book for Beginners

1200 Quick & Easy Keto Recipes and 4-Week Meal Plan for Everyone

Soledad Bruce

Table of Contents

Chapter 4 Poultry Mains 42

Chapter 5 Fish and Seafood 56

Introduction

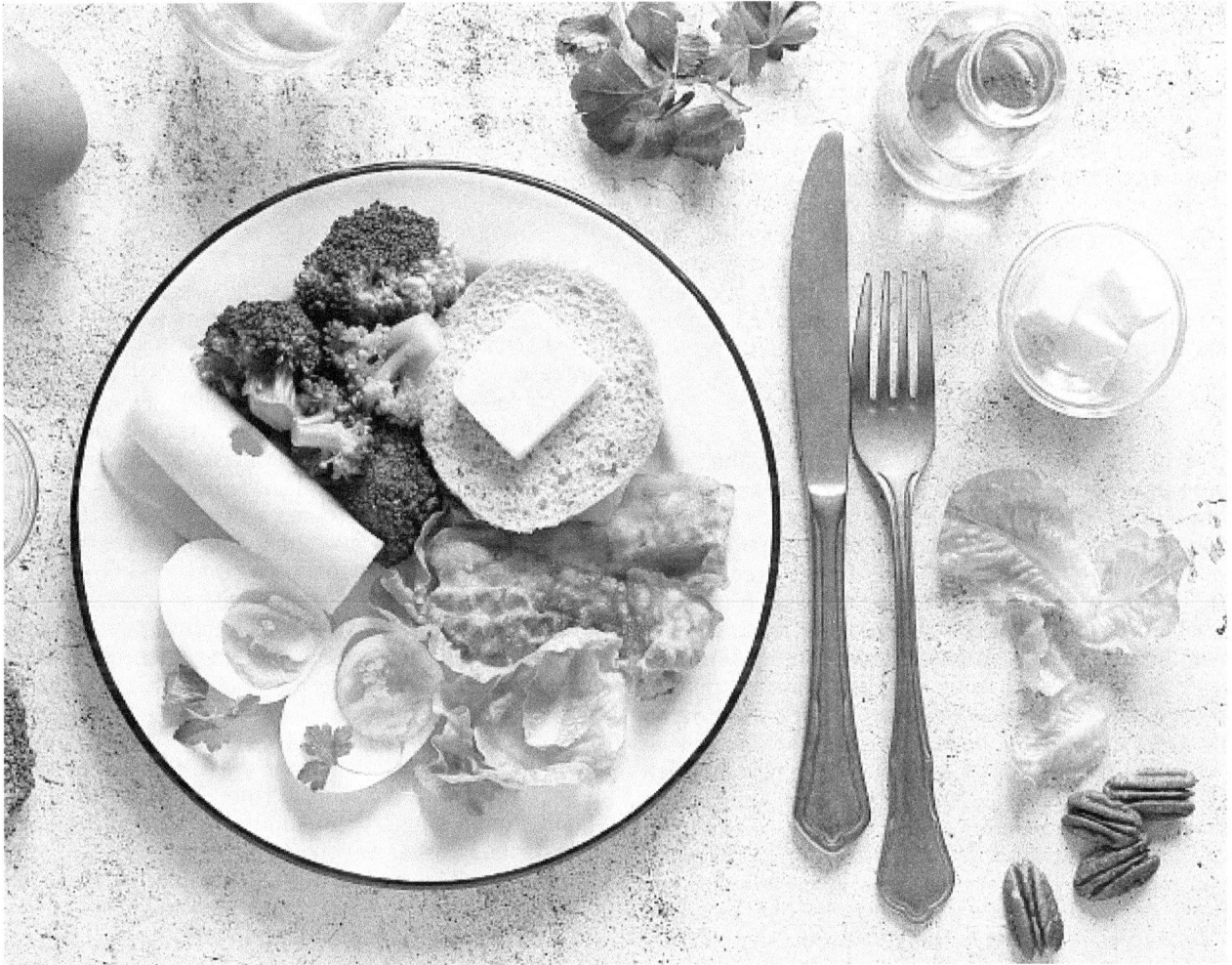

With the rise in the number of incurables diseases, obesity, and other health complexities, we all need to rethink our eating habits and bring about a difference in the daily intake of food. Thankfully, many experts have carried out research in this regard and discovered the rightful impact of food on the human body. Specialized diets are now being created to achieve the desired results. There are a number of ways to help improve health, your body immune system and metabolism. A ketogenic diet is one diet which offers all through the decreased intake of carbohydrates. There are many misperceptions that exist around the use of fats and carbohydrates, and through the text of this cookbook, we shall know how we can use fats for our own health advantage and shun the use of carbohydrates to avoid a variety of health problems. The ketogenic diet is all about cutting down your carb intake and taking a shift towards more use of fats. Along with a comprehensive ketogenic diet introduction, this cookbook will present a bunch of nutritious and luscious recipes to help you get started.

The ketogenic diet offers a solution to such a problem as it offers carb-restricted alternatives for a daily meal. According to this diet, the number of carbs per meal should not exceed 20 grams. Lesser the carbs and higher the fats; this is the standard guideline for a ketogenic diet. Excess fats allow better ketosis in the body. A process which is used to produce energy through the breakdown of fat molecules, releasing ketones and a high amount of energy.

The ketogenic diet came as a breakthrough in the field of nutritional sciences as it busted all the prevailing myths and misassumptions regarding the use of fats and carbohydrates. It basically challenged the existing norms and practices and propagated the idea of a carb-free lifestyle. Carbohydrates are known as an instant and cheapest source of energy, and even today, many millions of people rely on carb-rich food to meet their energy needs. However, the ketogenic diet provided an alternative which was earlier never thought of. The diet offers fats as a good and lasting means of energy, and when they are consumed in the absence of carbs, they can actually prove to be healthier.

History of the Ketogenic Diet

The rise of the ketogenic diet dates back to the 1920 to 1930s as a food therapy for epilepsy, a brain-related disease. Unlike other medicated treatments, ketogenic diet worked due to its long-lasting impact. It emerged as a good alternative to fasting, which was earlier used to treat epilepsy. But the idea of keto therapy soon faced failure due to a lack of research and extensive use of medications.

However, in 1921, Rollin Woodyatt revived the idea of the ketogenic diet and brought its benefits back into the spotlight when is spotted the three important compounds being produced in the bodies of those who either fast or eat low-carb and high-fat diet. Soon Russel Wilder termed such a diet "Ketogenic" due to its known effects of producing a high amount of ketones in the body. From that point on, the concept of ketosis prevailed. It was, however, got to the public attention as late as 1997 when Charlie Abraham's epilepsy was treated through the use of a complete Ketogenic Diet plan. The interest of the scientific community and ordinary individuals in the study of ketogenic study came to the rise by 2007; the idea spread to up to 45 countries around the world. People actively sought this diet plan not only to treat specific diseases but also to reduce weight and avoid cardiovascular disease.

The Phases of the Ketogenic Diet:

The dietary changes never come with quick results. Our body always takes enough to process the change and then work accordingly. Switching from a carb-dependent lifestyle to a low-carb one is one huge change for our bodies. That is why the ketogenic diet's result appears after at least three to four weeks. The early time period is utilized by the body to adapt to the changes, get into ketosis, and maintain sufficient energy levels. And once the ketosis is initiated and you have completely switched to the ketogenic diet, the real challenge starts from there! And then comes the next stage. A dieter experiences different effects on the body during these phases. So, here is how you can divide the whole keto journey!

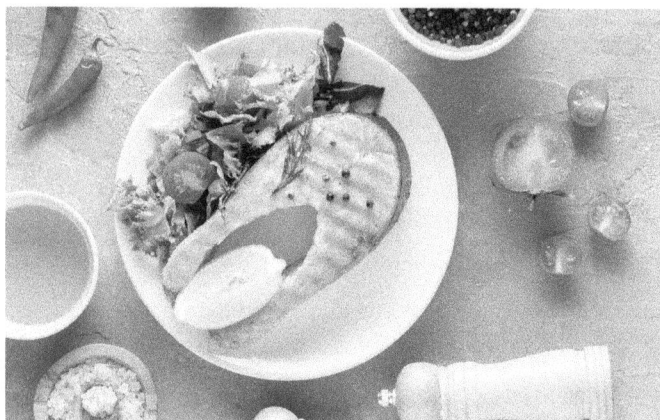

Stage 1: Getting into Ketosis

The first and primary goal of the ketogenic diet is to kick-start ketosis. So, the first phase only begins when you manage to initiate this process in the body. We have gone through all the ways to start ketosis. Let me just tell you how it will turn out for you in this first phase. Initially, it takes extra effort to force your liver to produce ketones. It is only possible when you burn and deplete the existing glycogen reserves. And that is the challenging part. Because to do so, you need to abandon all the carbs and adopt an active lifestyle to burn more calories every day. The phase is difficult, and some people even experience a condition known as "Keto Flu." The dieter may experience mild discomfort during this phase, but with determination, strong will, and an expert's opinion, he can get through this part once the dieter gets over this keto flu or the feeling of discomfort that marks the end of phase 1.

How to Get through Phase 1:

There are certain things that can make it easier for the dieter to get through this challenging time. Firstly, it is important to stay hydrated all the time. Add more fluids to the diet, and drink as much water as you can.

Since you will be having a lot of cravings for sugar or fast food, you can satisfy your craving by eating fresh berries and avocados in between meals. In this way, you can control your caloric intake as well.

To avoid developing an electrolyte imbalance in the body, add more minerals to your diet. Eat leafy green vegetables and low-carb juicy veggies to consume magnesium, potassium, and phosphorous.

Lastly, if you are not familiar with the keto substitutes and their taste, then it is best not to use them at this stage. Start with basic low-carb recipes that you already know and like in taste. Remember, the goal of this phase is to get you one step closer to the ketogenic lifestyle. So, if there is anything that can put you off track, you should probably avoid it.

Stage 2: Keto-Adaption

Once your body switches to ketosis for energy production, the keto-adaption phase starts. Up till now, the body only has taken a turn to ketogenesis to produce ketones and release energy, but it takes a little while for other systems and organs to start working on this new fuel. In this phase, the other parts of the body learn to live on ketosis. So, in this phase, you will need to do everything that will help each and every cell to metabolize according to the new lifestyle. During this phase, all those symptoms of ketosis that a person feels during the early days start to disappear. And he will start feeling better. A new positive energy kicks in, which makes the keto dieter feel more active and alive. Unlike the 'getting into ketosis' phase, the keto-adaptation is not short-lived; it all depends on your body and your effort. It can take a minimum of four weeks to even months to make yourself fully flexible. But once you get through this part, living on the ketogenic diet gets pretty easier.

The human body longs for stability, routine, and balance, and it makes that happen through homeostasis. So, when you externally change the conditions or dietary factors, the body gradually starts changing according to it, and a point comes when it fully moulds itself according to those changes. And that's what actually happens during this phase. So, to make your body more flexible to the keto lifestyle, you need to be strategic about your carb intake. Unlike the first phase, now you need to periodically shift in and out of ketosis. This will make your body more flexible to change. It will help to instantly switch to the available source of energy to meet its need. This is the phase in which adding a few carbs to the diet might not affect the metabolism. But this has to be done carefully in an organized manner. Here is how you can do it.

Carb Cycling

In the carb cycling technique, you can have some good quality carbs once a week. Select a day and pick some healthy carb sources like whole grains and sweet potatoes to have on this cheat day. By refeeding carbs once in a while, you can refill the depleted glycogen reserves in the muscles, and that can help strengthen them.

On this cheat day, you can eat roughly about 15-25 per cent of protein, 60-70 per cent of carbohydrates, and 15 per cent of fats in the diet. Whereas for the rest of the week, you need to get back on track and should only eat a low-carb diet. Remember that during this carb-cycling process, the quality of the carbohydrates is important. Yes, you can have some carb-rich fruits and vegetables on this day, but this day is not an excuse to stuff yourself with a pizza, cakes, or ice cream. Only enjoy low-sugar whole foods like whole grains, sweet potatoes, starchy vegetables, lentils and legumes, and berries.

Targeted Keto Diet

This technique is suitable for those who regularly carry out high-intensity exercises. The diet and the carbohydrate intake are then adjusted around the workout schedule. So, instead of carb cycling on a random, once-in-a-week basis, in this approach, you can get to have carbs on the day of your exercise. In this way, all the excess calories will be used by the muscles. A dieter can have up to 50 grams of carbohydrates about 30 minutes before the exercise. Unlike the cyclic ketogenic diet, in this approach, you need to look for simpler and refined carbs. So that they are broken down instantly, and the energy is then utilized by the muscle cells.

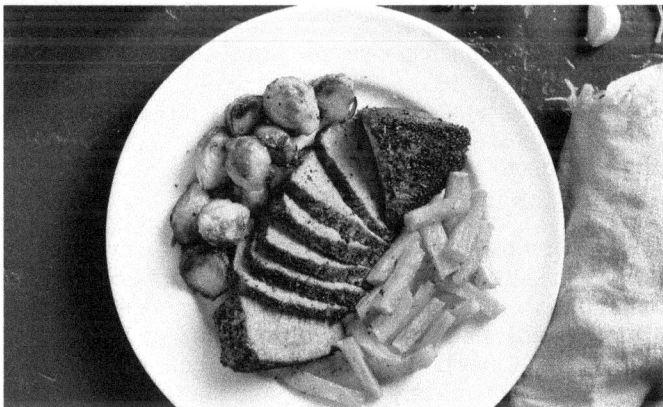

But set a limit to this intake and avoid over-consumption. This practice is only to provide a temporary break to your body from ketosis.

How you manage the keto-adaption period depends on your lifestyle. No matter which approach you select for yourself, remember that this going in and out of ketosis is as crucial as the diet itself in order to reach metabolic flexibility. At the end of the keto-adaption phase, you will start noticing prominent changes in your health, from weight to body mass index, your focus, attention span, memory, metabolism, everything gets better.

Stage 3: Metabolic Flexibility

The last of the ketogenic transition is termed the phase of metabolic flexibility. It is the time when your body overcomes all the challenges and actually masters the art of keto-adaptation. By this time, your body gets more flexible in adjusting itself according to the given fuel source. Now it knows how to work best through ketosis and how to use it for its own advantages. It also learns to adjust its metabolic pathways according to the energy source available, whether it's fat or glucose as a fuel. So now you don't need to stay strictly Keto all the time. You can continue with the carb-cycling while being on the ketogenic diet. Add exercise, healthy fats, and keto supplements to maintain the rate of ketosis in the body.

Even if you mistakenly consume some grains or carbs during this phase, your body won't even respond to it as it is adjusted itself to run on fat-sourced energy. However, a person can also lose metabolic flexibility when he starts eating a high-carb diet again on a regular basis. So, even when you are on a cyclic ketogenic diet, make sure to continue eating healthy and keep the balance of the nutrients in between the two consecutive keto-eating periods.

The Ketosis Process

The word ketosis comes from the word "ketone," it is described as the process during which fats are broken in the body to produce energy and Ketones. A high level of ketosis means a greater amount of ketones. In the absence of complex carbohydrates, the fats are forced to break down and produce ketones which are highly beneficial for active metabolism. To make this all happen, a special meal plan is required, known as the "Ketogenic diet." It describes a sum whole of all the eatables which are low in carbs and high in fats. Thus allowing the body to extract energy directly from fats and not from glucose. The diet plan is prescribed to treat a number of diseases like diabetes, epilepsy, obesity, and heart problems. However, there are certain complexities related to this diet, and it should always be opted with the guidance of a professional nutritionist, at least at the beginning when it is essential to learn about the basics of ketosis and the right approach to switch to a ketogenic balanced diet.

Potential Benefits of Ketogenic Diet

Being smart about our diet and health is the need of the hour. In today's ever-busy lifestyle quality of food and diet is greatly compromised. Thus having a good diet plan is crucial to maintain our health and prevent fatal diseases. There are many known benefits of the ketogenic diet that most of us are unaware of. From better mental condition to improved health, the diet plan has proven to be miraculous in effect.

Diabetes and Cholesterol Control

Sugar control is important for patients with type 2 diabetes, and Keto is complete abstention from sugars. Instead, special sweeteners are used to maintain the flavor. The diet is also effective in controlling the cholesterol level in the body.

Weight Loss

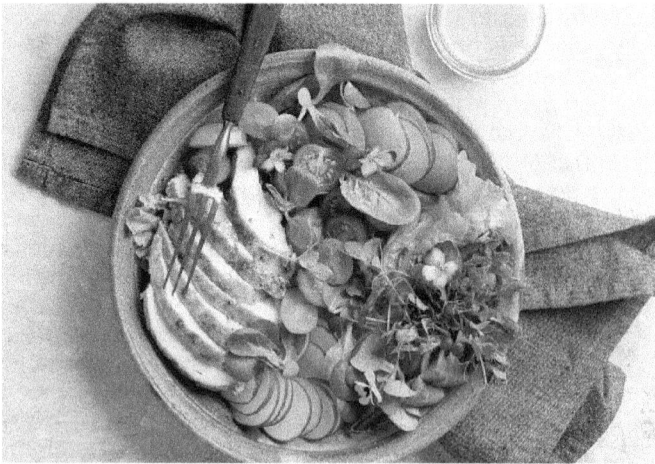

Weight loss is one of the major reasons many people opt for a ketogenic diet. And studies have proved that it does allow greater weight reduction in a much easier way.

Sound Mental Health

Ketones are knowns as the fuel for the mind, and ketosis ensures the production of ketones in a large amount in the body. Lesser intake of carbohydrates means an increased concentration of ketones.

Seizure Treatment

As the Ketogenic diet originally emerged to treat epileptic patients; it is known to control seizures or help to reduce them to some extent. Especially in children, it is effective alongside medications.

Controlled Blood Pressure

As a ketogenic diet helps to maintain high levels of triglyceride in the body, it is also effective in controlling blood pressure and cholesterol levels. This, in turn, saves us from many fatal diseases, like cardiovascular diseases

Reduced Skin Problems

For people having skin problems, especially acne, this diet is one good solution. In the absence of complex carbohydrates, there is minimal production of toxins in the blood, thus keeping our skin healthy and acne free.

What to Have on a Ketogenic Diet:

To make things simple and easier, let's break it down a little and try to understand the Keto vegetarian diet plan as a chart explaining what to have and what not to have. Down below is a brief list of all the items which can be used on a Ketogenic vegetarian diet.

Meat of All Types

There is no restriction on meat for a keto diet. Whether it is poultry, beef, pork, lamb or seafood, the meat of all kinds can be freely enjoyed on a keto diet, as they don't contain any extra carbs or sugars.

Vegetables

Keep in mind that not all vegetables are low on carbs. There are some who are full of starch, and they need to be avoided. A simple technique to access the suitability of the vegetables for a keto diet is to check if they are 'grown above the ground' or 'below it.' All vegetables which are grown underground are a no go for Keto, whereas vegetables which are grown above are best for Keto, and these mainly include cauliflower, broccoli, zucchini, etc.

Green Vegetables:

Among the vegetables, all the leafy green vegetables that can be added to this diet include spinach, kale, parsley, cilantro, etc.

Seeds and Dry Nuts

Nuts and seeds like sunflower seeds, pistachios, pumpkin seeds, almonds, etc., can all be used on a ketogenic diet.

Keto Fruits

Not all berries are Keto-friendly; only choose blackberries or raspberries and other low-carb berries. Similarly, not all fruits can be taken on a keto diet; avocado, coconut, etc., are Keto-friendly, whereas orange, apples, pineapple, etc., are high in carbohydrates.

Vegetable Fats

Following oils and fats can be used on a ketogenic diet: olive oil, coconut oil, palm oil, etc.

Dairy Products

Not every dairy product is allowed on a keto diet. For example, milk is a no-go for Keto, whereas hard cheeses, high-fat cream, butter, eggs, etc., can all be used.

Keto Sweeteners

As sugar is strictly forbidden for a ketogenic diet, may it be brown or white, there is a certain substitutes which can be used like stevia, erythritol, monk fruit, and other low-carb sweeteners.

Foods to Avoid on a Ketogenic Diet:

Avoiding carbohydrates is the main aim of following a ketogenic diet. While most vegetarians may take the following food items on a regular basis but they are considered keto-friendly. In fact, any amount of these items drastically increases the carbohydrate value of your meal. So it is best to avoid their use completely.

Sugar

Besides white and brown sugar, there are other forms of it which are also not keto-friendly; this list includes honey, agave, maple syrup, etc. Also, avoid chocolates which are high in sugar. Use special sweeteners and sugar-free chocolates only.

Legumes

Legumes are also the underground parts of the plants. Thus they are highly rich in carbohydrates. Make no mistake about using them in your diet. These include all sorts of beans, from Lima to chickpeas, Garbanzo, black, white, red beans, etc. cross all of them off your grocery list if you are about to go Keto. All types of lentils are also not allowed on a keto diet.

Grains

All types of grains are high in carbohydrates, whether it's rice or corn or wheat. And product extracted from them is equally high in carbs, like corn flour, wheat flour or rice flour. So while you need to avoid these grains for Keto, their flours should also be avoided. Coconut and almond flours are good substitutes for that.

Dairy

As stated above, not all dairy products can be freely used on a ketogenic diet. Animal milk should be strictly avoided.

Fruits

Certain fruits need to be avoided while on a keto diet. Apples, bananas, oranges, pineapples, etc., all fall into that category. Do not use them in any form. Avoid using their flesh, juice, and mash to keep your meal carb-free.

Tubers

Tubers are basically underground vegetables, and some of them are rich in carbs, including potatoes, yams, sweet potatoes, beets, etc.

Steps to Follow Before Going Keto!

Are you still planning to achieve all your health goals by giving this ketogenic diet a try? Then there is a certain thing that must need to do before actually starting with the diet. And if you recommend this diet to others as well, try to share these 5 basic steps to help them get started easily. Whenever it's the dietary changes, you need to work on the

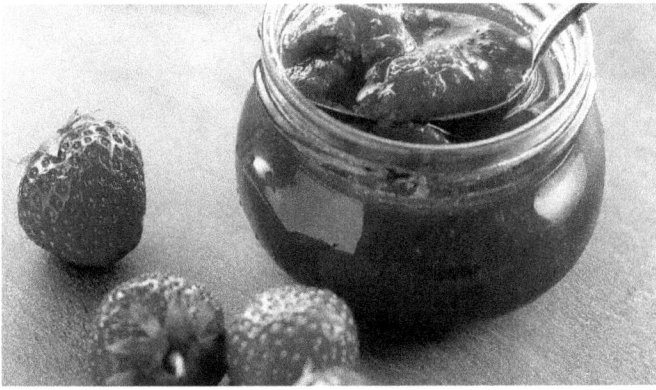

foundation first. In the case of the ketogenic diet, we have to fight against our long hold belief that carbs are friendly and fats are real enemies. So, it is difficult to stand against that unless you have a sound foundation and strongly believe in the science behind this diet. To do so, try doing the following things:

1.Do Your Research.

Reading this book is also your part of the research, but it is essential to learn every possible thing about the ketogenic diet through a number of sources. It is mainly to convince your mind and body about the effectiveness of the diet. Moreover, you must take a new start with a clear and well-aware mind. When you leave certain ambiguities in your mind and start practicing the new dietary regime, you are bound to make mistakes. Your research should include reading books and articles on the ketogenic diet, talking to health experts, asking about people's experiences with the diet, and discussing things with your dietician. And remember, never stop yourself from asking questions. When it comes to a diet as complicated as the ketogenic diet, the more you ask, the easier it will get for you to adapt to the ketogenic lifestyle.

2.Consult your Health Experts.

Then comes the point where you need to ask your health expert, like a personal physician or any doctor, whether you can switch to this diet. This may include a complete medical checkup. You must know what your body mass index is, what is blood sugar level normally, and during fasting, your triglyceride levels if there is any medical condition, etc. If the doctor suggests any special preferences or considerations for you to follow while being on this diet, then follow them accordingly.

3.Analyze your Health Problems.

Once you are aware of your existing health condition, start preparing according to it. For instance, if you have a very high body mass index, then you will need a rigorous exercise regime along with the ketogenic diet. Some people may need to resort to intermittent fasting along with the ketogenic diet to achieve the required level of ketosis in a quick time. So, listen to your body closely and respond according to your body's demands. If there are things that are recommended on the ketogenic diet, but you don't like them, then cross them off the list, at least for the early days of the diet. Set the pace of the change according to your own level of acceptance.

4.Find a Good Ketogenic Meal Plan

The next step is to find yourself a good ketogenic meal plan. By good, we can say that the meal plan should offer all the other nutrients in a balanced amount and in accordance with the ketogenic formula. It is not necessary to ask a meal planner to draw your diet plan; you can even do it yourself. But initially, it may be troublesome to look into all the keto-friendly ingredients and manage them in your diet, so ask

help from your dietician to create at least a three-week keto meal plan for you so that you can get started with it.

5.Get Rid of High Carb Food

The last basic step of the pre-diet regime is to remove all the carb-rich ingredients from your life. If you are living alone, then it will be easy to simply remove them from your home, but if you are living with your family, then asks them to keep the high-carb ingredients hidden from you or out of your sight so that you may not get distracted. Start eliminating the obvious carb-rich ingredients like fast food, desserts, flours, grains, sweets, candies, other processed food products, etc.

Tips to Succeed on the Keto Diet

The keto lifestyle, known for its low-carb and high-fat diet, will present you several health benefits, including weight loss, control of blood glucose levels, regulating metabolism, and prevention of serious conditions like diabetes, insulin resistance, epilepsy, and Alzheimer's, to name a few. Switching to a new fat-dependent lifestyle from carb dependent one is never easy. So here we bring you some basic principles and hacks to go Keto with ease:

Reduce Your Carbohydrates Intake.

It is only the absence of carbohydrates that can initiate ketosis in the body. And to achieve the state of ketosis, a dieter must consume less than 50 grams of carbohydrates in a day. To cut down the carb intake, the keto dieter needs to omit all the high-carb ingredients from his diet, like potatoes, yams, squash, sugar, milk, grains, legumes, etc. While doing so, he must replace the carb-rich ingredients with fat-rich ones like cheese, creams, butter, vegetable oil, and shortenings to keep the energy levels high.

Count the Calories.

The calorie count is the only parameter that can keep you on track. By practicing the habit of reading the food labels, a person can learn more about the nutritional values of the food and can better ensure if the food is suitable for health.

Keep Track of Your Macros.

Carbohydrates, proteins, and fats together make the most of the food we eat. Since carbs are not really an option on the ketogenic diet, their reduced intake must be balanced by the higher intake of fats and proteins. To do so, a dieter must also keep an eye on his macro intake.

Monitor Your Progress.

Whether you are achieving the claimed benefits of the keto diet or not, it is difficult without monitoring the progress. Constantly check your weight and body mass index to keep track of your progress.

Maintain Electrolyte Balance.

When you are on a ketogenic diet, frequent urination and increased hydrolysis during ketosis can lead to electrolyte imbalance in the body. This needs to be prevented by consuming more minerals and vitamins through food, drinks, and supplements.

Stay Hydrated All the Time.

Since ketosis can lead to loss of water from the body, it is important to keep yourself hydrated all the time. Constantly rink low carb, zero caloric drinks, or water on this diet.

Listen to Your Appetite.

Eating all the time is not going to help, especially when you are struggling to lose weight through your ketogenic diet. It is always recommended to eat only when your body shows clear signs of hunger. Avoid falling for your false alarms and cravings.

Prep Your Meal.

When you plan and prepare your meal beforehand, you can ensure a 100 per cent low carb diet. You can remove all the unwanted high-carb ingredients from your kitchen and

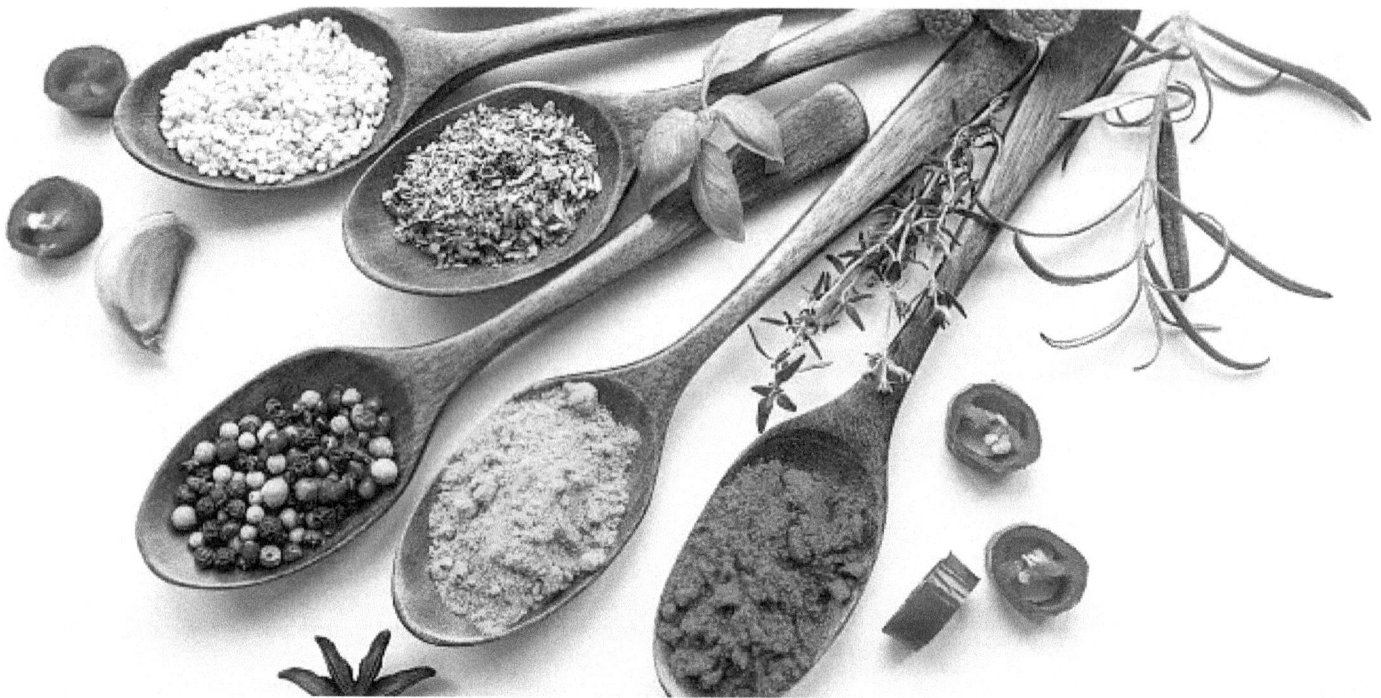

fridges and stuff them with healthy low-carb alternatives.

Look Out for Keto Flu.

Since switching to ketosis to run its metabolism is a major shift for the human body, it may show some symptoms like dizziness, weakness, headache, dry mouth, bad smells, etc. The condition is termed keto flu, and it can be prevented by drinking more water, eating rich low-carb food, and carrying out routine exercises.

Frequently Asked Questions

How to calculate daily carb intake?

Whenever you follow a recipe, look for its contents and the nutritional value available with the recipe. If it is not available, look for online nutrition calculators which enable you to calculate the nutritional value within a few minutes.

Do I need to count calories? Do calories matter?

Keeping track of caloric intake is important as it directly relates to weight gain. Whether on a low-carb diet or on a high one, it is necessary to keep a check on the calories.

Is there any difference between a low-carbohydrate diet and a ketogenic diet?

A low carbohydrate diet is a general term used to describe any diet containing 130 to 150 grams of the total. However, ketogenic diets are the subset of this general diet plan. It further restricts the number of carbohydrates to minimum levels and, at the same time, requires an increased intake of fat. Thus a ketogenic diet plan is more specific than a low carbohydrate plan.

After how much time does ketosis start to take place?

If you are a person of discipline and routine, then it usually takes 2 to 3 days to start a keto routine. However, it is a gradual process and goes through different stages. Exercise helps boost the speed of the process. For people with sedentary lifestyles, it can also take weeks.

What kind of dairy products is Keto-friendly?

Not all dairy products are keto-friendly, as raw dairy products are rich in carbohydrates. But those fermented or processed lose their carbohydrates and are good to use; these include butter, cheese, and yogurt.

Are fruits allowed on a ketogenic vegetarian diet?

Yes, fruits with low amounts of carbohydrates, like coconut, strawberries, raspberries, avocado, etc., are allowed. This list also includes tomato, which is also a keto-friendly fruit. However, fruits which are high in sugar should be avoided.

Can I use sugars?

No, sugars are strictly forbidden on a ketogenic diet. Sugars can, however, be replaced with special sweeteners available in the markets. Using sweeteners is a tricky part of the ketogenic diet. While there are many available in the market, there are few that are mostly used, like stevia, erythritol, swerve, etc. These sweeteners are a good substitute for any sugar when used in the right proportion. As the sweetness of these sweeteners varies, always compare the proportions and then add them to the recipe.

What kinds of fermented food products are allowed on a ketogenic diet?

Products like sauerkraut, plain yogurt, kombucha, and kimchi, are all fermented, and they are also Keto friendly. They help in better digestion and strengthen the immunity system of the body due to the large number of probiotics present in them. Their regular intake is vital for active metabolism.

Are peanuts allowed?

Not all legumes are non-ketogenic; peanuts are one of them. There is a great misconception that peanuts can't be taken on a keto diet, but it is clearly not true as they are low on carbs and high in fats. When taken in small amounts, they do not disrupt the balance of the ketogenic diet.

Is "ketosis" dangerous for human health?

There is no proven evidence which could suggest that ketosis is dangerous. Many people confuse ketosis with ketoacidosis; the latter is a health problem which only occurs in patients with diabetes type 1. During ketoacidosis, the ketone level in the blood exceeds a critical value. Ketosis, on the other hand, is completely normal and doesn't pose any danger to a person's health.

Aren't high-fat diets unhealthy? Isn't eating so much fat going to make me fat?

Most of us believe that high fats are unhealthy, but it is nothing but a myth. Fats can only be unhealthy if taken with a high amount of carbohydrates. However, when taken with low carbs or no carbs, these fats become a direct and active source of energy for the body. They easily break down and release essential compounds, including ketones.

4 Weeks Meal Plan

Week-1

Day 1:

Breakfast: Bacon Fritters
Lunch: Smashed Cauliflower
Snack: Pretzel Bites with Sauce
Dinner: Garlic Steak
Dessert: Espresso Cream

Day 2:

Breakfast: Jelly with Almond Butter
Lunch: Sweet Pepper Nachos
Snack: Ranch Chicken Bites
Dinner: Citrus-Marinated Tilapia
Dessert: Best Attempt Rice Pudding

Day 3:

Breakfast: Tasty Denver Eggs
Lunch: Cheesy Broccoli Sticks
Snack: Buffalo Cauliflower Bites
Dinner: Creamy Tangy Chicken
Dessert: Chocolate Chip Fat Bomb

Day 4:

Breakfast: Meatballs
Lunch: Roasted Asparagus
Snack: Fried Ranch Pickles
Dinner: Corn Dogs
Dessert: Strawberry Milkshake

Day 5:

Breakfast: Egg Cups with Jalapeno
Lunch: Crab Rangoons
Snack: Crispy Salami Roll-Ups
Dinner: Beef with Broccoli
Dessert: Blueberry Ice Cream

Day 6:

Breakfast: Kale Kiwi Smoothie
Lunch: Zucchini Boats
Snack: Bacon Cauliflower Skewers
Dinner: Coconut Saffron Mussels
Dessert: Chocolate Truffles

Day 7:

Breakfast: Low-Carb Pancakes
Lunch: Trot Mushroom Salad
Snack: Crispy Deviled Eggs
Dinner: Grandma Bev's Ahi Poke
Dessert: Sweet Iced Tea

Week-2

Day 1:

Breakfast: Zucchini Egg Bake
Lunch: Asparagus Fries
Snack: Pepperoni Chips
Dinner: White Chicken Casserole
Dessert: Strawberries Coconut Whip

Day 2:

Breakfast: Egg Casserole
Lunch: Garlic Spinach Stir-Fry
Snack: Broccoli and Carrot Bites
Dinner: Spicy Kung Pao
Dessert: Creamy Coconut Brownies

Day 3:

Breakfast: Meatballs with Apple Chutney
Lunch: Creamed Spinach
Snack: Creamy Salami Pinwheels
Dinner: Pan-Fried Tilapia
Dessert: Chocolate Macaroons

Day 4:

Breakfast: Deviled Mayo Eggs
Lunch: Oven-Safe Baking Dishes
Snack: Charcuterie Board
Dinner: Soy-Ginger Steak Roll-Ups
Dessert: Peanut Butter Bars

Day 5:

Breakfast: Ricotta Sausage Pie
Lunch: Dijon Roast Cabbage
Snack: Cheeseburgers
Dinner: Roast Beef
Dessert: Chocolate Almonds

Day 6:

Breakfast: Bacon Fritters
Lunch: Crispy Green Beans
Snack: Hot Chili-Garlic Wings
Dinner: Corn Dogs
Dessert: Snicker Bites

Day 7:

Breakfast: Green Citrus Smoothie
Lunch: Cauliflower Pizza Crust
Snack: Classy Crudités with Dip
Dinner: Pork Ribs
Dessert: Strawberry Milkshake

Day 1:

Breakfast: Zucchini Egg Bake
Lunch: Cauliflower Pizza Crust
Snack: Bacon Asparagus
Dinner: Grandma Bev's Ahi Poke
Dessert: Nuts Squares

Day 2:

Breakfast: Sausage Stuffed Peppers
Lunch: Spicy Bacon Cheeseburger Soup
Snack: Delicious Devil Eggs
Dinner: Chicken Piccata
Dessert: Chocolate Coconut Torts

Day 3:

Breakfast: Potato-Crusted Frittata
Lunch: Nutty Kale Tilapia
Snack: Popcorns
Dinner: Crab Fried Rice
Dessert: Nutty Chocolate Milkshake

Day 4:

Breakfast: Breakfast Pizza
Lunch: Simple Fish Curry
Snack: Crispy Wings
Dinner: Shredded Chicken
Dessert: Strawberry Cheesecakes

Day 5:

Breakfast: Avocado Breakfast Tacos
Lunch: Tuna Casserole
Snack: Red Pepper Edamame
Dinner: Loaded Taco Soup
Dessert: Delicious Chocolate Lava Cake

Day 6:

Breakfast: Bacon Fritters
Lunch: Crab Fried Rice
Snack: Ants On a Log
Dinner: Chicken Bacon Chowder
Dessert: Coconut Nut Cookies

Day 7:

Breakfast: Mushroom Quiche
Lunch: Pan-Fried Tilapia
Snack: Bake Kale Chips
Dinner: Grandma Bev's Ahi Poke
Dessert: Chocolate Coconut Torts

Day 1:

Breakfast: Whey Waffles
Lunch: Chili Haddock with Vegetables
Snack: Cheesy Hangover Homies
Dinner: Mac & Cheese Stew
Dessert: Nutty Chocolate Fudge

Day 2:

Breakfast: Kale Kiwi Smoothie
Lunch: Delicious Jerk Chicken
Snack: Delicious Caprese Skewers
Dinner: White Chicken Chili
Dessert: Healthy Almond Cookies

Day 3:

Breakfast: Low-Carb Pancakes
Lunch: Delicious Turkey Meatloaf
Snack: Broccoli and Carrot Bites
Dinner: Carnitas
Dessert: Delicious Swoop Cream

Day 4:

Breakfast: Morning Doughnuts
Lunch: Herbed Roasted Chicken
Snack: Bacon Cauliflower Skewers
Dinner: Tuna Casserole
Dessert: Caramel Macchiato

Day 5:

Breakfast: Mushroom Cream Crepes
Lunch: Oven-Fried Catfish
Snack: Spicy Turkey Meatballs
Dinner: Coconut Chicken
Dessert: Piña Colada

Day 6:

Breakfast: Egg Casserole
Lunch: Citrus-Marinated Tilapia
Snack: Chipotle Lime Kale Chips
Dinner: Keto Crusted Lamb Chops
Dessert: Hibiscus Tea

Day 7:

Breakfast: Mexican Breakfast Casserole
Lunch: Citrus-Marinated Tilapia
Snack: Ranch Chicken Bites
Dinner: Lemon Pork
Dessert: Chocolate Chip Cookies

Jelly with Almond Butter

Prep time: 5 minutes| Cook time: 0 minutes| Serves: 1

¼ teaspoon almond extract
10 drops liquid stevia
1 teaspoon vanilla extract
2 tablespoons unsweetened creamy almond butter
½ tablespoon milled golden flaxseed

⅛ teaspoon sea salt
1 cup ice cubes
1 teaspoon sugar-free strawberry jam
1 cup plain unsweetened almond milk

1. Add almond milk, almond butter, flaxseed, vanilla extract, almond extract, stevia and salt to the blender and puree until smooth. 2. Add ice cubes and pulsate to thicken and cream, squeeze as needed. 3. Pour into a glass, stir in the strawberry jam and serve immediately.
Per Serving: Calories 277; Fat 22g; Sodium 551mg; Carbs 13g; Fiber 4g; Sugar 3g; Protein 9g

Tropical Blackberry Coconut

Prep time: 5 minutes| Cook time: 0 minutes| Serves: 1

⅔ cup canned unsweetened full-fat coconut milk
¼ cup frozen blackberries
1 cup ice cubes
⅛ teaspoon sea salt

10 drops of liquid stevia
¾ teaspoon vanilla extract
½ tablespoon milled golden flaxseed
¼ teaspoon coconut extract

1. Add the coconut milk, flaxseed, vanilla extract, coconut extract, salt, and stevia to a blender and process until smooth. 2. Add the frozen blackberries and ice cubes and pulse until thick and creamy, tamping down as necessary. 3. Pour into a glass and serve immediately.
Per Serving: Calories 344; Fat 34g; Sodium 314mg; Carbs 9g; Fiber 4g; Sugar 2g; Protein 4g

Traditional Blackberry Mojito

Prep time: 5 minutes| Cook time: 0 minutes| Serves: 1

1 sprig mint
¼ cup water
1 tablespoon MCT oil
14 drops of liquid stevia

¼ cup frozen blackberries
1 tablespoon fresh lime juice
1 teaspoon fresh lime zest
½ cup crushed ice

1. Add the oil, lime juice, lime zest, stevia, mint, and water to a blender and process until smooth. 2. Add the frozen blackberries and ice, and pulse until thick and creamy, tamping down as necessary. 3. Pour into a glass and serve immediately.
Per Serving: Calories 136; Fat 14g; Sodium 4mg; Carbs 5g; Fiber 2g; Sugar 2g; Protein 1g

Breakfast Blueberry Cheesecake

Prep time: 5 minutes| Cook time: 0 minutes| Serves: 1

12 drops liquid stevia
1-ounce cream cheese
¼ teaspoon vanilla bean paste
⅛ teaspoon sea salt
¼ cup heavy whipping cream
½ cup water

¼ cup frozen blueberries
½ teaspoon milled golden flaxseed
1 teaspoon vanilla extract
1 cup ice cubes

1. Add the cream cheese, cream, water, flaxseed, vanilla extract, vanilla bean paste, salt, and stevia to a blender and process until smooth. 2. Add frozen blueberries and ice cubes and mix to thicken and cream, squeeze as needed. 3. Pour into a glass and serve immediately.
Per Serving: Calories 347; Fat 32g; Sodium 400mg; Carbs 10g; Fiber 1g; Sugar 8g; Protein 4g

Blueberry Lemon Drink

Prep time: 5 minutes| Cook time: 0 minutes| Serves: 1

14 drops liquid stevia
¼ cup water
1 tablespoon MCT oil
1 teaspoon fresh lemon zest

¼ cup frozen blueberries
½ cup crushed ice
¼ teaspoon vanilla extract
1 tablespoon fresh lemon juice

1. Add the oil, lemon juice, lemon zest, stevia, water, and vanilla extract to a blender and process until smooth. 2. Add the frozen blueberries and ice, and pulse until thick and creamy, tamping down as necessary. 3. Pour into a glass and serve immediately.
Per Serving: Calories 144; Fat 14g; Sodium 4mg; Carbs 7g; Fiber 1g; Sugar 4g; Protein 0g

Tangy Citrus Matcha

Prep time: 5 minutes| Cook time: 0 minutes| Serves: 1

⅛ teaspoon sea salt
10 drops of liquid stevia
1 teaspoon fresh lemon zest
½ teaspoon fresh lemon juice
⅔ cup canned unsweetened full-fat coconut milk

1 teaspoon fresh lime zest
½ tablespoon milled golden flaxseed
¾ teaspoon powdered matcha
1 cup ice cubes

1. Add coconut milk, flaxseed, matcha, lime peel, lemon peel, lemon juice, salt, and stevia to the blender and puree until smooth. 2. Add ice cubes and pulsate to thicken and creamy. 3. Pour into a glass and serve immediately.
Per Serving: Calories 322; Fat 34g; Sodium 314mg; Carbs 6g; Fiber 3g; Sugar 0g; Protein 5g

Dark Chocolate Matcha

Prep time: 5 minutes| Cook time: 0 minutes| Serves: 1

1 teaspoon vanilla extract
¼ teaspoon fresh lemon juice
⅛ teaspoon sea salt
⅔ cup canned unsweetened full-fat coconut milk
1 tablespoon unsweetened cocoa

powder
½ tablespoon milled golden flaxseed
1 cup ice cubes
¾ teaspoon powdered matcha
12 drops liquid stevia

1. Add coconut milk, cocoa powder, flaxseed, matcha, vanilla extract, lemon juice, salt, and stevia to the blender and process until smooth. 2. Add ice cubes and pulsate to thicken and creamy. 3. Pour into a glass and serve immediately.
Per Serving: Calories 359; Fat 35g; Sodium 315mg; Carbs 9g; Fiber 4g; Sugar 1g; Protein 6g

Breakfast Chocolate Chip Muffins

Prep time: 5 minutes| Cook time: 15 minutes| Yields: 6 muffins

1 tablespoon baking powder
½ cup low-carb chocolate chips
1½ cups blanched finely ground almond flour

2 large eggs, whisked
4 tablespoons salted butter, melted
⅓ cup granular brown erythritol

1. In a large bowl, combine all ingredients. Evenly pour batter into six silicone muffin cups greased with cooking spray. 2. Put the muffin cups in the basket of the air fryer. Set the temperature of air fryer to 320°F/160°C and timer to 15 minutes. When the muffins are ready, they turn golden. 3. Let muffins cool in cups for 15 minutes to avoid crumbling. Serve warm.
Per Serving (1 muffin): Calories 329; Fat 29g; Sodium 328mg; Carbs 28g; Fiber 8g; Sugar 1g; Protein 10g

Breakfast Blueberry Muffins

Prep time: 5 minutes| Cook time: 15 minutes| Yields: 6 muffins

2 teaspoons baking powder
1½ cups blanched finely ground almond flour
2 large eggs, whisked

⅓ cup fresh blueberries, chopped
½ cup granular erythritol
4 tablespoons salted butter, melted

1. In a large bowl, combine all ingredients. Evenly pour batter into six silicone muffin cups greased with cooking spray. 2. Put the muffin cups in the basket of the air fryer. Set the temperature of air fryer to 320°F/160°C and timer to 15 minutes. When the muffins are ready, they turn golden. 3. Let muffins cool in cups for 15 minutes to avoid crumbling. Serve warm.
Per Serving (1 muffin): Calories 269; Fat 24g; Sodium 165mg; Carbs 23g; Fiber 3g; Sugar 2g; Protein 8g

Traditional Spice Muffins

Prep time: 5 minutes| Cook time: 15 minutes| Yields: 6 muffins

1 cup blanched finely ground almond flour	1 large egg, whisked
2 tablespoons salted butter, melted	1 teaspoon ground allspice
	¼ cup granular erythritol
	2 teaspoons baking powder

1. In a large bowl, combine all ingredients. Evenly pour batter into six silicone muffin cups greased with cooking spray. 2. Put the muffin cups in the basket of the air fryer. Set the temperature of air fryer to 320°F/160°C and timer to 15 minutes. When the muffins are ready, they turn golden. 3. Let muffins cool in cups for 15 minutes to avoid crumbling. Serve warm.

Per Serving (1 muffin): Calories 160; Fat 14g; Sodium 123mg; Carbs 20g; Fiber 2g; Sugar 1g; Protein 5g

Bacon, Egg, With Cheese Calzones

Prep time: 15 minutes| Cook time: 12 minutes| Serves: 4

1 cup blanched finely ground almond flour	bacon, crumbled
2 ounces cream cheese, softened and broken into small pieces	2 cups shredded mozzarella cheese
4 slices of cooked sugar-free	2 large eggs

1. Beat eggs in a small bowl. Pour into a medium nonstick pan over medium heat and scramble. Set aside. 2. In a large microwave-safe bowl, mix flour and mozzarella. Add cream cheese to the bowl. 3. Microwave it for 45 seconds to dissolve the cheese, then stir with a fork until a soft ball of dough forms. Place the parchment paper in air fryer basket. Separate dough into two sections and press each out into an 8" round. 4. Place half of the scrambled eggs and crumbled bacon on half of each dough round. 5. Fill the other side of the dough and press to close the sides. 6. Place the dough pockets on unlubricated parchment and in an air fryer basket. Set the air fryer's temperature to 350°F/177°C and set the timer to 12 minutes, turning the dough pockets back in the middle of cooking. The crust will be golden and firm. 7. Let calzones cool on a cooking rack 5 minutes before serving.

Per Serving: Calories 477; Fat 35g; Sodium 665mg; Carbs 10g; Fiber 3g; Sugar 3g; Protein 28g

Tasty Denver Eggs

Prep time: 5 minutes| Cook time: 15 minutes| Serves: 2

¼ teaspoon salt	2 tablespoons peeled and chopped yellow onion
¼ teaspoon ground black pepper	1 tablespoon salted butter, melted
3 large eggs	¼ cup seeded and chopped green bell pepper
¼ cup chopped cooked no-sugar-added ham	

1. Crack eggs into an ungreased 6" round nonstick baking dish. Mix in butter, bell pepper, onion, ham, salt, and black pepper. 2. Place the dish in the air fryer's basket. Set the temperature of air fryer to 320°F/160°C and timer to 15 minutes. The eggs will be fully cooked and firm in the middle when done. 3. Slice in half and serve warm on two medium plates.

Per Serving: Calories 201; Fat 14g; Sodium 650mg; Carbs 3g; Fiber 1g; Sugar 1g; Protein 13g

Classic Cinnamon Rolls

Prep time: 10 minutes| Cook time: 20 minutes| Yields: 12 rolls

½ cup confectioners' erythritol	2 ounces cream cheese, softened
1 tablespoon ground cinnamon	½ teaspoon vanilla extract
2½ cups shredded mozzarella cheese	1 cup blanched finely ground almond flour

1. In a bowl, combine mozzarella cheese, cream cheese, and flour. Microwave the cheese mixture on high for 90 seconds until the cheese is melted. 2. Add vanilla extract and erythritol to the cheese mixture, and mix 2 minutes until a dough forms. 3. Once the dough is cool to work with your hands, for about 2 minutes, spread it out into a 12" × 4" rectangle on ungreased parchment paper. Evenly sprinkle the dough with cinnamon. 4. Roll the dough into a log. Slice the log into twelve even pieces. 5. Divide rolls between two ungreased 6" round nonstick baking dishes. Place one dish into the air fryer basket. Set the temperature to 375°F/191°C and the timer for 10 minutes. 6. When rolls are firm and golden from the edges, its done. Repeat with the second cinnamon roll dish. Allow rolls to cool in dishes 10 minutes before serving.

Per Serving (1 roll): Calories 145; Fat 10g; Sodium 177mg; Carbs 10g; Fiber 1g; Sugar 1g; Protein 8g

Cheesy Eggs with Bell Peppers

Prep time: 10 minutes| Cook time: 15 minutes| Serves: 4

3 ounces chopped cooked no-sugar-added ham	removed, seeded
¼ cup peeled and chopped white onion	1 cup shredded mild Cheddar cheese
4 large eggs	1 tablespoon coconut oil
4 green bell peppers, tops	½ teaspoon salt

1. Place peppers upright into an ungreased air fryer basket. Drizzle each pepper with coconut oil. Divide ham and onion evenly among peppers. 2. In a medium bowl, whisk eggs, then sprinkle with salt. Pour mixture evenly into each pepper. Top each with ¼ cup Cheddar. 3. Set the temperature of air fryer to 320°F/160°C for 15 minutes. Peppers will be tender, and eggs will be firm when done. 4. Serve warm on four medium plates.

Per Serving: Calories 281; Fat 18g; Sodium 767mg; Carbs 8g; Fiber 2g; Sugar 4g; Protein 18g

Egg Cups

Prep time: 10 minutes| Cook time: 15 minutes| Serves: 4

3 tablespoons salted butter, melted	and diced
¼ teaspoon salt	½ cup chopped fresh spinach leaves
¼ teaspoon onion powder	2 cups 100% liquid egg whites
½ medium Roma tomato, cored	

1. Whisk egg whites with butter, salt, and onion powder. Stir in tomato and spinach, then pour evenly into four 4" ramekins greased with cooking spray. 2. Place ramekins into the air fryer basket. Set the temperature to 300°F/149°C and the timer for 15 minutes. Eggs will be fully cooked and firm in the center when done. Serve warm.

Per Serving: Calories 146; Fat 8g; Sodium 416mg; Carbs 1g; Fiber 0g; Sugar 0g; Protein 14g

Healthy Spinach Omelet

Prep time: 5 minutes| Cook time: 12 minutes| Serves: 2

¼ teaspoon salt	yellow onion
4 large eggs	½ cup shredded mild Cheddar cheese
1½ cups chopped fresh spinach leaves	2 tablespoons salted butter, melted
2 tablespoons peeled and chopped	

1. In an ungreased 6" round nonstick baking dish, whisk eggs. Stir in spinach, onion, butter, Cheddar, and salt. 2. Place dish into air fryer basket. Set the temperature of air fryer to 320°F/160°C and the timer for 12 minutes. Omelet will be done when browned on the top and firm in the middle. 3. Slice in half and serve warm on two medium plates.

Per Serving: Calories 368; Fat 28g; Sodium 722mg; Carbs 3g; Fiber 1g; Sugar 1g; Protein 20g

Cheesy Keto "Hash Browns"

Prep time: 30 minutes| Cook time: 24 minutes| Serves: 6

1 large egg	½ cup shredded sharp Cheddar cheese
1 (12-ounce) steamer bag cauliflower, cooked according to package instructions	2 ounces 100% cheese crisps
	½ teaspoon salt

1. Let cooked cauliflower cool for 10 minutes. 2. Place cheese crisps into a food processor and pulse on low for 30 seconds until crisps are finely ground. 3. Using a kitchen towel, wash excess moisture from cauliflower and place it into the food processor. 4. Add egg to the food processor and sprinkle with Cheddar and salt. Pulse five times until the mixture is mostly smooth. 5. Prepare the air fryer basket with parchment paper. Separate mixture into six scoops and place three on each piece of ungreased parchment, keeping at least 2" of space between each scoop. Press each into a hash brown shape, about ¼" thick. 6. Place one batch on parchment into the air fryer basket. Set the temperature of air fryer to 375°F/191°C for 12 minutes, turning hash browns halfway through cooking. Hash browns will be golden brown when done. Repeat with the second batch. 7. Allow 5 minutes to cool. Serve warm.

Per Serving: Calories 120; Fat 8g; Sodium 390mg; Carbs 3g; Fiber 1g; Sugar 1g; Protein 8g

Cheesy Cheddar Soufflés

Prep time: 15 minutes| Cook time: 12 minutes| Serves: 4

¼ teaspoon cream of tartar
3 ounces cream cheese, softened
½ cup shredded sharp Cheddar
cheese
3 large eggs, whites, and yolks
separated

1. Beat egg whites with ¼ teaspoon cream of tartar until soft peaks form, about 2 minutes. 2. In a separate bowl, beat egg yolks, Cheddar, and cream cheese together until frothy, about 1 minute. Add egg yolk mixture to whites, gently folding until combined. 3. Pour mixture evenly into four 4" ramekins greased with cooking spray—place ramekins into air fryer basket. Set the temperature to 350°F/177°C and the timer for 12 minutes. When done, eggs will be browned on the top and firm in the center. Serve warm.
Per Serving: Calories 183; Fat 14g; Sodium 221mg; Carbs 1g; Fiber 0g; Sugar 1g; Protein 9g

Keto Pancakes

Prep time: 10 minutes| Cook time: 5 to 10 minutes| Serves: 4

1 cup almond flour
¼ cup full-fat, plain yogurt
½ cup fresh blueberries
4 large eggs
1 teaspoon cream of tartar
¼ cup coconut oil, melted
½ teaspoon baking soda
1 teaspoon vanilla extract
¼ cup sugar substitute
Additional coconut oil to grease the pan

1. Whisk the eggs until frothy in a bowl. In a separate bowl, mix the almond flour, sugar substitute, baking soda, and cream of tartar until well combined. 2. Stir the vanilla extract and the melted coconut oil into the eggs. 3. Add the dry ingredients to the wet and mix well. 4. Grease a large pan with a teaspoon of coconut oil and spoon 2–3 small pancakes for every serving. 5. Cook on medium for about 5 minutes until the pancake firm up. Flip and cook the other side for about a minute. 6. Cook pancake for about 5 minutes until firm up. Flip and cook the other side for about a minute. Top each serving of pancakes with yogurt and berries. 6. Serve and enjoy!
Per Serving: Calories 368; Fat 33g; Sodium 412mg; Carbs 9g; Fiber 3g; Sugar 2g; Protein 12g

Cheesy Bacon Quiche

Prep time: 5 minutes| Cook time: 12 minutes| Serves: 2

3 large eggs
2 tablespoons heavy whipping cream
4 slices of cooked sugar-free
bacon, crumbled
½ cup shredded mild Cheddar cheese
¼ teaspoon salt

1. Whisk eggs, cream, and salt until combined. Mix in bacon and Cheddar. 2. Pour mixture evenly into two ungreased 4" ramekins. Place into air fryer basket. Set the temperature of air fryer to 320°F/160°C and the timer for 12 minutes. Quiche will be fluffy and set in the middle when done. 3. Let quiche cool in ramekins for 5 minutes. Serve warm.
Per Serving: Calories 380; Fat 28g; Sodium 971mg; Carbs 2g; Fiber 0g; Sugar 1g; Protein 24g

Meatballs

Prep time: 10 minutes| Cook time: 15 minutes| Serves: 6

½ cup shredded sharp Cheddar cheese
1 pound ground pork breakfast sausage
¼ teaspoon ground black pepper
1 large egg, whisked
½ teaspoon salt
1-ounce cream cheese softened

1. Combine all ingredients in a large bowl—form the mixture into eighteen 1" meatballs. 2. Place meatballs into an air fryer basket. Select the temperature to 400°F/205°C and the timer for 15 minutes, shaking the basket three times during cooking. Meatballs will be browned on the outside and have an internal temperature of at least 145°F/63°C when thoroughly cooked. Serve warm.
Per Serving: Calories 288; Fat 24g; Sodium 742mg; Carbs 1g; Fiber 0g; Sugar 1g; Protein 11g

Bunless Turkey Burgers

Prep time: 5 minutes| Cook time: 15 minutes| Serves: 4

1 pound ground turkey breakfast sausage
¼ teaspoon ground black pepper
¼ cup seeded and chopped green bell pepper
1 medium avocado, peeled, pitted, and sliced
½ teaspoon salt
2 tablespoons mayonnaise

1. Mix sausage with salt, black pepper, bell pepper, and mayonnaise—form the meat into four patties. 2. Place patties into an ungreased air fryer basket. Set the temperature of air fryer to 370°F/188°C and the timer for 15 minutes, turning the cakes halfway through cooking. Burgers will be done when dark brown and have an internal temperature of at least 165°F/74°C. 3. Serve burgers topped with avocado slices on four medium plates.
Per Serving: Calories 276; Fat 17g; Sodium 917mg; Carbs 4g; Fiber 3g; Sugar 0g; Protein 22g

Egg Cups with Sausage-Crust

Prep time: 10 minutes| Cook time: 15 minutes| Serves: 6

¼ teaspoon ground black pepper
6 large eggs
12 ounces ground pork breakfast sausage
½ teaspoon salt
½ teaspoon crushed red pepper flakes

1. Place sausage in six 4" ramekins (about 2 ounces per ramekin) greased with cooking oil. Press sausage down to cover the bottom and about ½" up the sides of ramekins. Crack one egg into each ramekin and sprinkle evenly with salt, black pepper, and red pepper flakes. 2. Place ramekins into the air fryer basket. Set the temperature to 350°F/177°C and the timer for 15 minutes. Egg cups will be done when the sausage is fully cooked to at least 145°F/63°C, and the egg is firm. Serve warm.
Per Serving: Calories 267; Fat 21g; Sodium 679mg; Carbs 1g; Fiber 0g; Sugar 0g; Protein 14g

Mini Breakfast Bagels

Prep time: 5 minutes| Cook time: 10 minutes| Serves: 6

1½ teaspoons baking powder
2 cups shredded mozzarella cheese
3 tablespoons salted butter, divided
2 cups blanched finely ground almond flour
2 large eggs, divided
1 teaspoon apple cider vinegar

1. To make the dough: Mix together the mozzarella cheese, flour, and 1 tablespoon butter and microwave for 90 seconds on high. Form the mixture into a soft ball. Then add the vinegar, 1 egg, and the baking powder and stir until well combined. When dough is cool, divide evenly into six balls. Poke a hole in each rough dough ball with your finger and gently stretch each ball out to be 2" in diameter. 2. In a microwave, melt 2 tablespoons butter for 30 seconds, and cool for 1 minute. Whisk with remaining egg, then brush mixture over each bagel. 3. Prepare the basket with parchment paper and place bagels onto ungreased parchment, working in batches if needed. 4. Set the temperature to 350°F/177°C and the timer for 10 minutes. Halfway through, use tongs to flip bagels for even cooking. 5. Allow bagels to set and cool thoroughly, about 15 minutes, before serving.
Per Serving: Calories 415; Fat 33g; Sodium 447mg; Carbs 10g; Fiber 4g; Sugar 2g; Protein 19g

Sausage Gravy with Biscuits

Prep time: 10 minutes. | Cooking time: 0 minutes. | Serves: 8

½ pound mild Italian turkey sausage
4 ounces cream cheese
½ cup heavy whipping cream
½ cup chicken broth
½ teaspoon garlic powder
½ teaspoon onion powder
¼ teaspoon black pepper
⅛ teaspoon salt
1 batch basic biscuits
1 tablespoon fresh minced parsley, for garnish

1. In a suitable saucepan over medium-high heat, add the sausage. Cook until browned. for almost 5 minutes, using a wooden spoon to break up the meat. 2. Add the cream cheese, cream, chicken broth, garlic powder, onion powder, black pepper, and salt. Turn the heat down to medium and bring to a simmer, whisking to incorporate the cream cheese. 3. Simmer until the sauce is thickened. for almost 5–10 minutes, stirring frequently. 4. Serve each biscuit warm, split open with a ¼ cup sausage gravy spooned inside, topped with fresh parsley.
Per Serving: Calories 222; Total Fat 3.8g; Sodium 193mg; Total Carbs 8.2g; Fiber 7.1g; Sugars 35.5g; Protein 2.3g

Jalapeño and Bacon Pizza

Prep time: 5 minutes| Cook time: 10 minutes| Serves: 2

1 cup shredded mozzarella cheese
¼ cup chopped pickled jalapeños
1-ounce cream cheese, broken into small pieces
4 slices cooked sugar-free bacon, chopped
¼ teaspoon salt
1 large egg, whisked

1. Place mozzarella in a single layer on the bottom of an ungreased 6" round nonstick baking dish. Scatter cream cheese pieces, bacon, and jalapeños over mozzarella, then pour egg evenly around the baking dish. 2. Sprinkle with salt and place into the air fryer basket. Set the temperature to 330°F/165°C and the timer for 10 minutes. the pizza will be done when the cheese is brown, and the egg is set. 3. Let cool on a large plate for 5 minutes before serving.
Per Serving: Calories 361; Fat 24g; Sodium 1324mg; Carbs 5g; Fiber 0g; Sugar 2g; Protein 26g

Traditional Pancake with Keto Twist

Prep time: 5 minutes| Cook time: 30 minutes| Serves: 2

½ teaspoon vanilla extract
1 cup blanched finely ground almond flour
⅓ cup unsweetened almond milk
2 tablespoons granular erythritol
1 large egg
1 tablespoon salted butter, melted

1. In a bowl, mix all ingredients, then pour half the batter into an ungreased 6" round nonstick baking dish. 2. Place dish into air fryer basket. Set the temperature of air fryer to 320°F/160°C for 15 minutes. The pancake will be golden brown on top and firm, and a toothpick inserted in the center will come out clean when done. Repeat with the remaining batter. 3. Slice in half in a dish and serve warm.
Per Serving: Calories 434; Fat 38g; Sodium 111mg; Carbs 23g; Fiber 6g; Sugar 2g; Protein 15g

Golden Coconut Smoothie

Prep time: 10 minutes. | Cooking time: 0 minutes. | Serves: 1

⅔ cup canned unsweetened full-fat coconut milk
½ tablespoon milled golden flaxseed
¾ teaspoon vanilla extract
¼ teaspoon coconut extract
½ teaspoon ground turmeric
⅛ teaspoon ground black pepper
⅛ teaspoon sea salt
10 drops liquid stevia
1 cup ice cubes

1. Add the coconut milk, flaxseed, vanilla extract, coconut extract, turmeric, black pepper, salt, and stevia to your high-speed blender and process until smooth. 2. Add the ice cubes and pulse until thick and creamy, tamping down as necessary. 3. Pour into a glass and serve immediately.
Per Serving: Calories 180; Total Fat 6.5g; Sodium 92mg; Total Carbs 2g; Fiber 0.8g; Sugars 14.7g; Protein 5.6g

Delicious Scotch Eggs

Prep time: 10 minutes| Cook time: 12 minutes| Serves: 8

¼ teaspoon ground black pepper
1 large egg, whisked
½ teaspoon salt
8 large hard-boiled eggs, shells removed
½ cup blanched finely ground almond flour
1 pound ground pork breakfast sausage

1. Mix raw egg with sausage, flour, salt, and pepper. 2. Form ¼ cup of the mixture around 1 hard-boiled egg, thoroughly covering the egg. Repeat with the remaining mixture and hard-boiled eggs. 3. Place eggs into an air fryer basket. Set the temperature to 400°F/205°C and timer for 12 minutes, turning halfway through cooking. Eggs will be done when browned. Let eggs cool for 5 minutes before serving.
Per Serving: Calories 325; Fat 25g; Sodium 630mg; Carbs 2g; Fiber 1g; Sugar 1g; Protein 17g

Chocolaty Chia Pudding

Prep time: 2 minutes| Cook time: 3 minutes| Serves: 2

½ cup almond flour
1 cup canned coconut milk
2 tablespoons chia seeds
2 tablespoons ground flax seeds
4 tablespoons hemp hearts
¼ tablespoon ground cinnamon
4 scoops chocolate protein powder
⅔ cup water
¼ tablespoon ground nutmeg

Toppings
Toasted almonds
Toasted coconut
Almond butter

1. Mix the coconut milk with water in a bowl. Combine the chia seeds, protein powder, flax seeds, almond flour, cinnamon, and nutmeg in a separate bowl. 2. Make a well shape in the dry ingredients and pour the milk/water mixture into the dry ingredients while continuously mixing. Repeat until the ingredients are thoroughly mixed together. Cover the bowl and place it in the fridge overnight. 3. Pour the mix in a saucepan and use gentle heat. Bring the mixture to a simmer and frequently stir until it thickens. The thickness should not be too runny but not solid either. This can be to your personal preference. 4. Stir in the hemp hearts just before serving. 5. Divide evenly between two bowls and add your favorite healthy toppings.
Per Serving: Calories 486; Fat 32g; Sodium 256mg; Carbs 20g; Fiber 10g; Sugar 6g; Protein 38g

Healthy Cinnamon Granola

Prep time: 10 minutes| Cook time: 7 minutes| Serves: 6

1 cup unsweetened coconut flakes
2 cups shelled pecans, chopped
1 teaspoon ground cinnamon
2 tablespoons granular erythritol
1 cup slivered almonds

1. In a large bowl, mix all ingredients. Place mixture into an ungreased 6" round nonstick baking dish. 2. Place dish into air fryer basket. Set the temperature of air fryer to 320°F/160°C for 7 minutes, stirring halfway through cooking. 3. Let cool in a dish for 10 minutes before serving. Store in an airtight container at room temperature for up to 5 days.
Per Serving: Calories 445; Fat 42g; Sodium 0mg; Carbs 17g; Fiber 9g; Sugar 3g; Protein 8g

Egg Cups with Jalapeno

Prep time: 10 minutes| Cook time: 14 minutes| Serves: 4

¼ teaspoon garlic powder
4 large eggs
½ teaspoon salt
½ cup shredded sharp Cheddar
cheese
2 ounces cream cheese, softened
¼ teaspoon ground black pepper
¼ cup chopped pickled jalapeños

1. Beat eggs with salt and pepper, then pour evenly into four 4" ramekins greased with cooking spray. 2. Mix jalapeños, cream cheese, garlic powder, and Cheddar in a separate large bowl. Pour ¼ of the mixture into the center of one ramekin. Repeat with the remaining mixture and ramekins. 3. Place ramekins in the air fryer basket. Set the temperature of air fryer to 320°F/160°C for 14 minutes. Eggs will be set when done. Serve warm.
Per Serving: Calories 177; Fat 13g; Sodium 591mg; Carbs 1g; Fiber 0g; Sugar 1g; Protein 11g

Prosciutto Eggs Benedict

Prep time: 10 minutes. | Cooking time: 30 minutes. | Serves: 4

8 ham or prosciutto slices
8 large eggs
Bun
3 eggs, separated
¼ cup unflavored protein powder
2 tablespoons coconut flour
Hollandaise sauce
3 egg yolks
¼ cup lemon juice
1 tablespoon Dijon mustard
½ cup butter, melted
black pepper and sea salt to taste

To make the buns: 1. At 325°F/163°C, preheat your oven. 2. Separate the eggs (reserve the egg yolks) and whip the egg whites until stiff peaks form. 3. Gently mix in the protein powder and coconut flour. 4. Grease a suitable baking sheet and evenly divide the prepared mixture into 4 mounds, for almost the size of a hamburger bun, onto the sheet. Bake for almost 15–20 minutes or until golden brown. 5. Allow to cool completely before slicing in half lengthwise.
To prepare the hollandaise sauce: 1. Place the reserved egg yolks, lemon juice, and Dijon mustard in the top of a double boiler set over simmering water. Whisk to blend. 2. Whisking constantly, add the melted butter in a slow, steady stream. Cook the sauce, whisking constantly, until thickened. Season with black pepper and salt and remove from heat.
To assemble: 1. Slice a bun in half, plate, and top each half with a slice of ham or prosciutto. 2. Top each half with poached egg and 2-3 tablespoons hollandaise sauce. Serve immediately.
Per Serving: Calories 612 Fat 47g; Sodium 1103mg; Carbs 14.4g; Fiber 1.4g; Sugar 6.6g; Protein 33g

Egg Pizza

Prep time: 5 minutes| Cook time: 10 minutes| Serves: 2

1 cup shredded mozzarella cheese
7 slices pepperoni, chopped
1 large egg, whisked
¼ teaspoon dried oregano
¼ teaspoon salt
¼ teaspoon dried parsley
¼ teaspoon garlic powder

1. Place mozzarella in a single layer on the bottom of an ungreased 6" round nonstick baking dish. Scatter pepperoni over cheese, then pour egg evenly around the baking dish. 2. Sprinkle with remaining ingredients and place into air fryer basket. Set the temperature to 330°F/166°C and the timer for 10 minutes. The dish will be done when the cheese is brown and the egg is set. 3. Let cool in dish for 5 minutes before serving.
Per Serving: Calories 241; Fat 15g; Sodium 834mg; Carbs 4g; Fiber 0g; Sugar 1g; Protein 19g

Chia Pudding with Mocha and Coconut

Prep time: 5 minutes plus 30 minutes for refrigerating| Cook time: 0 minutes| Serves: 4

½ cup coconut cream
2 tablespoons cocoa powder
½ cup chia seeds
4 tablespoons instant coffee
4 tablespoons cacao nibs
1 tablespoon vanilla extract
2 tablespoons sugar substitute
2 cups water

1. Prepare a strong cup of coffee by simmering the instant coffee with 2 cups of water for 15 minutes until the liquid has reduced to about 1 cup. Whisk the cocoa powder, coconut cream, vanilla extract, and sugar substitute into the coffee. 2. Mixing in the chia seeds and cacao nibs. Mix well. 3. Divide into 4 small serving dishes and allow to set for at least 30 minutes. 4. Remove from refrigerator, garnish with a few additional cacao nibs, and serve!
Per Serving: Calories 257; Fat 21g; Sodium 697mg; Carbs 14g; Fiber 11g; Sugar 1g; Protein 7g

Blue Cheese Omelet

Prep time: 5 minutes| Cook time: 10 minutes| Serves: 4

2 tablespoons hot sauce
4 ounces cream cheese, softened
4 tablespoons blue cheese
6 eggs
2 tablespoons coconut oil
2 tablespoons water
Garnishes: chopped fresh parsley and chives

1. Warm the cream cheese, blue cheese, and hot sauce in a small bowl in the microwave for about 15 seconds. Stir until smooth and combined. 2. Whisk the eggs until frothy. 3. Heat about half a tablespoon coconut oil in a non-stick pan over medium heat. Pour the eggs into the pan. Drop one-quarter of the cream cheese mixture by spoonful over half of the eggs. 4. Once the eggs have firmed up, fold the empty half over the half with filling. Cook on low heat for another minute. 5. Carefully remove from pan, cover with tin foil to keep warm, and repeat with the remaining eggs and filling. Then garnish and serve.
Per Serving: Calories 282; Fat 26g; Sodium 689mg; Carbs 2g; Fiber 0g; Sugar 1g; Protein 12g

Avocado Smoothie

Prep time: 10 minutes. | Cooking time: 0 minutes. | Serves: 1

⅔ cup canned unsweetened full-fat coconut milk
1 teaspoon lemon juice
1 teaspoon lemon zest
⅛ teaspoon sea salt
10 drops liquid stevia
1 cup chopped kale
¼ medium avocado, peeled, pitted, and sliced
3 sprigs fresh parsley
1 sprig fresh mint
1 cup ice cubes

1. Add the coconut milk, lemon juice, lemon zest, salt, stevia, kale, avocado, parsley, and mint to your high-speed blender and process until smooth. 2. Add the ice cubes and pulse until thick and creamy, tamping down as necessary. 3. Pour into a glass and serve immediately.
Per Serving: Calories 448; Total Fat 31.1g; Sodium 35mg; Total Carbs 2.9g; Fiber 12.8g; Sugars 8.5g; Protein 9g

Cheesy Scrambled Eggs with Greens

Prep time: 5 minutes| Cook time: 10 minutes| Serves: 4

1 cup shredded mozzarella cheese
6 cups kale, baby spinach, or

Swiss Chard
2 tablespoons heavy cream
2 tablespoons olive oil
8 large eggs
Sea salt and pepper to taste

1. Crack the eggs into a medium bowl. Add the heavy cream to the eggs and season with salt and pepper. Whisk until well combined. 2. Roughly chop your greens. 3. Heat the olive oil in a pan. Add the baby spinach to the pan. Stir frequently, being careful not to burn. Once the spinach has wilted, reduce heat to low. 4. Add the egg mixture to the spinach and slowly stir until the eggs are almost set. 5. Add the mozzarella cheese and stir until well combined. 6. Once the cheese has melted, divide it onto four plates and serve!
Per Serving: Calories 251; Fat 19g; Sodium 784mg; Carbs 4g; Fiber 2g; Sugar 2g; Protein 16g

Flaxseed Piña Colada

Prep time: 10 minutes. | Cooking time: 0 minutes. | Serves: 1

¼ cup chopped fresh pineapple
⅔ cup canned unsweetened full-fat coconut milk
1 teaspoon milled golden flaxseed
1 teaspoon vanilla extract
¼ teaspoon coconut extract
⅛ teaspoon sea salt
6 drops liquid stevia
1 cup ice cubes

1. Add the pineapple, coconut milk, flaxseed, vanilla extract, coconut extract, salt, and stevia to your high-speed blender and process until smooth. 2. Add the ice cubes and pulse until thick and creamy, tamping down as necessary. 3. Pour into a glass and serve immediately.
Per Serving: Calories 365; Total Fat 33.6g; Sodium 195mg; Total Carbs 3.6g; Fiber 7g; Sugars 1.8g; Protein 9.7g

Traditional Pumpkin Muffins

Prep time: 10 minutes| Cook time: 30 minutes| Serves: 6

⅔ cup sugar substitute
1½ cups almond flour
1 tablespoon pumpkin pie spice mix
1 teaspoon baking powder
⅔ cup pumpkin puree
4 large eggs

1. Preheat the oven to 300°F/149°C. Prepare a muffin pan with 6 muffin paper liners. 2. Combine the almond flour, pumpkin pie spice, and sugar substitute in a large bowl. Mix well. 3. Add the pumpkin puree and eggs. Beat with an electric mixer until smooth. 4. Evenly divide the batter among the 6 paper liners and bake for 30–40 minutes. 5. Remove from the oven and allow to cool on a wire rack.
Per Serving: Calories 168; Fat 13g; Sodium 623mg; Carbs 9g; Fiber 6g; Sugar 2g; Protein 9g

Matcha Smoothie

Prep time: 10 minutes. | Cooking time: 0 minutes. | Serves: 1

½ cup canned unsweetened full-fat coconut milk
¼ cup water
1 cup fresh baby spinach leaves
¼ medium avocado, peeled, pitted, and sliced
¾ teaspoon powdered matcha
½ teaspoon fresh lemon juice
⅛ teaspoon sea salt
12 drops liquid stevia
1 cup ice cubes

1. Add the coconut milk, water, spinach, avocado, matcha, lemon juice, salt, and stevia to your high-speed blender and process until smooth. 2. Add the ice cubes and pulse until thick and creamy, tamping down as necessary. 3. Pour into a glass and serve immediately.
Per Serving: Calories 356; Total Fat 35.1g; Sodium 18mg; Total Carbs 2.1g; Fiber 4.6g; Sugars 6.9g; Protein 3.7g

Salmon-Avocado Boats

Prep time: 10 minutes| Cook time: 0 minutes| Serves: 4

4 ounces wild-caught smoked salmon
2 ripe avocados
2 limes for juice and garnish
Sea salt and pepper to taste
8 cherry tomatoes, halved

1. Marinate the salmon in the juice of one lime for about an hour. 2. Cut the avocados in half lengthwise and remove the seeds. 3. Cut the salmon into strips and place it into the avocado center. 4. Top each avocado half with a lime wedge and several cherry tomato halves. 5. Serve immediately.
Per Serving: Calories 263; Fat 24g; Sodium 987mg; Carbs 4g; Fiber 2g; Sugar 1g; Protein 10g

Monkey Bread

Prep time: 10 minutes. | Cooking time: 50 minutes. | Serves: 16

2 teaspoons instant yeast
3 tablespoons warm water
2 cups almond flour
4 tablespoons powdered erythritol
4 teaspoons baking powder
2 teaspoons psyllium husk powder
1 teaspoon ground cinnamon
¼ teaspoon salt
3 cups shredded low-moisture part-skim mozzarella cheese

2 ounces cream cheese
2 large eggs, lightly beaten
2 teaspoons vanilla bean paste
½ teaspoon almond extract
¼ teaspoon stevia glycerite
Coconut oil, for your hands
3 tablespoons unsalted butter, melted
10 tablespoons granulated monk fruit/erythritol blend

1. At 375°F/191°C, preheat your oven. 2. In a suitable bowl, add the yeast and warm water and stir to combine. Keep it aside until foamy. for almost 5–10 minutes. 3. In a suitable bowl, beat the almond flour, powdered erythritol, baking powder, psyllium husk powder, cinnamon, and salt. Keep it aside. 4. In a suitable microwave-safe bowl, add the mozzarella and cream cheese. Microwave for almost 60 seconds and then give it a stir, and continue microwaving in 20-second increments until the cheese is melted. 5. Mix the foamy yeast mixture into the melted cheese until well-mixed. 6. Stir in the beaten eggs, vanilla bean paste, almond extract, and stevia glycerite until well-mixed. 7. Stir in the flour mixture until it forms a dough. 8. Oil your hands with coconut oil, and knead the prepared dough until it comes as a ball. Cover and refrigerate 10 minutes. 9. Divide the prepared dough into sixteen equal pieces and roll each piece into a ball. Roll each ball in melted butter and then in the granulated monk fruit/erythritol blend to coat. 10. Arrange the coated balls of dough in a Bundt cake pan; refrigerate 15 minutes. 11. Bake for 30 minutes uncovered, and then cover the Bundt pan with foil and bake for about 5–10 minutes more. 12. Carefully invert onto a platter while still hot. Serve hot.
Per Serving: Calories 194; Total Fat 10.4g; Sodium 2576mg; Total Carbs 5.2g; Fiber 2.5g; Sugars 1.2g; Protein 21.1g

Tropical Coconut Smoothie

Prep time: 10 minutes. | Cooking time: 0 minutes. | Serves: 1

1 tablespoon unsalted macadamia nuts
⅔ cup canned unsweetened full-fat coconut milk
¾ teaspoon vanilla extract

¼ teaspoon coconut extract
⅛ teaspoon sea salt
10 drops liquid stevia
1 cup ice cubes

1. Add the macadamia nuts to your high-speed blender and pulse until powdery. 2. Add the coconut milk, vanilla extract, coconut extract, salt, and stevia to the blender and process until smooth. 3. Add the ice cubes and pulse until thick and creamy, tamping down as necessary. 4. Pour into a glass and serve immediately.
Per Serving: Calories 304; Total Fat 30.9g; Sodium 181mg; Total Carbs 8.2g; Fiber 2g; Sugars 3.9g; Protein 1.4g

Creamy French Toast

Prep time: 10 minutes. | Cooking time: 0 minutes. | Serves: 2

1 large egg
2 tablespoons heavy cream
1 tablespoon plus 2 teaspoons powdered erythritol
3 drops liquid stevia

¾teaspoon pure vanilla extract
¾ teaspoon ground cinnamon
4 slices bread
1 tablespoon coconut oil
4 tablespoons red raspberries

1. In a suitable shallow bowl, lightly beat the egg, cream, 1 tablespoon powdered erythritol, liquid stevia, vanilla, and cinnamon. Dip each slice of bread in the egg mixture, letting it soak in. 2. Heat a suitable nonstick skillet over medium heat. Once hot, add the coconut oil. Once the oil is melted, add the dipped bread slices. 3. Cook until the bread is golden on both sides, for almost 4–5 minutes on the first side and 2–3 minutes on the second side. 4. Sift the remaining 2 teaspoons powdered erythritol on top, sprinkle on the raspberries, and serve.
Per Serving: Calories 282; Total Fat 9.8g; Sodium 162mg; Total Carbs 1.9g; Fiber 5.7g; Sugars 4.3g; Protein 7.8g

Cheesy Fat Bombs

Prep time: 10 minutes plus 45 minutes for refrigerating| Cook time: 0 minutes| Serves: 5

⅓ cup butter, softened
3 large eggs, hard-boiled

¼ cup shredded cheddar cheese
5 slices bacon

Sea salt and pepper to taste   3 tablespoons mayonnaise

1. Preheat the oven to 375°F/191°C. Prepare a baking sheet with parchment paper. Lay the bacon flat and bake for 10–15 minutes until golden brown. Reserve any bacon grease for later use. 2. Peel and quarter the hard-boiled eggs. 3. Add thinly pieced butter to the eggs and mix well. Mash well with a fork. 4. Stir in the shredded cheese, mayonnaise, and any leftover bacon grease—season with salt and pepper. Mix well and place in the refrigerator for about 30–45 minutes until firm. 5. Form 5 balls from the cold egg mixture. 6. Wrap bacon on every ball and store in an airtight container until ready to serve.
Per Serving: Calories 292; Fat 28g; Sodium 689mg; Carbs 2g; Fiber 0g; Sugar 1g; Protein 8g

Egg Cheese Muffin Sandwiches

Prep time: 10 minutes. | Cooking time: 0 minutes. | Serves: 4

4 large eggs
1 tablespoon ghee
4 (1-ounce) slices gouda cheese
¾ cup arugula

4 English muffins, split in half and toasted
⅛ teaspoon black pepper

1. In a suitable skillet over medium heat, fry the eggs in the ghee any way you like. Add 1 slice gouda on top of each fried egg. 2. Divide the arugula between four English muffin bottoms, top each with a fried egg, a sprinkle of black pepper, and then the English muffin top. 3. Serve immediately.
Per Serving: Calories 222; Total Fat 13.6g; Sodium 738mg; Total Carbs 2g; Fiber 2g; Sugars 4.4g; Protein 13.7g

Chocolate Macadamia Smoothie

Prep time: 10 minutes. | Cooking time: 0 minutes. | Serves: 1

1 tablespoon unsalted macadamia nuts
⅔ cup canned unsweetened full-fat coconut milk
1 tablespoon unsweetened cocoa powder

¾ teaspoon vanilla extract
¼ teaspoon coconut extract
⅛ teaspoon sea salt
12 drops liquid stevia
1 cup ice cubes
Pinch flaky sea salt, for garnish

1. Add the macadamia nuts to your high-speed blender and pulse until powdery. 2. Add the coconut milk, cocoa powder, vanilla extract, coconut extract, salt, and stevia to the blender and process until smooth. 3. Add the ice cubes and pulse until thick and creamy, tamping down as necessary. 4. Pour into a glass, sprinkle the flaky sea salt on top, and serve immediately.
Per Serving: Calories 487; Total Fat 45.7g; Sodium 199mg; Total Carbs 0.3g; Fiber 14.5g; Sugars 1.3g; Protein 5.2g

Spiced Pear Bars

Prep time: 5 minutes| Cook time: 22 minutes| Serves: 6

1 large pear, cored and peeled
½ teaspoon nutmeg
¼ teaspoon cloves
¼ cup coconut flour
1 teaspoon cinnamon

3 large eggs
½ teaspoon baking soda
2 tablespoons coconut oil
2 tablespoons maple syrup
¼ teaspoon salt

1. Preheat the oven to 350°F/177°C. Grease an 8x8 baking tray with cooking spray. 2. In a food processor, pulse the pear until pureed. Add the eggs, maple syrup, along with coconut oil. Blend until well combined. 3. Add the salt, baking soda, cinnamon, nutmeg, cloves, and coconut flour. Mix until just combined. 4. Pour the batter into the prepared pan. Sprinkle with additional cinnamon, if desired. 5. Bake for 22–25 minutes until a toothpick test comes out clean. 6. Allow cooling on a wire rack. Cut into 6 squares.
Per Serving: Calories 127; Fat 9g; Sodium 489mg; Carbs 10g; Fiber 1g; Sugar 2g; Protein 4g

Chicken with Waffles

Prep time: 10 minutes. | Cooking time: 0 minutes. | Serves: 4

1 batch oven-fried chicken tenders
1 batch waffles
¼ cup sugar-free maple-flavored

syrup (preferably stevia-sweetened maple syrup), for serving

1. Serve half of each waffle topped with a quarter of the chicken tenders and 1 tablespoon of syrup.
Per Serving: Calories 334; Total Fat 3.4g; Sodium 211mg; Total Carbs 5.9g; Fiber 4.9g; Sugars 21.4g; Protein 11.5g

Low-Carb Pancakes

Prep time: 10 minutes. | Cooking time: 0 minutes. | Serves: 2

6 tablespoons almond flour
4 tablespoons golden milled flaxseed
1 tablespoon granulated erythritol
1 teaspoon baking powder
⅛ teaspoon salt

2 large eggs
3 tablespoons half-and-half
1 teaspoon pure vanilla extract
7 drops liquid stevia
4 teaspoons ghee

1. In a suitable bowl, beat the almond flour, flaxseed, granulated erythritol, baking powder, and salt. Beat in the eggs, half-and-half, vanilla, and liquid stevia. Let the batter rest for almost 3 minutes. 2. Preheat a suitable cast-iron skillet over high heat. Once hot, turn the heat down to medium to medium-high. 3. Add the ghee, and use a ¼-cup measure to pour out this pancake batter into the hot skillet. 4. Cook until this pancakes are light golden on both sides, flipping once. for almost 2–3 minutes on the first side and 1–2 minutes on the second side.
Per Serving: Calories 344; Total Fat 17g; Sodium 66mg; Total Carbs 8.9g; Fiber 12.2g; Sugars 27g; Protein 5.6g

Green Citrus Smoothie

Prep time: 10 minutes. | Cooking time: 0 minutes. | Serves: 1

⅔ cup canned unsweetened full-fat coconut milk
½ tablespoon milled golden flaxseed
½ teaspoon lemon juice
1 teaspoon lemon zest

1 teaspoon orange zest
¾ teaspoon grated fresh ginger
⅛ teaspoon sea salt
10 drops liquid stevia
1 cup fresh baby spinach leaves
1 cup ice cubes

1. Add the coconut milk, lemon juice, flaxseed, lemon zest, orange zest, ginger, salt, stevia, and spinach to your high-speed blender and process until smooth. 2. Add the ice cubes and pulse until thick and creamy, tamping down as necessary. 3. Pour into a glass and serve immediately.
Per Serving: Calories 482; Total Fat 43.1g; Sodium 255mg; Total Carbs 5.1g; Fiber 1.3g; Sugars 2.9g; Protein 21.4g

Whey Waffles

Prep time: 10 minutes. | Cooking time: 0 minutes. | Serves: 2

Nonstick spray
6 tablespoons almond flour
4 tablespoons ground flaxseed
1 scoop (26 g) unflavored whey protein powder
1 teaspoon baking powder
1 tablespoon granulated erythritol

8 drops liquid stevia
⅛ teaspoon salt
1 teaspoon pure vanilla extract
3 large eggs
2 tablespoons heavy whipping cream

1. Plug in your waffle iron. Once heated, coat with nonstick spray. 2. In a suitable bowl, beat all the recipe ingredients until well combined, making sure there are no lumps. Alternatively, you can put all the recipe ingredients into your high-speed blender and blend until smooth. 3. Pour half of the batter into the heated and sprayed waffle iron. The waffle is done when it starts to steam. for almost 2 minutes. Carefully remove the waffle and repeat with the remaining waffle batter.
Per Serving: Calories 257; Total Fat 17.9g; Sodium 1062mg; Total Carbs 1.2g; Fiber 0.1g; Sugars 1.2g; Protein 22.2g

Morning Doughnuts

Prep time: 15 minutes. | Cooking time: 30 minutes. | Serves: 6

Doughnuts
Coconut oil spray, for your hands and this pan
1 teaspoon instant yeast
1½ tablespoons warm water
1 cup almond flour
2 tablespoons powdered erythritol
2 teaspoons baking powder
1 teaspoon psyllium husk powder
1½ teaspoons ground cinnamon
⅛ teaspoon salt
1½ cups shredded low-moisture part-skim mozzarella cheese
1 ounce cream cheese
1 large egg, lightly beaten

1 teaspoon vanilla bean paste
¼ teaspoon almond extract
⅛ teaspoon stevia glycerite
3 tablespoons granulated monk fruit/erythritol blend
2 tablespoons unsalted butter, melted
Vanilla glaze
8 tablespoons powdered erythritol
1 tablespoon heavy whipping cream
2 teaspoons water
½ teaspoon pure vanilla extract
Pinch salt
3 drops almond extract

To prepare the doughnuts: 1. At 350°F/177°C, preheat your oven. Spray the inside of a doughnut pan with coconut oil. 2. In a suitable bowl, add the yeast and warm water and stir to combine. Keep it aside until foamy. for almost 5–10 minutes. 3. In a suitable bowl, beat the almond flour, powdered erythritol, baking powder, psyllium husk powder, ½ teaspoon cinnamon, and salt. Keep it aside. 4. In a suitable microwave-safe bowl, add the mozzarella and cream cheese. Microwave for almost 60 seconds and then give it a stir, and continue microwaving in 20-second until the cheese is melted. 5. Mix the foamy yeast mixture into the melted cheese until well-mixed, and then stir in the beaten egg, vanilla bean paste, almond extract, and stevia glycerite until well-mixed. 6. Stir in the flour mixture until it forms a dough. Oil your hands with coconut oil, and knead the prepared dough a couple times until it comes as a ball. Cover the prepared dough with a piece of plastic wrap and let it sit at room temperature for almost 15 minutes. 7. In a shallow bowl, stir the granulated monk fruit/erythritol blend and remaining 1 teaspoon cinnamon to make a cinnamon sugar. 8. Divide the prepared dough into six equal pieces and roll each piece into a ball. Roll a ball in the melted butter, and then roll it in the cinnamon sugar. Poke a mini hole in the center of the ball and shape it into a doughnut shape. Place the prepared doughnut into the prepared doughnut pan. Repeat with the remaining five balls of dough. 9. Bake the prepared doughnuts until golden and a toothpick inserted in the center comes out clean or with just a couple crumbs, for almost 15 minutes. 10. Let the prepared doughnuts cool in this pan 5 minutes before removing.
For the vanilla glaze: 1. In a suitable shallow bowl, stir all the recipe ingredients for the glaze. 2. Dip each doughnut in the glaze, and let the glaze harden before serving.
Per Serving: Calories 123; Total Fat 8.6g; Sodium 762mg; Total Carbs 2.1g; Fiber 0.6g; Sugars 0.7g; Protein 9.8g

Mushroom Quiche

Prep time: 10 minutes. | Cooking time: 50 minutes. | Serves: 10

1 press-in crust, pressed into a 7" springform pan
2 tablespoons unsalted butter
8 ounces button mushrooms, sliced
5 ounces baby spinach
2 large cloves garlic, minced
¼ cup chopped roasted red bell

pepper
4 large eggs
½ cup heavy whipping cream
½ teaspoon salt
¼ teaspoon black pepper
1 cup shredded sharp white cheddar cheese

1. At 350°F/177°C, preheat your oven. Pre-bake the press-in crust for almost 5 minutes. 2. Add the butter to a suitable, deep skillet over medium heat. Once melted, add the mushrooms and cook until softened, for almost 8–10 minutes, stirring occasionally. Add the spinach and garlic and cook until the spinach is wilted and the liquid is evaporated off, for almost 2–3 minutes, stirring continuously. Turn off the heat, stir in the roasted red bell pepper, and cool slightly. 3. In a suitable bowl, beat the eggs, cream, salt, and black pepper. Stir in the cooled vegetable mixture and the cheddar. 4. Pour the egg mixture into the pre-baked crust. 5. Bake until the quiche is set, for almost 40–50 minutes.
Per Serving: Calories 384; Total Fat 24.7g; Sodium 1130mg; Total Carbs 1.9g; Fiber 2g; Sugars 3.4g; Protein 19.3g

Bacon Fritters

Prep time: 10 minutes. | Cooking time: 15 minutes. | Serves: 6

⅔ cup cooked and crumbled bacon
1½ cups grated cheddar cheese
1 medium head cauliflower
3 large eggs

3 tablespoons coconut flour
2 cloves garlic, minced
black pepper and sea salt to taste
Coconut oil for this pan

1. Chop the cauliflower into ½-inch pieces and steam for almost 10–15 minutes, until soft. Drain well and mash with a fork or potato masher, pressing to release as much liquid as possible. 2. Transfer the cauliflower to a suitable bowl. Add the eggs, cheese, bacon, garlic, and coconut flour. Season with black pepper and salt and mix well. 3. Heat a suitable skillet over medium heat and add about a tablespoon of coconut oil. 4. Form the cauliflower mixture into flat patties, using about 2–3 tablespoons per patty. 5. Once this pan is hot, add a few of the patties and cook for almost 3–5 minutes, until browned on the bottom. Flip carefully and cook another 3–5 minutes. 6. Transfer the patty to a paper towel-lined plate and repeat with the remaining patties. Serve hot.
Per Serving: Calories 322; Total Fat 21.1g; Sodium 1469mg; Total Carbs 7.5g; Fiber 5.9g; Sugars 10.8g; Protein 8.7g

Pecan French Toast

Prep time: 10 minutes. | Cooking time: 55 minutes. | Serves: 8

1 tablespoon unsalted butter, at room temperature	1 teaspoon ground nutmeg
10 large egg yolks	¼ teaspoon salt
1½ cups half-and-half	4 cups cubed white bread
½ cup heavy whipped cream	¼ cup chopped pecans
⅓ cup granulated erythritol	¼ cup sugar-free maple-flavored
20 drops liquid stevia	syrup (preferably stevia-
1 tablespoon pure vanilla extract	sweetened maple syrup), for
2 teaspoons ground cinnamon	serving

1. Spread the butter on the inside of a 1½-quart casserole dish. 2. In a suitable bowl, beat the egg yolks, half-and-half, cream, granulated erythritol, liquid stevia, vanilla, cinnamon, nutmeg, and salt. Add the bread cubes and toss gently to coat. 3. Pour the prepared mixture into the prepared casserole dish, lightly pushing down the bread so it's mostly submerged in the liquid. Cover this dish with foil and refrigerate overnight. 4. At 375°F/191°C, preheat your oven. Take the casserole dish out of the refrigerator and let it sit at room temperature for almost 20 minutes while your oven is preheating. 5. Bake the casserole (covered with foil) for almost 50 minutes, and then remove the foil, sprinkle the pecans on top, and bake 5 more minutes. 6. Serve warm along with maple-flavored syrup to drizzle on top.
Per Serving: Calories 378; Total Fat 16.2g; Sodium 369mg; Total Carbs 5.8g; Fiber 1.9g; Sugars 15.6g; Protein 7.6g

Sausage Bread Pudding

Prep time: 10 minutes. | Cooking time: 1 hour 10 minutes. | Serves: 9

6 cornbread muffins	1 cup heavy whipping cream
1 pound Italian turkey sausage	¼ cup water
2 leeks, white parts only, sliced	1 cup shredded gruyere cheese
2 large cloves garlic, crushed or minced	¼ teaspoon salt
1 teaspoon minced fresh thyme	¼ teaspoon black pepper
7 large eggs	Olive oil spray

1. At 350°F/177°C, preheat your oven. Layer a suitable baking tray with parchment paper or a Silpat liner. 2. Cut each cornbread muffin into cubes, spread the cubes out on the prepared baking tray, and bake until golden, for almost 20 minutes. Cool. 3. Heat a suitable skillet over medium-high heat. Once hot, add the sausage, leeks, and garlic and cook until the meat is browned and the liquid is evaporated. for almost 8 minutes, stirring occasionally. Stir in the thyme. Cool. 4. In a suitable bowl, beat the eggs, cream, water, gruyere, salt, and black pepper. Stir in the sausage mixture, and then gently stir in the cornbread cubes. 5. Spray the inside of a 9" × 13" casserole dish with olive oil. Pour the egg mixture into the dish. Cover the dish with foil. 6. Bake (covered) 40 minutes, and then bake (uncovered) 10 minutes more. 7. Let the casserole sit for almost 10–15 minutes before serving. Serve warm.
Per Serving: Calories 383; Total Fat 25.2g; Sodium 184mg; Total Carbs 5g; Fiber 0.9g; Sugars 14.7g; Protein 5.1g

Mascarpone Pancakes

Prep time: 5 minutes. | Cooking time: 10 minutes. | Serves: 2

6 eggs	Suggested toppings
1 cup mascarpone cheese	Butter
¼ cup ground flaxseeds	Low-carb syrup
¼ cup chia seeds	Sour cream
1½ teaspoons baking powder	Berries
½ teaspoon salt	

1. Mix the flaxseeds, chia seeds, baking powder, and salt in a bowl. Add the eggs to the dry ingredients one at a time, whisking well after each egg. 2. Add the mascarpone cheese and whisk until smooth. Alternatively, put all of the ingredients into your high-speed blender to achieve the same results. If you want to sweeten the batter, add about a teaspoon of sugar substitute at this point and mix well. 3. Spray a griddle or nonstick skillet with cooking oil spray and set over medium-high heat. 4. Use a suitable spoon or, preferably, a ladle (this is the perfect size for cooking pancakes) to pour this pancake batter into the skillet once the skillet is hot. 5. Allow this pancake to cook for almost 2 minutes before carefully flipping it over with a spatula. Cook the other side for almost 2 minutes. Set the timing accordingly if you would prefer your pancakes more or less browned.
Per Serving: Calories 117; Total Fat 8.2g; Sodium 354mg; Total

Carbs 4.1g; Fiber 1.7g; Sugars 1.1g; Protein 7.3g

Italian Breakfast

Prep time: 15 minutes. | Cooking time: 10 minutes. | Serves: 2

2 large eggs	10 cherry tomatoes, halved
3-4 slices prosciutto ham	Celtic sea salt
1 clove garlic, peeled	Black pepper
½ cup arugula	4 tablespoons butter

1. Heat 1 tablespoon of butter in a suitable skillet over a medium to high heat. 2. Crack and fry the eggs, preferably sunny-side up, until the edges are golden (usually around 3-4 minutes). Remove from this pan and set to one side for the moment. 3. Next, crush the garlic clove. Add more butter, if needed, then add the garlic to the skillet and sauté until it begins to turn a golden brown. Add a dash of black pepper and salt. 4. Sauté the halved tomatoes for almost 2-3 minutes, turning halfway through.
Per Serving: Calories 233; Total Fat 18.5g; Sodium 97mg; Total Carbs 1.4g; Fiber 1.8g; Sugars 0.2g; Protein 8.3g

Ham Frittata

Prep time: 10 minutes. | Cooking time: 30 minutes. | Serves: 6

8 ounces diced ham	10 large eggs
2 bell peppers, any color, diced	2 egg whites
½ red onion, diced	½ cup milk
8-10 cherry tomatoes, quartered	black pepper and sea salt to taste
½ cup fresh cilantro, chopped	Optional garnishes: diced green
⅔ cup shredded pepper jack cheese	onions, salsa, sour cream

1. At 350°F/177°C, preheat your oven. Grease a 9-inch glass pie pan. 2. Brown the ham in a suitable skillet until golden brown. Remove from pan and keep it aside. 3. Using the same skillet, cook the peppers, onion and cherry tomatoes until softened. 4. In a suitable bowl, beat the eggs, egg whites and milk. 5. Evenly sprinkle the sausage and veggies into the prepared pie pan. Top with the chopped cilantro. Pour the egg mixture on top and season with black pepper and salt. 6. Top with the shredded cheese and bake for almost 25–30 minutes, or until set. 7. Allow to cool for almost 5–10 minutes and slice into 6 servings. 8. Top with optional garnishes and enjoy!
Per Serving: Calories 125; Total Fat 3.2g; Sodium 16mg; Total Carbs 0.4g; Fiber 6.9g; Sugars 11.1g; Protein 5.1g

Kale Kiwi Smoothie

Prep time: 10 minutes. | Cooking time: 0 minutes. | Serves: 1

1 cup chopped kale	1 teaspoon fresh lemon zest
½ medium kiwi, peeled and chopped	½ teaspoon fresh lemon juice
⅔ cup canned unsweetened full-fat coconut milk	⅛ teaspoon sea salt
	12 drops liquid stevia
	1 cup ice cubes

1. Add the kale, kiwi, coconut milk, lemon zest, lemon juice, salt, and stevia to your high-speed blender and process until smooth. 2. Add the ice cubes and pulse until thick and creamy, tamping down as necessary. 3. Pour into a glass and serve immediately.
Per Serving: Calories 213; Total Fat 13.1g; Sodium 1194mg; Total Carbs 9.3g; Fiber 3.3g; Sugars 4g; Protein 19.4g

Grain-Free Breakfast Cereal

Prep time: 5 minutes | Cook time: 8 minutes | Serves: 4

4 cups unsweetened almond milk	sliced almonds
6 tablespoons butter	Blueberries or raisins for topping
1 cup unsweetened, shredded coconut	Liquid stevia to taste (if desired)
	Pinch of salt
1 ⅓ cups crushed walnut pieces,	

1. Preheat the oven to 250°F/121°C. Toast the nuts and shredded coconut (keep separate from each other) until golden brown. 2. In a saucepan over medium heat, melt the butter. 3. Add the toasted nuts and a pinch of salt. Let cook for 1–2 whites, stirring constantly. Add the toasted coconut and continue stirring. 4. Add the milk and liquid stevia if using. Allow cooking for 5–7 minutes, until heated throughout. 5. Remove from heat, divide into 4 bowls and serve immediately.
Per Serving: Calories 603; Fat 62g; Sodium 697mg; Carbs 10g; Fiber 6g; Sugar 2g; Protein 9g

Delicious Carrot Cake Pudding

Prep time: 5 minutes| Cook time: 20 minutes| Serves: 4

½ teaspoon nutmeg
2 cups peeled and chopped carrots
½ teaspoon cinnamon
2 tablespoons coconut cream
¼ teaspoon cloves
2 tablespoons almond butter

1 teaspoon vanilla extract
Pinch of sea salt
Garnish: whipped to stiff peaks and/or toasted nuts, heavy cream, optional

1. Cover the carrots in a medium pot with water. Cook the carrots on a medium flame for 10-15 minutes until the fork soft. 2. Drain the water from cooked carrots and put them in a food processor. Add the remaining ingredients in blender and puree until smooth and creamy. 3. Divide into 4 serving dishes, garnish with whipped cream if desired, and enjoy! Sometimes, I like to top with nuts; the nutty flavor complements the pudding.
Per Serving: Calories 108; Fat 7g; Sodium 541mg; Carbs 11g; Fiber 4g; Sugar 3g; Protein 3g

Zucchini Egg Bake

Prep time: 10 minutes. | Cooking time: 25 minutes. | Serves: 6

4 small zucchinis, cut into ½-inch thick rounds
6 slices ham or Canadian bacon
½ cup grated asiago cheese

6 large eggs
1 small bunch parsley, chopped
black pepper and sea salt to taste

1. At 350°F/177°C, preheat your oven. Prepare an 8x8 baking dish with non-stick spray. 2. Cut the ham slices in half, then cut each half lengthwise into ¼-inch thick strips. 3. Cook the ham strips in a suitable skillet over medium heat for almost 3 minutes, until golden brown. Add the zucchini and continue to cook for almost 5 minutes, until softened. 4. In a suitable bowl, whisk the eggs until frothy. Season with black pepper and salt. 5. Mix the ham and zucchini into the eggs. Add the chopped parsley and mix until well combined. 6. Pour the prepared mixture into the prepared baking dish. Sprinkle the asiago cheese evenly over the top and bake for almost 20–25 minutes, until the eggs are set. 7. Allow to rest for almost 5 minutes before serving.
Per Serving: Calories 353; Total Fat 21.4g; Sodium 119mg; Total Carbs 3.6g; Fiber 12.6g; Sugars 20.2g; Protein 11.7g

Egg-Stuffed Bell Peppers

Prep time: 10 minutes. | Cooking time: 45 minutes. | Serves: 4

4 yellow bell peppers, halved lengthwise and seeded
5 large eggs
1 cup shredded cheddar cheese
4 slices bacon, cooked and crumbled

¼ cup heavy cream
¼ cup chopped frozen spinach, thawed
3 green onions, chopped
black pepper and sea salt to taste

1. At 350°F/177°C, preheat your oven. 2. In a suitable bowl, whisk the eggs and heavy cream until frothy. Add the sliced green onions, spinach, half of the shredded cheese and bacon. Mix until well combined and season with black pepper and salt. 3. Place the bell pepper halves in a lightly greased baking dish and divide the egg mixture between the peppers. Sprinkle with the remaining cheese. 4. Cover with foil and bake for almost 45 minutes, until the eggs are set. Serve immediately.
Per Serving: Calories 391; Total Fat 21.2g; Sodium 58mg; Total Carbs 4.6g; Fiber 3.5g; Sugars 24.5g; Protein 13.2g

Spinach Mushroom Quiche

Prep time: 10 minutes. | Cooking time: 50 minutes. | Serves: 6

1 (10-ounce) box frozen spinach, thawed and drained
2 (4-ounce) cans sliced mushrooms, drained
1 cup shredded mozzarella cheese
⅓ cup grated parmesan cheese

6 large eggs
½ cup heavy cream
½ cup water
½ teaspoon garlic powder
black pepper and sea salt to taste

1. At 350°F/177°C, preheat your oven. Grease a 9-inch pie pan. 2. Evenly spread the thawed and drained spinach into the bottom of the pie pan. Top with the mushroom slices. 3. Whisk the eggs with the heavy cream and water. Mix in the parmesan cheese, garlic powder, salt, and pepper. 4. Pour the egg mixture into this pan. 5. Sprinkle with mozzarella cheese and bake for almost 40–50 minutes, until the center

is set and the edges are golden brown. 6. Remove from oven and allow to cool for almost 5–10 minutes. Slice and serve!
Per Serving: Calories 316; Total Fat 18.4g; Sodium 235mg; Total Carbs 7.1g; Fiber 10.6g; Sugars 6.9g; Protein 8.2g

Mushroom Cream Crepes

Prep time: 10 minutes. | Cooking time: 25 minutes. | Serves: 4

1 boneless, skinless chicken breast, cut into ½-inch pieces
1 cup sliced mushrooms
2 cups heavy cream
4 large eggs
1 yellow onion, sliced

4 slices bacon, cooked and chopped
black pepper and sea salt to taste
Olive oil for this pan
Optional garnish: chopped parsley and/or chives

1. Whisk the eggs with about a tablespoon of heavy cream and season with black pepper and salt. 2. Heat a suitable pan over medium heat and add a bit of olive oil to it. 3. Pour approximately ½ cup of the egg mixture to this pan and swirl to evenly coat this pan. 4. Once the eggs have set, flip and cook for almost 1 minute. Transfer to a paper towel and repeat 3 times with the remaining egg mixture. 5. In a suitable pan, sauté the chicken, onions, and mushrooms until the chicken is cooked through. Season with black pepper and salt. 6. Stir in the bacon and the heavy cream. Cook about 4 minutes, until slightly thickened. 7. Divide most the chicken mixture between the 4 egg crepes, fold, and top with the remaining cream. Serve and enjoy!
Per Serving: Calories 302; Total Fat 21.3g; Sodium 354mg; Total Carbs 6g; Fiber 2.3g; Sugars 2.5g; Protein 23.1g

Ricotta Sausage Pie

Prep time: 10 minutes. | Cooking time: 35 minutes. | Serves: 6

6 cups kale, chopped
1½ cups ricotta cheese
1 pound breakfast sausage
4 eggs
1 cup shredded cheddar cheese

½ yellow onion, diced
3 cloves garlic, minced
2 tablespoons olive oil
black pepper and sea salt to taste

1. At 350°F/177°C, preheat your oven. 2. Heat the olive oil in a suitable skillet and add the onions and garlic. 3. Cook until softened. Add the kale and cook for almost 5 minutes, until wilted. 4. Rub with black pepper and salt and remove from heat. 5. Beat the eggs in a suitable bowl. Add the ricotta and shredded cheddar. 6. Stir in the sautéed kale. 7. Roll out the breakfast sausage and press it into a 9-inch pie pan, making sure to go up the sides of this pan. 8. Pour in the filling and place on a suitable baking sheet to catch any drippings from the sausage. 9. Bake for almost 30–35 minutes, until the eggs are set. 10. Allow to rest for almost 5–10 minutes, slice into 6 pieces and serve!
Per Serving: Calories 158; Total Fat 2.1g; Sodium 90mg; Total Carbs 4.4g; Fiber 7.5g; Sugars 26.1g; Protein 3.1g

Eggs with Hollandaise Sauce

Prep time: 10 minutes. | Cooking time: 20 minutes. | Serves: 4

4 strips of bacon, chopped
2 cups baby spinach or kale
8 large eggs
Optional garnish: fresh basil
Hollandaise sauce

2 egg yolks
¼ cup butter, melted
1 tablespoon lemon juice
¼ teaspoon salt

To prepare the hollandaise sauce: 1. In a high speed blender, blend the egg yolks with the lemon juice and salt. 2. Slowly pour the melted butter into the blender while it's running. Blend for almost 30 seconds, until thickened. Pour into a suitable bowl set over a sauce pan of simmering water to keep warm until ready to use.
For the baked eggs: 1. At 400°F/204°C, preheat your oven. 2. Set the rack in the top third of your oven. 3. Heat a suitable skillet over medium heat. Cook the bacon until crisp. 4. Add the greens and sauté until wilted. 3. Divide the prepared mixture evenly between 4 large ramekins or gratin dishes. 4. Gently crack 2 eggs onto the filling of each ramekin. Place on a suitable baking sheet and into your oven for almost 10–12 minutes, until the white is set, but the yolk is still runny. 5. Drizzle with hollandaise sauce, garnish with fresh basil, if desired, and serve immediately.
Per Serving: Calories 397; Total Fat 37.7g; Sodium 595mg; Total Carbs 5.1g; Fiber 7.3g; Sugars 4.5g; Protein 5.3g

Sausage Stuffed Peppers

Prep time: 10 minutes. | Cooking time: 6 hours. | Serves: 4

1 pound Italian sausage
4 bell peppers
½ head of cauliflower
1 (8-ounce) can tomato paste

1 small yellow onion, diced
3 garlic cloves, minced
2 teaspoons oregano
black pepper and sea salt to taste

1. Chop the tops off of the bell peppers and discard the seeds. Save the tops. 2. Grate the cauliflower into "rice" with a cheese grater or food processor and transfer to a suitable mixing bowl. 3. Add the minced garlic, oregano, and onion. Mix well to combine. 4. Add the sausage and tomato paste to the cauliflower mixture and mix well with your hands. Season with black pepper and salt. 5. Evenly divide the sausage mixture between the peppers. Cover each pepper with their tops and gently place into your slow cooker. 6. Cook on low for almost 6 hours. Serve and enjoy!
Per Serving: Calories 306; Total Fat 29.6g; Sodium 987mg; Total Carbs 1g; Fiber 4.2g; Sugars 2.9g; Protein 5.8g

Blueberry Cake

Prep time: 10 minutes. | Cooking time: 30 minutes. | Serves: 6

1 cup fresh or frozen blueberries
(or other berry of choice)
4 large eggs, separated
½ cup coconut flour
¼ cup coconut oil
¼ cup sugar substitute
2 teaspoons vanilla extract

¼ teaspoon baking soda
1 teaspoon cream of tartar
Topping
¼ cup coconut sugar
¼ cup coconut oil
2 tablespoons coconut flour
½ teaspoon cinnamon

1. At 350°F/177°C, preheat your oven. Prepare an 8x8 baking pan with non-stick spray. 2. In a suitable bowl, mix the egg whites and cream of tartar. Whisk until stiff peaks form. 3. In another bowl, cream the sugar substitute and coconut oil. Mix in the egg yolks. 4. Slowly stir in the coconut flour, vanilla, and baking soda. Mix until just combined. 5. Gently fold the egg whites into the batter. Pour into the prepared pan. Evenly scatter the blueberries on top. 6. In a suitable bowl, mix the ingredients for the topping. 7. Spread the prepared mixture over the batter. 8. Bake for almost 30 minutes, or until a toothpick inserted comes out clean. 9. Allow to cool to room temperature before cutting into squares.
Per Serving: Calories 348; Total Fat 32.6g; Sodium 595mg; Total Carbs 6.5g; Fiber 8.8g; Sugars 5.5g; Protein 3.4g

Meatballs with Apple Chutney

Prep time: 10 minutes. | Cooking time: 30 minutes. | Serves: 4

For the meatballs
½ pound lean ground pork
1 teaspoon onion powder
1 teaspoon salt
1 teaspoon garam masala
For the apple chutney
2 medium tart apples (such as

granny smith)
¼ cup raisins
2 tablespoons butter
½ teaspoon garam masala
1 tablespoon maple syrup
2 tablespoons water
1 tablespoon apple cider vinegar

1. At 400°F/204°C, preheat your oven. Layer a suitable baking sheet with parchment paper. 2. In a suitable bowl, mix all of the meatball the recipe ingredients. Mix well with hands. 3. Portion into small balls and bake for almost 15–20 minutes, until cooked through.
To prepare the chutney: 1 Mix all of the ingredients into a suitable saucepan over medium heat. 2 Cook to a simmer, cover, and allow to cook for almost 6–8 minutes, stirring occasionally. 3 Mash the chutney with a potato masher or fork until few chunks remain.
Top the meatballs with the chutney and enjoy.
Per Serving: Calories 343; Total Fat 26.6g; Sodium 924mg; Total Carbs 1.2g; Fiber 7.1g; Sugars 0.6g; Protein 20.3g

Egg-Stuffed Meatloaf

Prep time: 10 minutes. | Cooking time: 35 minutes. | Serves: 6

4 hard-boiled eggs, peeled
1 cup baby spinach or kale
1½ pounds ground pork
1 teaspoon smoked paprika
1 teaspoon fennel seeds

½ teaspoon salt
½ teaspoon pepper
½ teaspoon sage
¼ teaspoon cayenne pepper

1. At 400°F/204°C, preheat your oven. 2. Grease a 9x5-inch loaf pan with non-stick spray. 3. In a suitable mixing bowl, mix the ground pork with the spices and mix well with hands. 4. Place a thin layer of pork in the bottom of the prepared pan. 5. Line the baby spinach down the center of this pan and top with the hard-boiled eggs. 6. Place the remaining pork on top and press gently. 7. Bake for almost 35 minutes, or until golden brown. 8. Allow to cool for almost 5–10 minutes. Slice and serve.
Per Serving: Calories 354; Total Fat 31.8g; Sodium 320mg; Total Carbs 9.7g; Fiber 1.7g; Sugars 6.6g; Protein 10.5g

Potato-Crusted Frittata

Prep time: 10 minutes. | Cooking time: 60 minutes. | Serves: 6

2 sweet potatoes, peeled and very sliced
1 medium zucchini, sliced
1 bell pepper, sliced
2 cups baby spinach
3 bacon slices, cooked and

crumbled
1 small onion, sliced
5 eggs, beaten
2 tablespoons olive oil
2 cloves garlic, minced
Sea black pepper and salt to taste

1. At 400°F/204°C, preheat your oven. 2. Toss the sweet potato slices with olive oil and season with black pepper and salt. 3. Arrange the slices in a 9" pie dish to form a crust for the quiche. Bake for almost 15–20 minutes. 4. While the crust bakes, add the reserved bacon fat to a suitable skillet over medium heat. 5. Sauté the garlic, zucchini, bell pepper, and onion until translucent. Add the spinach and cook until wilted. Remove from heat. 6. Once the sweet potatoes are done, lower the heat to 375°F/191°C. 7. Layer the spinach mixture into the crust, top with the beaten eggs and crumbled bacon. Season with black pepper and salt and bake for almost 30–35 minutes, until the eggs are set. Serve warm.
Per Serving: Calories 198; Total Fat 19g; Sodium 1035mg; Total Carbs 5.7g; Fiber 2g; Sugars 1g; Protein 4g

Breakfast Pizza

Prep time: 10 minutes. | Cooking time: 30 minutes. | Serves: 6

Pizza dough
½ cup coconut flour
3 eggs
1 cup canned coconut milk
1 teaspoon onion powder
1 teaspoon garlic powder
½ teaspoon baking powder
½ teaspoon baking soda
¼ teaspoon dried basil

¼ teaspoon dried oregano
Pizza toppings
9 eggs, beaten
½ pound breakfast sausage
1 red onion, sliced
6 garlic cloves, minced
8 sun-dried tomatoes
2 tablespoons olive oil
1 cup baby spinach, chopped

1. At 425°F/218°C, preheat your oven. 2. In a suitable bowl, mix the coconut flour with the baking powder, baking soda, and spices. 3. Add the coconut milk and eggs and mix well. Keep it aside to rest for almost 5 minutes. 4. Layer a suitable baking sheet with parchment paper and spread the pizza dough over it evenly. 5. Bake for almost 25 minutes, or until golden brown. 6. In a suitable skillet over medium heat, brown the breakfast sausage until golden brown. 7. Transfer to a plate. 8. Add the olive oil to this pan and cook the onion, garlic, and sun-dried tomatoes until softened. 9. For the eggs, you can either add them to this pan and scramble with the other ingredients, or fry them and put them on top after. 10. Top the pizza crust evenly with the eggs and sausage. 11. Place back in your oven and bake for almost 5–7 minutes. Remove from oven, slice, and serve.
Per Serving: Calories 335; Fat 21.8g; Sodium 581mg; Carbs 14.6g; Fiber 2.5g; Sugar 3g; Protein 21.6g

Cheddar Breakfast Bake

Prep time: 10 minutes. | Cooking time: 45 minutes. | Serves: 6

1 pound chorizo sausage
1 (8-ounce) can green chilies
1 cup shredded cheddar cheese
1 yellow onion, diced
½ head cauliflower

4 eggs, beaten
½ teaspoon garlic powder
black pepper and sea salt to taste
Optional garnish: sliced green onions

1. At 375°F/191°C, preheat your oven. Grease a 9x13 glass baking dish with olive oil. 2. In a suitable skillet over medium heat, cook the chorizo and onion until golden brown. 3. Add the chilies to this pan and mix well. Transfer to a suitable mixing bowl and allow to cool slightly. 4. Shred the cauliflower into "rice" using a food processor or cheese grater. Add to the bowl. 5. Stir in the beaten eggs and half of the cheese. Season with salt, pepper, and garlic powder. Pour into the prepared dish. Top with the remaining cheese. 6. Bake for almost 45 minutes, until the eggs are set and the cheese is golden brown. 7. Let rest for almost 5 minutes. Top with green onions, if desired. Serve!
Per Serving: Calories 216; Total Fat 20.6g; Sodium 639mg; Total Carbs 8.7g; Fiber 4.3g; Sugars 2.9g; Protein 3.1g

Deviled Mayo Eggs

Prep time: 10 minutes. | Cooking time: 10 minutes. | Serves: 4

8 hard-boiled eggs, peeled and sliced in half	1 tablespoon olive oil
1 tablespoon mayonnaise	1 clove garlic, minced
1 teaspoon Dijon mustard	1 tablespoon green onion, minced
1 tablespoon heavy cream	1 teaspoon lemon juice
	2 tablespoons parsley, chopped

1. Gently remove the yolks from the hard-boiled eggs and place in a suitable bowl. Place the egg whites on a serving tray. 2. Add the mayonnaise, mustard, heavy cream, olive oil, garlic, green onion, lemon juice, and parsley. 3. Mash everything until a thick paste forms. Spoon the prepared mixture back into the egg whites. 4. Serve over a bed of salad greens.
Per Serving: Calories 210; Total Fat 13.4g; Sodium 708mg; Total Carbs 3.3g; Fiber 4.3g; Sugars 6.6g; Protein 11.7g

Eggs with Avocado Salsa

Prep time: 10 minutes. | Cooking time: 30 minutes. | Serves: 4

8 large eggs	½ a jalapeño, minced
1 avocado, diced	¼ cup feta cheese
1 cup cherry tomatoes, quartered	½ teaspoon sea salt
¼ cup red onion, diced	Juice of 1 lime
½ cup cilantro, chopped	

1To prepare the avocado salsa: Mix everything except the eggs in a suitable bowl and mix well. Cover and refrigerate until ready to serve. 2. To soft boil the eggs: Fill a suitable saucepan with water and cook to a boil. Reduce its heat to a simmer and add the eggs to the pot. Cook 5 minutes for a runny yolk, or 7 minutes for a soft-set yolk. Remove it from the heat and run the eggs under cold water for almost 1 minute, or until cool enough to peel. 3. Gently peel the eggs and plate with a big scoop of the avocado salsa. Enjoy!
Per Serving: Calories 223; Total Fat 12g; Sodium 845mg; Total Carbs 5.4g; Fiber 3.8g; Sugars 4.8g; Protein 17.4g

Egg Casserole

Prep time: 10 minutes. | Cooking time: 30 minutes. | Serves: 6

12 large eggs	½ cup shredded cheddar cheese
1 pound breakfast sausage	¼ teaspoon thyme
1 zucchini, sliced	black pepper and sea salt to taste
½ red onion, diced	Optional garnish: chopped fresh basil leaves
½ green pepper, diced	
1 cup half & half	

1. At 350°F/177°C, preheat your oven. 2. Prepare an 8x8 baking dish with non-stick spray.
In a suitable skillet over medium heat, brown the sausage. 3. Once the sausage is cooked through, add the onions, peppers, and zucchini. 4. Cook until tender. Remove from heat. 5. In a suitable bowl, whisk the eggs until frothy. Season with salt, pepper, and thyme. 6. Add the vegetables to the eggs and pour into the prepared baking dish. Sprinkle evenly with the shredded cheese. 7. Bake for almost 30 minutes, until the eggs are set. 8. Garnish with chopped basil, if desired and serve.
Per Serving: Calories 335; Total Fat 26.5g; Sodium 52mg; Total Carbs 3.4g; Fiber 8.6g; Sugars 2.4g; Protein 16g

Broccoli Frittata

Prep time: 10 minutes. | Cooking time: 25 minutes. | Serves: 6

8 eggs	1 large carrot, grated
1 small red onion, sliced	3 cloves garlic, minced
1 small head of broccoli, cut into small florets	¼ cup feta cheese
	black pepper and sea salt to taste
2 cups baby spinach or kale	2 tablespoons olive oil
2 tomatoes, sliced	

1. At 350°F/177°C, preheat your oven. 2. Prepare a 9-inch pie plate with non-stick spray. 3. Heat the olive oil in a suitable skillet over medium-high heat. 4.Sauté the onions and garlic until translucent. 5. Add the broccoli florets and reduce heat to medium-low. 6. Cover and cook for almost 5 minutes, until the broccoli is tender. 7. Add the spinach and cook until slightly wilted. Remove from heat and transfer to your prepared pie plate. 8. In a suitable bowl, whisk the eggs with the carrot and feta cheese. 9. Season with black pepper and salt and carefully pour over the vegetable mixture. 10. Top with the sliced tomatoes and bake for almost 20 minutes, or until the eggs are set. 11.

Allow to rest for almost 10 minutes before slicing and serving.
Per Serving: Calories 200; Total Fat 14.7g; Sodium 893mg; Total Carbs 4.7g; Fiber 3.2g; Sugars 5.4g; Protein 4.5g

Avocado Breakfast Tacos

Prep time: 10 minutes. | Cooking time: 15 minutes. | Serves: 4

4 eggs	black pepper and sea salt
1 (10-ounce) can Rotel tomatoes	½ cup fresh cilantro, chopped
1 ripe avocado, sliced	4 low-carb tortillas

1. At 400°F/204°C, preheat your oven. Spray a suitable sized, oven-proof skillet with non-stick spray. 2. Pour the tomatoes into the skillet and place over medium heat. 3. Once almost all of the liquid has evaporated from the tomatoes, crack the eggs on top and season with black pepper and salt. 4. Transfer the skillet to your oven and bake for almost 10–12 minutes, until the egg whites are set. 5. Serve each egg alongside sliced avocado and fresh cilantro, with a low-carb tortilla.
Per Serving: Calories 231; Total Fat 21.3g; Sodium 710mg; Total Carbs 7.7g; Fiber 2.5g; Sugars 2.3g; Protein 5g

Zucchini Frittata

Prep time: 10 minutes. | Cooking time: 25 minutes. | Serves: 6

8 large eggs	2 tablespoons olive oil
2 medium zucchinis, sliced	black pepper and sea salt to taste
1 red onion, sliced	Optional topping: Pico de Gallo or salsa
2 green peppers, sliced	
2 cloves garlic, minced	

1. At 400°F/204°C, preheat your oven. 2. Preheat 1 tablespoon oil in a 9-inch oven-proof pan. Add the onion, zucchini slices, bell pepper, and garlic. Cook for almost 5 minutes, until softened. 3. While the veggies cook, whisk the eggs with the black pepper and salt in a suitable bowl. 4. Add the zucchini mixture to the eggs and mix well. 5. Heat the remaining tablespoon of olive oil in this pan and add the egg mixture. Cook over medium heat for almost 5 minutes. 6. Transfer pan to your oven and bake for almost 20 minutes, until the eggs are set. 7. Remove from oven; allow to cool for almost 10 minutes. Carefully flip onto a serving platter and slice into wedges. 7. Top with Pico de Gallo or salsa, if desired, and serve!
Per Serving: Calories 219; Total Fat 18.8g; Sodium 590mg; Total Carbs 1.7g; Fiber 5.7g; Sugars 2.2g; Protein 4.9g

Mexican Breakfast Casserole

Prep time: 10 minutes. | Cooking time: 25 minutes. | Serves: 6

8 eggs, beaten	8 ounces mushrooms, sliced
½ cup broccoli florets	1 sweet potato, peeled and diced
½ pound bacon	2 tablespoons taco seasoning
1 yellow onion, diced	Garnish: guacamole, salsa, and fresh cilantro
1 red bell pepper, diced	

1. Cook the bacon in a suitable skillet until crispy. Keep it aside. Crumble once cooled. 2. In the same skillet, cook the onions until translucent. 3. Transfer the crumbled bacon, onions, sweet potato, bell pepper, mushrooms, broccoli florets and eggs to a slow cooker. Stir to combine. 4. Sprinkle with taco seasoning and mix well. Cook on low for almost 6 hours. 5. Scoop into serving bowls, top with guacamole, salsa, and/or fresh cilantro.
Per Serving: Calories 579; Total Fat 18.3g; Sodium 689mg; Total Carbs 6.7g; Fiber 35.5g; Sugars 11g; Protein 30.2g

Traditional Pho

Prep time: 15 minutes| Cook time: 15 minutes| Serves: 4

½ cup chopped green onions, divided
1 tablespoon minced fresh ginger
6 cups beef broth
½ tablespoon minced garlic
1 tablespoon soy sauce
2 (8-ounce) packages shirataki noodles

1 pound flank steak, thinly sliced
¼ cup bean sprouts
1 medium jalapeño pepper, seeded, deveined, and sliced in rings
½ tablespoon chopped fresh cilantro
½ tablespoon chopped fresh basil

1. In a nonstick pan, add ¼ cup onion and ginger. Cook for 5 minutes while stirring until brown. Transfer to a large soup pot. 2. Place soup pot over medium heat. Add broth, garlic, and soy sauce. Boil it and lower the heat to low and simmer for 10 minutes. 3. Divide the remaining ingredients evenly among four bowls. 4. Carefully ladle broth mixture into bowls. The near-boiling broth will cook meat as well as other vegetables. 5. Enjoy when cool enough to taste.
Per Serving: Calories 221; Fat 8g; Sodium 1632mg; Carbs 5g; Fiber 4g; Sugar 1g; Protein 29g

Zoodle Soup

Prep time: 10 minutes| Cook time: 20 minutes| Serves: 6

1 tablespoon olive oil
1½ cups chopped celery
2 tablespoons chopped green onion
½ tablespoon minced garlic
4 cups chicken broth

2 tablespoons white vinegar
¼ teaspoon salt
⅛ teaspoon ground black pepper
1 pound boneless, skinless chicken breasts
1½ cups spiralized zucchini

1. Heat the oil in Instant Pot using the Sauté function at the Less setting. Stir in celery, green onions, and garlic and cook for 5 minutes while stirring. 2. Stir in broth, vinegar, salt, and pepper until combined. Arrange chicken breasts evenly over the mixture. 3. Put on lid and close pressure release. Cook on High Pressure for 10 minutes. Carefully quick-release pressure and remove the lid to cool. 4. Using two forks, shred cooked chicken in Instant Pot. 5. Add zucchini and stir to combine. Using the Sauté function at the Normal setting, cook for 5 minutes while stirring. 6. Turn off heat and let cool with lid off. Serve warm.
Per Serving: Calories 132; Fat 4g; Sodium 769mg; Carbs 3g; Fiber 1g; Sugar 2g; Protein 19g

Lasagna Soup

Prep time: 20 minutes| Cook time: 6 hours| Serves: 6

3 tablespoons extra-virgin olive oil, divided
1 pound ground beef
½ sweet onion, chopped
2 teaspoons minced garlic
4 cups beef broth
1 (28-ounce) can diced tomatoes,

undrained
1 zucchini, diced
1½ tablespoons dried basil
2 teaspoons dried oregano
4 ounces cream cheese
1 cup shredded mozzarella

1. Lightly grease the slow cooker with 1 tablespoon of olive oil. 2. In a large pan over medium-high heat, heat the remaining 2 tablespoons of the olive oil. Add the ground beef and sauté until it is cooked through about 6 minutes. 3. Sauté the onion and garlic for an additional 3 minutes. 4. Transfer the meat mixture to the insert. Stir in the broth, tomatoes, zucchini, basil, and oregano. 5. Cover it and cook on low temperature setting for 6 hours. Stir in the cream cheese and mozzarella and serve.
Per Serving: Calories 472; Fat 36g; Sodium 111mg; Carbs 9g; Fiber 3g; Sugar 3g; Protein 30g

Cheesy Bacon Keto Soup

Prep time: 15 minutes| Cook time: 6 hours| Serves: 6

1 tablespoon extra-virgin olive oil
4 cups chicken broth
2 cups coconut milk
2 cups chopped cooked chicken
1 cup chopped cooked bacon

2 cups chopped cauliflower
1 sweet onion, chopped
3 teaspoons minced garlic
½ cup cream cheese, cubed
2 cups shredded cheddar cheese

1. Lightly oil the slow cooker with olive oil. 2. Place the broth, coconut milk, chicken, bacon, cauliflower, onion, and garlic in the insert. 3. Cover it and cook on low temp setting for 6 hours. 4. Stir in the cream cheese and Cheddar, and serve.
Per Serving: Calories 540; Fat 44g; Sodium 120mg; Carbs 6g; Fiber 1g; Sugar 2g; Protein 35g

Bacon It Up Chicken Soup

Prep time: 15 minutes| Cook time: 8 hours| Serves: 8

1 tablespoon extra-virgin olive oil
6 cups chicken broth
3 cups cooked chicken, chopped
1 sweet onion, chopped
2 celery stalks, chopped
1 carrot, diced

2 teaspoons minced garlic
1½ cups heavy (whipping) cream
1 cup cream cheese
1 cup cooked chopped bacon
1 tablespoon chopped fresh parsley, for garnish

1. Lightly oil the slow cooker with olive oil. 2. Add the broth, chicken, onion, celery, carrot, and garlic. Cover it and cook on low temperature setting for 8 hours. 3. Stir in the heavy cream, cream cheese, and bacon. 4. Serve topped with the parsley.
Per Serving: Calories 488; Fat 37g; Sodium 156mg; Carbs 10g; Fiber 1g; Sugar 1g; Protein 27g

Crunchy Slaw

Prep time: 10 minutes| Cook time: 0 minutes| Serves: 5

1 (16-ounce) bag coleslaw mix
⅓ cup full-fat mayonnaise
1 tablespoon apple cider vinegar
1 teaspoon 100% lemon juice

1 tablespoon 0g net carbs sweetener
¼ teaspoon salt
⅛ teaspoon ground black pepper

1. In a large bowl, add coleslaw mix. 2. In a bowl, mix all ingredients. Stir to mix thoroughly. Stir to mix thoroughly. 3. Using a spatula, add dressing to the coleslaw mix. Stir to combine. 4. Cover and put in refrigerator until ready to serve. Serve chilled.
Per Serving: Calories 124; Fat 11g; Sodium 225mg; Carbs 7g; Fiber 2g; Sugar 3g; Protein 1g

"Potato" Soup

Prep time: 5 minutes| Cook time: 25 minutes| Serves: 6

1 (12-ounce) bag frozen cauliflower pieces, broken into bite-sized florets
2 tablespoons unsalted butter
1 cup finely chopped radishes
1 cup sliced zucchini
½ cup chopped green onions, divided

1 tablespoon minced garlic
4 cups chicken broth
½ cup full-fat cream cheese
2 (3.7-gram) chicken-flavored bouillon cubes
⅛ teaspoon ground black pepper
2 cups shredded cheddar cheese
¼ cup cooked bacon bits

1. In a large microwave-safe dish, add cauliflower. Cover the bowl and microwave on high 4–5 minutes until tender. 2. While cauliflower cooks melt butter in a large soup pot over medium heat. Add radishes, zucchini, ¼ cup onion, and garlic. Sauté for 3–4 minutes until softened. 3. Add cauliflower, broth, cream cheese, bouillon, and pepper to soup pot. Bring covered pot to a boil, then simmer on low heat for 20 minutes while stirring. 4. Using an immersion blender, pulse soup ingredients 1–2 minutes to desired consistency. 5. Add cheddar to soup and fold in. 6. Pour into six small bowls and top with equal amounts bacon bits and remaining green onion. Serve immediately.
Per Serving: Calories 310; Fat 22g; Sodium 1354mg; Carbs 7g; Fiber 2g; Sugar 4g; Protein 15g

Quick Cream of Asparagus Soup

Prep time: 10 minutes. | Cooking time: 30 minutes. | Serves: 4

4 cups vegetable broth
1 cup heavy cream
1 bunch asparagus, chopped into

1-inch pieces
2 cloves garlic, chopped
1 pinch of sea salt

1. Add all the recipe ingredients to a stockpot over medium heat minus the heavy cream and cook to a boil. 2. Reduce its heat to a simmer and cook for almost 30 minutes. 3. Warm the heavy cream, and then stir into the soup. 4. Use an immersion blender and blend until smooth.
Per Serving: Calories 353; Total Fat 28.2g; Sodium 472mg; Total Carbs 4.9g; Fiber 9.9g; Sugars 1.2g; Protein 14.6g

Italian Soup

Prep time: 10 minutes| Cook time: 4 hours| Serves: 6

6 cups chicken broth	1 cup shredded mozzarella cheese
3 boneless, skinless chicken breasts	1 jalapeno pepper, seeded and sliced
1 cup canned diced tomatoes	1 teaspoon dried thyme
1 yellow onion, chopped	1 teaspoon dried oregano
2 cloves garlic, chopped	Salt & black pepper to taste

1. Add all the ingredients excluding the salt and black pepper to the base of a slow cooker instead of the cheese and cook on high for 4 hours. 2. Stir in the cheese and season with salt and black pepper. 3. Shred the chicken and served.
Per Serving: Calories 125; Fat 4g; Sodium 74mg; Carbs 5g; Fiber 1g; Sugar 1g; Protein 17g

Pollo Soup

Prep time: 10 minutes| Cook time: 20 minutes| Serves: 4

1 pound boneless, skinless chicken thighs, sliced	½ teaspoon ground cumin
1 (10-ounce) can no-sugar-added diced tomatoes and green chiles	½ tablespoon paprika
	½ medium jalapeño pepper, seeded, deveined, and diced
2 cups chicken broth	½ teaspoon salt
2 tablespoons unsalted butter	1 medium avocado, peeled, pitted, and sliced
¼ cup chopped green onion	
2 teaspoons minced garlic	1 tablespoon chopped fresh cilantro
½ tablespoon onion powder	
1 teaspoon chili powder	

1. In Instant Pot, combine all ingredients except avocado and cilantro. Stir to mix. 2. Put on lid and close pressure release. Cook on High Pressure for 20 minutes. Carefully quick-release pressure and remove cover. Stir to mix well. 3. Serve warm, top with avocado slices and a sprinkle of cilantro.
Per Serving: Calories 317; Fat 18g; Sodium 1060mg; Carbs 9g; Fiber 4g; Sugar 3g; Protein 25g

Turkey Soup

Prep time: 20 minutes| Cook time: 7 to 8 hours| Serves: 8

1 tablespoon extra-virgin olive oil	2 teaspoons chopped fresh thyme
4 cups chicken broth	1 cup cream cheese, diced
½ pound skinless turkey breast, cut into ½-inch chunks	2 cups heavy (whipping) cream
	1 cup green beans, chopped into 1-inch bites
2 celery stalks, chopped	
1 carrot, diced	Salt, for seasoning
1 sweet onion, chopped	Freshly ground black pepper, for seasoning
2 teaspoons minced garlic	

1. Lightly oil the slow cooker with olive oil. 2. Place the broth, turkey, celery, carrot, onion, garlic, and thyme in the insert. 3. Cover it and cook on low temperature setting for 7 to 8 hours. 4. Stir in the cream cheese, heavy cream, and green beans. 5. Season with salt and pepper, and serve.
Per Serving: Calories 415; Fat 35g; Sodium 231mg; Carbs 5g; Fiber 2g; Sugar 2g; Protein 20g

Chicken and nacho Soup

Prep time: 15 minutes| Cook time: 6 hours| Serves: 8

3 tablespoons extra-virgin olive oil, divided	4 cups chicken broth
	2 cups coconut milk
1 pound ground chicken	1 tomato, diced
1 sweet onion, diced	1 jalapeño pepper, chopped
1 red bell pepper, chopped	2 cups shredded cheddar cheese
2 teaspoons minced garlic	½ cup sour cream, for garnish
2 tablespoons taco seasoning	scallion, chopped, for garnish

1. Lightly grease the slow cooker with 1 tablespoon of olive oil. 2. In a pan, heat the remaining 2 tablespoons of the olive oil. Add the chicken and sauté until it is cooked through about 6 minutes. 3. Add the onion, red bell pepper, garlic, taco seasoning, and sauté for 3 minutes. 4. Transfer the chicken mixture to the insert, and stir in the broth, coconut milk, tomato, and jalapeño pepper. 5. Cover it and cook on low temp setting for 6 hours. 6. Stir in the cheese. Serve topped with sour cream and scallion.
Per Serving: Calories 434; Fat 35g; Sodium 189mg; Carbs 7g; Fiber 2g; Sugar 3g; Protein 22g

Spiced-Pumpkin with Chicken Soup

Prep time: 15 minutes| Cook time: 6 hours| Serves: 6

1 tablespoon extra-virgin olive oil	¼ teaspoon ground nutmeg
4 cups chicken broth	¼ teaspoon freshly ground black pepper
2 cups coconut milk	
1 pound pumpkin, diced	¼ teaspoon salt
½ sweet onion, chopped	Pinch ground allspice
1 tablespoon grated fresh ginger	1 cup heavy (whipping) cream
2 teaspoons minced garlic	2 cups chopped cooked chicken
½ teaspoon ground cinnamon	

1. Lightly oil the slow cooker with olive oil. 2. Place the broth, coconut milk, pumpkin, onion, ginger, garlic, cinnamon, nutmeg, pepper, salt, and allspice in the insert. 3. Cover it and cook on low temp setting for 6 hours. Using an immersion blender or a regular blender, purée the soup. 4. If you removed the soup from the insert to purée, add it back to the pot, and stir in the cream and chicken. 5. Keep heating the soup on low for 15 minutes to heat the chicken through, and then serve warm.
Per Serving: Calories 389; Fat 32g; Sodium 52mg; Carbs 10g; Fiber 5g; Sugar 3g; Protein 16g

Sausage Soup

Prep time: 15 minutes| Cook time: 6 hours| Serves: 6

3 tablespoons olive oil, divided	1 leek, thoroughly cleaned and chopped
1½ pounds sausage, without casing	
	2 teaspoons minced garlic
6 cups chicken broth	2 cups chopped kale
2 celery stalks, chopped	1 tablespoon chopped fresh parsley, for garnish
1 carrot, diced	

1. Lightly grease the slow cooker with 1 tablespoon of olive oil. 2. In a large pan over medium-high heat, heat the remaining 2 tablespoons of the olive oil. Add the sausage and sauté until it is cooked through for about 7 minutes. 3. Transfer the sausage to the insert, and stir in the broth, celery, carrot, leek, and garlic. 4. Cover it and cook on low temperature setting for 6 hours. 5. Stir in the kale. Serve topped with the parsley.
Per Serving: Calories 383; Fat 31g; Sodium 171mg; Carbs 5g; Fiber 1g; Sugar 2g; Protein 21g

Amazing Cheeseburger Soup

Prep time: 15 minutes| Cook time: 6 hours| Serves: 8

3 tablespoons olive oil, divided	1 carrot, chopped
1 pound ground beef	1 cup heavy (whipping) cream
1 sweet onion, chopped	2 cups shredded cheddar cheese
2 teaspoons minced garlic	½ teaspoon freshly ground black pepper
6 cups beef broth	
1 (28-ounce) can diced tomatoes	1 scallion, white and green parts, chopped, for garnish
2 celery stalks, chopped	

1. Lightly grease the slow cooker with 1 tablespoon of olive oil. 2. In a large pan over medium-high heat, heat the remaining 2 tablespoons of the olive oil. Add the ground beef and sauté until it is cooked through about 6 minutes. 3. Sauté the onion and garlic for an additional 3 minutes. 4. Transfer the beef mixture to the insert, and stir in the broth, tomatoes, celery, and carrot. 5. Cover it and cook on low temperature setting for 6 hours. 6. Stir in the heavy cream, cheese, and pepper. Serve hot, top with the scallion.
Per Serving: Calories 413; Fat 32g; Sodium 101mg; Carbs 8g; Fiber 2g; Sugar 3g; Protein 26g

Cheddar Cheesy Soup

Prep time: 15 minutes| Cook time: 6 hours| Serves: 6

1 tablespoon butter	8 ounces cream cheese, cubed
5 cups chicken broth	2 cups shredded cheddar cheese
1 cup coconut milk	Salt, for seasoning
2 celery stalks, chopped	Freshly ground black pepper, for seasoning
1 carrot, chopped	
½ sweet onion, chopped	1 tablespoon chopped fresh thyme for garnish
Pinch cayenne pepper	

1. Lightly grease the slow cooker with the butter. 2. Place the broth, coconut milk, celery, carrot, onion, and cayenne pepper in the insert. 3. Cover it and cook on low temperature setting for 6 hours. 4. Stir in the cream cheese and cheddar, then season with salt and pepper. 5. Serve topped with thyme.
Per Serving: Calories 406; Fat 36g; Sodium 88mg; Carbs 7g; Fiber 1g; Sugar 2g; Protein 15g

Healthy Jambalaya Soup

Prep time: 15 minutes| Cook time: 6 to 7 hours| Serves: 8

1 tablespoon extra-virgin olive oil	2 teaspoons minced garlic
6 cups chicken broth	3 tablespoons Cajun seasoning
1 (28-ounce) can diced tomatoes	½ pound medium shrimp, peeled,
1 pound spicy organic sausage, sliced	deveined, and chopped
	½ cup sour cream, for garnish
1 cup chopped cooked chicken	1 avocado, diced, for garnish
1 red bell pepper, chopped	2 tablespoons chopped cilantro,
½ sweet onion, chopped	for garnish
1 jalapeño pepper, chopped	

1. Lightly oil the slow cooker with olive oil. 2. Add the broth, tomatoes, sausage, chicken, red bell pepper, onion, jalapeño pepper, garlic, and Cajun seasoning. 3. Cover it and cook on low temperature setting for 6 to 7 hours. 4. Stir in the shrimp and leave on low for 30 minutes, or until the shrimp are cooked through. 5. Serve topped with avocado, sour cream, and cilantro.
Per Serving: Calories 400; Fat 31g; Sodium 1783mg; Carbs 9g; Fiber 4g; Sugar 1g; Protein 24g

Chicken-Vegetable Soup

Prep time: 15 minutes| Cook time: 7 to 8 hours| Serves: 6

1 tablespoon extra-virgin olive oil	½ cup chopped cauliflower
4 cups chicken broth	2 teaspoons minced garlic
2 cups coconut milk	1 teaspoon chopped thyme
2 cups diced chicken breast	1 teaspoon chopped oregano
½ sweet onion, chopped	¼ teaspoon freshly ground black
2 celery stalks, chopped	pepper
1 carrot, diced	

1. Lightly oil the slow cooker with olive oil. 2. Add the broth, coconut milk, chicken, onion, celery, carrot, cauliflower, garlic, thyme, oregano, and pepper. 3. Cover it and cook on low temperature setting for 7 to 8 hours. 4. Serve warm.
Per Serving: Calories 187; Fat 11g; Sodium 720mg; Carbs 8.8g; Fiber 1g; Sugar 6.9g; Protein 13g

Regular Beef Stew

Prep time: 15 minutes| Cook time: 8 hours| Serves: 6

3 tablespoons extra-virgin olive oil, divided	¼ cup apple cider vinegar
	1½ cups cubed pumpkin, cut into
1 (2-pound) beef chuck roast, cut into 1-inch chunks	1-inch chunks
	½ sweet onion, chopped
½ teaspoon salt	2 teaspoons minced garlic
¼ teaspoon freshly ground black pepper	1 teaspoon dried thyme
	1 tablespoon chopped fresh
2 cups beef broth	parsley, for garnish
1 cup diced tomatoes	

1. Lightly grease the slow cooker with 1 tablespoon of olive oil. 2. Lightly season the beef chucks with salt and pepper. 3. In a pan heat 2 tablespoons of the olive oil. Add the meat and brown on all sides for about 7 minutes. 4. Transfer the beef to the insert and stir in the broth, tomatoes, apple cider vinegar, pumpkin, onion, garlic, and thyme. 5. Cover it and cook on low temperature setting heat for about 8 hours until the beef is very tender. 6. Serve topped with the parsley.
Per Serving: Calories 461; Fat 24g; Sodium 100mg; Carbs 10g; Fiber 3g; Sugar 2g; Protein 32g

Chicken Stew with Coconut Cream

Prep time: 20 minutes| Cook time: 6 hours | Serves: 6

3 tablespoons extra-virgin olive oil, divided	1 carrot, diced
	1 teaspoon dried thyme
1 pound boneless chicken thighs, diced into 1½-inch pieces	1 cup shredded kale
	1 cup coconut cream
½ sweet onion, chopped	Salt, for seasoning
2 teaspoons minced garlic	Freshly ground black pepper, for
2 cups chicken broth	seasoning
2 celery stalks, diced	

1. Lightly grease the slow cooker with 1 tablespoon of olive oil. 2. In a large pan over medium-high heat, heat the remaining 2 tablespoons of the olive oil. Add the chicken and sauté until it is just cooked through about 7 minutes. 3. Sauté the onion and garlic for an additional 3 minutes. Sauté the onion and garlic for an additional 3 minutes.

Transfer the chicken mixture to the insert, and stir in the broth, celery, carrot, and thyme. 4. Cover it and cook on low temperature setting for 6 hours. 5. Stir in the kale and coconut cream. 6. Sprinkle salt and pepper, and serve warm.
Per Serving: Calories 276; Fat 22g; Sodium 0mg; Carbs 4g; Fiber 2g; Sugar 1g; Protein 17g

Asian Vegetable Stew

Prep time: 15 minutes| Cook time: 7 to 8 hours| Serves: 6

1 tablespoon extra-virgin olive oil	1 sweet onion, chopped
4 cups coconut milk	2 teaspoons grated fresh ginger
1 cup diced pumpkin	2 teaspoons minced garlic
1 cup cauliflower florets	1 tablespoon curry powder
1 red bell pepper, diced	2 cups shredded spinach
1 zucchini, diced	1 avocado, diced, for garnish

1. Lightly oil the slow cooker with olive oil. 2. Add the coconut milk, pumpkin, cauliflower, bell pepper, zucchini, onion, ginger, garlic, and curry powder. 3. Cover it and cook on low temperature setting for 7 to 8 hours. Stir in the spinach. 4. Garnish each bowl with a spoonful of avocado and serve.
Per Serving: Calories 502; Fat 44g; Sodium 235mg; Carbs 19g; Fiber 10g; Sugar 6g; Protein 7g

Meat with Vegetable Stew

Prep time: 20 minutes| Cook time: 7 to 8 hours| Serves: 6

3 tablespoons extra-virgin olive oil, divided	2 celery stalks, chopped
	2 cups diced pumpkin
1 pound turkey breast, boneless, cut into 1-inch pieces	1 carrot, diced
	2 teaspoons chopped thyme
1 leek, thoroughly cleaned and sliced	Salt, for seasoning
	Freshly ground black pepper, for
2 teaspoons minced garlic	seasoning
2 cups chicken broth	1 scallion, chopped, for garnish
1 cup coconut milk	

1. Grease the slow cooker with olive oil. In a pan, heat the remaining 2 tablespoons of the olive oil. Add the turkey and sauté until browned, about 5 minutes. 2. Add the leek and garlic and sauté for an additional 3 minutes. Transfer the turkey mixture to the insert and stir in the broth, coconut milk, celery, pumpkin, carrot, and thyme. Cover it and cook on low temperature setting for 7 to 8 hours. 3. Season with salt and pepper. 4. Serve topped with the scallion.
Per Serving: Calories 356; Fat 27g; Sodium 580mg; Carbs 11g; Fiber 4g; Sugar 2g; Protein 21g

Turmeric Stew

Prep time: 10 minutes. | Cooking time: 40 minutes. | Serves: 6

4 cups vegetable broth	2 teaspoons ground turmeric
1 cauliflower head, cut into florets	1 teaspoon ground cinnamon
1 cup full-fat coconut milk	1 teaspoon dried oregano
2 cloves garlic, chopped	Salt & black pepper, to taste
1 yellow onion, chopped	

1. Add all the recipe ingredients minus the salt, black pepper, and coconut milk to a stockpot and cook to a boil. 2. Reduce its heat to a simmer and cook for almost 40 minutes. 3. Stir in the coconut milk. 4. Season with salt and black pepper and serve.
Per Serving: Calories 460; Total Fat 10.1g; Sodium 332mg; Total Carbs 3.9g; Fiber 20.3g; Sugars 14.5g; Protein 21.7g

Spicy Cilantro Soup

Prep time: 10 minutes| Cook time: 4 hours| Serves: 6

6 cups chicken broth	2 cloves garlic, chopped
3 boneless, skinless chicken breasts	1 jalapeno pepper, seeded and sliced
Juice from 1 lime	1 handful fresh cilantro
1 yellow onion, chopped	Salt & black pepper, to taste

1. Add all the ingredients excluding the cilantro, salt, and black pepper to the base of a slow cooker. 2. Cook on high setting for 4 hours. Add the cilantro and season with salt and black pepper. 3. Shred the chicken and served.
Per Serving: Calories 108; Fat 3g; Sodium 689mg; Carbs 4g; Fiber 1g; Sugar 2g; Protein 16g

Cilantro & Lime Soup

Prep time: 15 minutes plus 1 hour for chilling| Cook time: 0 minutes| Serves: 6

4 cups vegetable broth
1 cup heavy cream
2 ripe avocados, pitted and sliced
½ cup freshly chopped cilantro

2 tablespoons freshly squeezed lime juice
½ teaspoon sea salt

1. Add all the ingredients in a blender. 2. Blend until smooth. 3. Chill for 1 hour before serving.
Per Serving: Calories 232; Fat 21g; Sodium 689mg; Carbs 7g; Fiber 5g; Sugar 3g; Protein 5g

Spicy Chipotle Chicken Chili

Prep time: 20 minutes| Cook time: 7 to 8 hours| Serves: 6

3 tablespoons extra-virgin olive oil, divided
1 pound ground chicken
½ sweet onion, chopped
2 teaspoons minced garlic
1 (28-ounce) can diced tomatoes
1 cup chicken broth

1 cup diced pumpkin
1 green bell pepper, diced
3 tablespoons chili powder
1 teaspoon chipotle chili powder
1 cup sour cream, for garnish
1 cup shredded cheddar cheese, for garnish

1. Lightly grease the slow cooker with 1 tablespoon of olive oil. 2. In a large pan over medium-high heat, heat the remaining 2 tablespoons of the olive oil. Add the chicken and sauté until it is cooked through about 6 minutes. Sauté the onion and garlic for an additional 3 minutes. 3. Transfer the chicken mixture to the insert and stir in the tomatoes, broth, pumpkin, bell pepper, chili powder, and chipotle chili powder. 4. Cover it and cook on low temperature setting for 7 to 8 hours. 5. Serve topped with sour cream and cheese.
Per Serving: Calories 390; Fat 30g; Sodium 102mg; Carbs 14g; Fiber 5g; Sugar 3g; Protein 22g

Jalapeno & Lime in Shrimp Soup

Prep time: 10 minutes| Cook time: 35 minutes| Serves: 6

4 cups chicken broth
Juice from 1 lime
1 pound peeled, deveined shrimp
1 yellow onion, chopped
1 shallot, chopped
3 cloves garlic, chopped

1 jalapeno pepper, seeded and sliced
Salt & black pepper, to taste
1 tablespoon coconut oil for cooking

1. Heat the coconut oil in a stockpot. Add the shrimp, onion, shallot, and garlic and cook until the shrimp are pink. 2. Add the remaining ingredients instead of the salt and black pepper, and bring to a boil. 3. Simmer on low for 30 minutes. 4. Spice with salt and black pepper, and serve.
Per Serving: Calories 153; Fat 5g; Sodium 69mg; Carbs 6g; Fiber 1g; Sugar 2g; Protein 21g

Regular Italian Beef Soup

Prep time: 10 minutes| Cook time: 4 hours| Serves: 6

1 pound lean ground beef
1 cup beef broth
1 cup heavy cream
½ cup shredded mozzarella cheese

½ cup diced tomatoes
1 yellow onion, chopped
2 cloves garlic, chopped
1 tablespoon Italian seasoning
Salt & pepper to taste

1. Put in all the ingredients to a slow cooker excluding the heavy cream and mozzarella cheese—cook on high for 4 hours. 2. Warm the heavy cream, and then add the warmed cream and cheese to the soup. Stir well and serve.
Per Serving: Calories 241; Fat 14g; Sodium 111mg; Carbs 4g; Fiber 1g; Sugar 1.6g; Protein 25g

Cheesy Bacon Soup

Prep time: 15 minutes| Cook time: 40 minutes| Serves: 6

1 pound of lean ground beef
6 slices uncured bacon
6 cups beef broth
1 cup heavy cream
1 cup shredded cheddar cheese
1 yellow onion, chopped
1 teaspoon garlic powder

½ teaspoon onion powder
½ teaspoon cumin
½ teaspoon paprika
½ cup sour cream, for serving
1 tablespoon coconut oil, for cooking

1. Add the coconut oil to a pan and cook the bacon. 2. Chop the cooked crispy bacon into small chunks. 3. Add the ground beef to the pan with the bacon fat and cook until well browned and cooked. 4. Add the onions and cook it for another 2 to 3 minutes. 5. In a stockpot, add all the ingredients instead of the bacon, heavy cream, sour cream, and cheese to a stockpot and stir—cook for 25 minutes. 6. Warm the heavy cream, and then add the warmed cream and cheese and serve with the bacon and a dollop of sour cream.
Per Serving: Calories 498; Fat 34g; Sodium 145mg; Carbs 5g; Fiber 1g; Sugar 1g; Protein 41g

Texas Chili

Prep time: 20 minutes| Cook time: 7 to 8 hours| Serves: 4

¼ cup extra-virgin olive oil
1½ pounds beef sirloin, cut into 1-inch chunks
1 sweet onion, chopped
2 green bell peppers, chopped
1 jalapeño pepper, seeded, finely chopped
2 teaspoons minced garlic
1 (28-ounce) can diced tomatoes

1 cup beef broth
3 tablespoons chili powder
½ teaspoon ground cumin
¼ teaspoon ground coriander
1 cup sour cream, for garnish
1 avocado, diced, for garnish
1 tablespoon cilantro, chopped, for garnish

1. Lightly grease the slow cooker with 1 tablespoon of olive oil. 2. In a large pan over medium-high heat, heat the remaining 2 tablespoons of the olive oil. Add the beef and sauté until it is cooked through about 8 minutes. 3. Add the onion, bell peppers, jalapeño pepper, garlic, and sauté for 4 minutes. 4. Transfer the beef mixture to the insert and stir in the tomatoes, broth, chili powder, cumin, and coriander. 5. Cover it and cook on low temperature setting for 7 to 8 hours. 6. Serve topped with the sour cream, avocado, and cilantro.
Per Serving: Calories 752; Fat 50g; Sodium 826mg; Carbs 34g; Fiber 11g; Sugar 13g; Protein 45g

Red Chili

Prep time: 10 minutes. | Cooking time: 35 minutes. | Serves: 6

4 slices bacon
½ pound 85% lean ground beef
½ pound 84% lean ground pork
1 green pepper, diced
½ medium onion, diced
2 cups beef broth
1 (14.5-ounce) can diced tomatoes

1 (6-ounce) can tomato paste
1 tablespoon chili powder
2 teaspoons salt
½ teaspoon pepper
⅛ teaspoon cayenne
¼ teaspoon xanthan gum

1. Hit the sauté button on the Instant Pot and cook bacon. Remove bacon, crumble, and keep it aside. In bacon grease, brown beef and pork until fully cooked. Add green pepper and onion to Instant Pot and allow to soften for almost 1 minute. 2. Hit the cancel button and add remaining ingredients except xanthan gum to pot. Turn the pot's lid to close. Hit the soup button and adjust time for almost 30 minutes. Allow a 10-minute natural release and then quick-release the remaining pressure. Stir in cooked bacon and xanthan gum then allow to thicken for almost 10 minutes. Serve warm with favorite chili toppings. 3. For thicker chili, remove lid when timer goes off and hit the sauté button. Add xanthan gum and reduce chili, stirring frequently, until desired thickness. Top with additional diced onions or other toppings.
Per Serving: Calories 285; Total Fat 7.5g; Sodium 1367mg; Total Carbs 5.6g; Fiber 9.6g; Sugars 18.2g; Protein 4.4g

Easy Jalapeño Popper Soup

Prep time: 10 minutes. | Cooking time: 25 minutes. | Serves: 4

2 tablespoons butter
½ medium diced onion
¼ cup sliced pickled jalapeños
¼ cup cooked crumbled bacon
2 cups chicken broth
2 cups cooked diced chicken
4 ounces cream cheese

1 teaspoon salt
½ teaspoon pepper
¼ teaspoon garlic powder
⅓ cup heavy cream
1 cup shredded sharp cheddar cheese

1. Hit the sauté button. Add butter, onion, and sliced jalapeños to Instant Pot. Sauté for almost 5 minutes, until onions are translucent. Add bacon and hit the cancel button. 2. Add broth, cooked chicken, cream cheese, salt, pepper, and garlic to Instant Pot. Turn the pot's lid to close. Hit the soup button and adjust time for almost 20 minutes. 3. When the pot beeps, quick-release the steam. Stir in heavy cream and cheddar. Continue stirring until cheese is fully melted. Serve warm.
Per Serving: Calories 137; Total Fat 7.1g; Sodium 1067mg; Total Carbs 6.2g; Fiber 3.8g; Sugars 4.7g; Protein 3.1g

Zesty Chicken Soup

Prep time: 10 minutes | Cook time: 4 hours | Serves: 6

6 cups chicken broth
3 boneless, skinless chicken breasts
Juice from 1 lemon
1 yellow onion, chopped

2 cloves garlic, chopped
1 teaspoon cayenne pepper
1 teaspoon dried thyme
1 handful of fresh parsley, minced
Salt & black pepper, to taste

1. Add all the ingredients excluding the salt, black pepper, and parsley to the base of a slow cooker instead of the parsley and cook on high for 4 hours. 2. Add the parsley and spiced with salt and black pepper. Shred the chicken and served.
Per Serving: Calories 108; Fat 3g; Sodium 365mg; Carbs 4g; Fiber 1g; Sugar 2g; Protein 16g

Chicken Cheese Soup

Prep time: 20 minutes | Cook time: 33 to 40 minutes | Serves: 6

2 boneless, skinless chicken breasts
2 cups chicken broth
2 cups water
1 cup whipped cream cheese
½ cup shredded cheddar cheese
1 yellow onion, chopped

2 cloves garlic, chopped
1 teaspoon chili powder
½ teaspoon cumin
½ teaspoon salt
¼ teaspoon black pepper
1 tablespoon coconut oil, for cooking

1. Heat a ½ tablespoon coconut oil in a pan. Sear the chicken breasts until cooked through. Set aside. 2. Sauté the garlic and onion to a large stockpot with the remaining 1 tablespoon of the coconut oil until translucent over low to medium heat. 3. Add this chicken broth and water. 4. On low heat whisk in the cream cheese and keep whisking until combined. 5. Add the spices and boil. Cut the chicken into bite-sized pieces and add to the stockpot. Simmer on low heat for 30 to 35 minutes. 6. Stir in the cheddar cheese and serve.
Per Serving: Calories 157; Fat 7g; Sodium 463mg; Carbs 5g; Fiber 1g; Sugar 1g; Protein 17g

Beef Veggie Broth

Prep time: 10 minutes. | Cooking time: 120 minutes. | Serves: 6

2 pounds beef bones
2 celery stalks, chopped
2 medium halved carrots
1 medium onion, peeled and

halved
2 bay leaves
2 sprigs fresh thyme
6 cups water

1. Add all the recipe ingredients to Instant Pot. Turn the pot's lid to close. 2. Hit the manual button and adjust time for almost 120 minutes. 3. When the pot beeps, allow a full natural release. When pressure valve drops, remove large pieces of vegetables. Pour broth through fine-mesh strainer and store in closed containers in fridge or freezer.
Per Serving: Calories 52; Total Fat 2.1g; Sodium 766mg; Total Carbs 1.8g; Fiber 0.3g; Sugars 0.9g; Protein 6.3g

Chicken Veggie Broth

Prep time: 10 minutes. | Cooking time: 120 minutes. | Serves: 6

2 pounds chicken bones
2 celery stalks, chopped
2 medium halved carrots
1 medium onion, peeled and

halved
2 bay leaves
2 sprigs fresh thyme
6 cups water

1. Add all the recipe ingredients to Instant Pot. Turn the pot's lid to close. Hit the manual button and adjust time for almost 120 minutes. 2. When the pot beeps, allow a full natural release. When pressure valve drops, remove large pieces of vegetables. Pour broth through fine-mesh strainer and store in closed containers in fridge or freezer.
Per Serving: Calories 367; Total Fat 28.6g; Sodium 663mg; Total Carbs 8.5g; Fiber 4.8g; Sugars 1.1g; Protein 22.7g

Leftover Bone Broth

Prep time: 10 minutes. | Cooking time: 3 hours. | Serves: 6

2–3 pounds leftover chicken bones
3 tablespoons coconut oil
2 medium halved carrots
2 celery stalks, chopped

2 tablespoons apple cider vinegar
1 medium onion, large dice
2 whole cloves garlic
2 bay leaves
8 cups water

1. Hit the sauté button on the Instant Pot and add meat bones and coconut oil to Instant Pot. Sauté for almost 5 minutes. Hit the cancel button. 2. Add remaining ingredients to pot and hit the soup button. Hit the adjust button to set heat to more. Set time for almost 3 hours. When the pot beeps, allow a 20-minute natural release. Quick-release the remaining pressure. 3. Strain liquid and store in sealed jars in fridge up to 5 days.
Per Serving: Calories 311; Total Fat 15.9g; Sodium 610mg; Total Carbs 4.4g; Fiber 9.7g; Sugars 6g; Protein 10.6g

Shellfish Stock

Prep time: 10 minutes. | Cooking time: 120 minutes. | Serves: 6

4 cups shellfish shells
6 cups water
1 medium onion, peeled and chopped

2 tablespoons apple cider vinegar
2 bay leaves
2 celery stalks, chopped

1. Add all the recipe ingredients to Instant Pot. Turn the pot's lid to close. Hit the manual button and adjust time for almost 120 minutes. 2. Allow a 30-minute natural release, then quick-release the remaining pressure. When pressure valve drops, strain stock and store in sealed containers in fridge for almost 1–2 days or freeze.
Per Serving: Calories 328; Total Fat 25.9g; Sodium 9mg; Total Carbs 4.5g; Fiber 9.8g; Sugars 12.6g; Protein 5.3g

Greek Egg Soup

Prep time: 10 minutes. | Cooking time: 15 minutes. | Serves: 4

4 cups store-bought chicken broth   1 lemon
4 eggs, separated

1. Hit the sauté button. Add chicken broth to Instant Pot to warm. 2. In two suitable bowls, separate egg yolks and egg whites. Beat egg yolks and stir into broth. Hit the cancel button so Instant Pot switches to stay warm mode. 3. Using whisk or hand mixer, whisk egg whites until they form soft peaks. Add into Instant Pot. Squeeze in juice from lemon. Foam may stay at the top of soup initially, but with continued occasional stirring, will dissipate by the end of cooking.
Per Serving: Calories 354; Total Fat 19.2g; Sodium 318mg; Total Carbs 0.3g; Fiber 3.5g; Sugars 5g; Protein 26.3g

Chicken Cordon Bleu Soup

Prep time: 10 minutes. | Cooking time: 15 minutes. | Serves: 6

2 (6-ounce) boneless, skinless chicken breasts, cubed
4 cups chicken broth
½ cup cubed ham
8 ounces cream cheese
1 teaspoon salt

½ teaspoon pepper
½ teaspoon garlic powder
½ cup heavy cream
2 cups grated Swiss cheese
2 teaspoons Dijon mustard

1. Place all the recipe ingredients except heavy cream, cream cheese, and mustard into Instant Pot. Turn the pot's lid to close. 2. Hit the soup button and adjust time for almost 15 minutes. When the pot beeps, quick-release the pressure. Stir in heavy cream, cheese, and mustard. Serve warm.
Per Serving: Calories 136; Total Fat 14.3g; Sodium 9mg; Total Carbs 3.5g; Fiber 0g; Sugars 0g; Protein 0.3g

Buffalo Chicken Soup

Prep time: 10 minutes. | Cooking time: 25 minutes. | Serves: 4

2 tablespoons diced onion
2 tablespoons butter
3 cups store-bought chicken broth
2 (6-ounce) boneless, skinless chicken breasts, cubed
1 teaspoon salt
¼ teaspoon garlic powder

¼ teaspoon pepper
2 celery stalks, chopped
½ cup hot sauce
4 ounces cream cheese
½ cup shredded cheddar cheese
¼ teaspoon xanthan gum

1. Hit the sauté button on the Instant Pot and add onion and butter to Instant Pot. Sauté 2–3 minutes until onions begin to soften. Hit the cancel button. 2. Add broth and chicken to Instant Pot. Sprinkle salt, garlic powder, and pepper on chicken. Add celery and hot sauce and place cream cheese on top of chicken. Turn the pot's lid to close. 3. Hit the manual button and adjust time for almost 25 minutes. When the pot beeps, quick-release the pressure and stir in cheddar and xanthan gum. Serve warm.
Per Serving: Calories 270; Total Fat 8.4g; Sodium 1761mg; Total Carbs 5.7g; Fiber 13.3g; Sugars 24.1g; Protein 14.8g

Chicken Zucchini Noodle Soup

Prep time: 10 minutes. | Cooking time: 20 minutes. | Serves: 6

3 stalks celery, diced
2 tablespoons diced pickled jalapeño
1 cup bok choy, sliced into strips
½ cup fresh spinach
3 zucchinis, spiralized
1 tablespoon coconut oil
¼ cup button mushrooms, diced

¼ medium onion, diced
2 cups cooked diced chicken
3 cups store-bought chicken broth
1 bay leaf
1 teaspoon salt
½ teaspoon garlic powder
⅛ teaspoon cayenne pepper

1. Place celery, jalapeño, bok choy, and spinach into suitable bowl. Spiralize zucchini; keep it aside in a separate suitable bowl. (the zucchini will not go in the pot during the pressure cooking.) 2. Hit the sauté button on the Instant Pot and add the coconut oil to Instant Pot. Once the oil is hot, add mushrooms and onion. Sauté for almost 4–6 minutes until onion is translucent and fragrant. Add celery, jalapeños, bok choy, and spinach to Instant Pot. Cook for additional 4 minutes. Hit the cancel button. 3. Add cooked diced chicken, broth, bay leaf, and seasoning to Instant Pot. Turn the pot's lid to close. Hit the soup button and set time for almost 20 minutes. 4. When the pot beeps, allow a 10-minute natural release, and quick-release the remaining pressure. Add spiralized zucchini on keep warm mode and cook for additional 10 minutes or until tender. Serve warm.
Per Serving: Calories 568; Total Fat 20.8g; Sodium 1493mg; Total Carbs 1.8g; Fiber 3.8g; Sugars 10.2g; Protein 75.8g

Garlic Chicken Soup

Prep time: 10 minutes. | Cooking time: 20 minutes. | Serves: 6

10 roasted garlic cloves
½ medium onion, diced
4 tablespoons butter
4 cups chicken broth
½ teaspoon salt
¼ teaspoon pepper

1 teaspoon thyme
1 pound boneless, skinless chicken thighs, cubed
½ cup heavy cream
2 ounces cream cheese

1. In suitable bowl, mash roasted garlic into paste. Hit the sauté button on the Instant Pot and add garlic, onion, and butter to Instant Pot. Sauté for almost 2–3 minutes until onion begins to soften. Hit the cancel button. 2. Add chicken broth, salt, pepper, thyme, and chicken to Instant Pot. Turn the pot's lid to close. Hit the manual button and adjust time for almost 20 minutes. 3. When the pot beeps, quick-release the pressure. Stir in heavy cream and cream cheese until smooth. Serve warm.
Per Serving: Calories 291; Total Fat 10.8g; Sodium 2153mg; Total Carbs 2.1g; Fiber 1.6g; Sugars 5.6g; Protein 37g

Creamy Mushroom Soup

Prep time: 10 minutes. | Cooking time: 10 minutes. | Serves: 4

1 pound sliced button mushrooms
3 tablespoons butter
2 tablespoons diced onion
2 cloves garlic, minced
2 cups chicken broth

½ teaspoon salt
¼ teaspoon pepper
½ cup heavy cream
¼ teaspoon xanthan gum

1. Hit the sauté button on the Instant Pot and then hit the adjust button to set heat to less. Add mushrooms, butter, and onion to pot. Sauté for almost 5–8 minutes or until onions and mushrooms begin to brown. Add garlic and sauté until fragrant. Hit the cancel button. 2. Add broth, salt, and pepper. Turn the pot's lid to close. Hit the manual button and adjust time for almost 3 minutes. When the pot beeps, quick-release the pressure. Stir in heavy cream and xanthan gum. Allow a few minutes to thicken and serve warm.
Per Serving: Calories 330; Total Fat 29.1g; Sodium 348mg; Total Carbs 2.6g; Fiber 1.6g; Sugars 0g; Protein 7.7g

Cabbage Roll Soup

Prep time: 10 minutes. | Cooking time: 8 minutes. | Serves: 4

½ pound 84% lean ground pork
½ pound 85% lean ground beef
½ medium onion, diced
½ medium head of cabbage, sliced
2 tablespoons tomato paste

½ cup diced tomatoes
2 cups chicken broth
1 teaspoon salt
½ teaspoon thyme
½ teaspoon garlic powder
¼ teaspoon pepper

1. Hit the sauté button on the Instant Pot and add beef and pork to Instant Pot. Brown meat until no pink remains. Add onion and continue cooking until onions are fragrant and soft. Hit the cancel button. 2. Add remaining ingredients to Instant Pot. Hit the manual button and adjust time for almost 8 minutes. 3. When the pot beeps, allow a 15-minute natural release and then quick-release the remaining pressure. Serve warm.
Per Serving: Calories 194; Total Fat 10.9g; Sodium 292mg; Total Carbs 1.7g; Fiber 6.4g; Sugars 9g; Protein 6.4g

White Chicken Chili

Prep time: 10 minutes. | Cooking time: 20 minutes. | Serves: 6

4 tablespoons butter
¼ cup chopped onions
1 (4-ounce) can green chilies, drained
2 cloves garlic, minced
1 green pepper, chopped
1½ cups store-bought chicken

broth
1 pound boneless, skinless chicken breasts, cubed
1 teaspoon salt
¼ teaspoon pepper
4 ounces cream cheese
¼ cup heavy cream

1. Hit the sauté button on the Instant Pot and place butter and onions into Instant Pot. Sauté until onions are fragrant and translucent. Add chilies, garlic, and green pepper. Sauté for almost 3 minutes, stirring frequently. 2. Hit the cancel button and add broth, chicken, seasoning, and cream cheese to pot. Hit the manual button and adjust time for almost 30 minutes. 3. When the pot beeps allow a 10-minute natural release and quick-release the remaining pressure. Stir in heavy cream. 4. Top it with avocado!
Per Serving: Calories 110; Total Fat 4.3g; Sodium 81mg; Total Carbs 6.4g; Fiber 5.4g; Sugars 6.1g; Protein 3.8g

Chicken Bacon Chowder

Prep time: 10 minutes. | Cooking time: 20 minutes. | Serves: 6

½ pound bacon
1 teaspoon salt
½ teaspoon pepper
½ teaspoon garlic powder
¼ teaspoon dried thyme
3 (6 ounces) boneless, skinless chicken breasts

½ cup button mushrooms, sliced
½ medium onion, diced
1 cup broccoli florets
½ cup cauliflower florets
4 ounces cream cheese
3 cups store-bought chicken broth
½ cup heavy cream

1. Hit the sauté button on the Instant Pot and then hit the adjust button to lower heat to less. Add bacon to Instant Pot and fry for a few minutes until fat begins to render, working in multiple batches if necessary. Hit the cancel button. 2. Hit the sauté button on the Instant Pot and then hit the adjust button to set heat to normal. Continue frying bacon until fully cooked and crispy. Remove from pot and keep it aside. Sprinkle salt, pepper, garlic powder, and thyme over chicken breasts. Sear each side of the chicken for almost 3–5 minutes or until dark and golden. Hit the cancel button. 3. Add mushrooms, onion, broccoli, cauliflower, cream cheese, and broth to pot with chicken. Turn the pot's lid to close. Hit the manual button and adjust time for almost 12 minutes. When the pot beeps, quick-release the pressure. Remove chicken and shred or dice; add to pot. Crumble cooked bacon and stir into pot with heavy cream. Serve warm.
Per Serving: Calories 176; Total Fat 9.6g; Sodium 122mg; Total Carbs 5.7g; Fiber 4.5g; Sugars 3.8g; Protein 7.8g

Creamy Enchilada Soup

Prep time: 10 minutes. | Cooking time: 40 minutes. | Serves: 6

2 (6-ounce) boneless, skinless chicken breasts
½ tablespoon chili powder
½ teaspoon salt
½ teaspoon garlic powder
¼ teaspoon pepper
½ cup red enchilada sauce
½ medium onion, diced
1 (4-ounce) can green chilies

2 cups chicken broth
⅛ cup pickled jalapeños
4 ounces cream cheese
1 cup uncooked cauliflower rice
1 avocado, diced
1 cup shredded mild cheddar cheese
½ cup sour cream

1. Sprinkle seasoning over chicken breasts and keep it aside. Pour enchilada sauce into Instant Pot and place chicken on top. 2. Add onion, chilies, broth, and jalapeños to the pot, then place cream cheese on top of chicken breasts. Turn the pot's lid to close. Adjust time for almost 25 minutes. When the pot beeps, quick-release the pressure and shred chicken with forks. 3. Mix soup and add cauliflower rice, with pot on keep warm setting. Replace lid and let pot sit for almost 15 minutes, still on keep warm. This will cook cauliflower rice. Serve with avocado, cheddar, and sour cream.
Per Serving: Calories 236; Total Fat 8.1g; Sodium 14mg; Total Carbs 2.1g; Fiber 6.3g; Sugars 0.8g; Protein 2.3g

Lobster Bisque

Prep time: 10 minutes. | Cooking time: 10 minutes. | Serves: 4

4 tablespoons butter	¼ teaspoon paprika
½ medium onion, diced	⅛ teaspoon cayenne
1 clove garlic, finely minced	2 tablespoons tomato paste
1 pound cooked lump lobster meat	1 cup store-bought seafood stock
	1 cup store-bought chicken broth
½ teaspoon salt	½ cup heavy cream
¼ teaspoon pepper	½ teaspoon xanthan gum

1. Hit the sauté button on the Instant Pot and add butter and onions to Instant Pot. Sauté for almost 2–3 minutes until onions begin to soften. Add garlic and sauté 30 seconds. Hit the cancel button. 2. Add lobster, seasonings, tomato paste, and broths. Hit the manual button and adjust time for almost 7 minutes. When the pot beeps, quick-release the pressure. Stir in heavy cream and xanthan gum. Allow a few minutes to thicken. Serve warm.
Per Serving: Calories 171; Total Fat 10g; Sodium 2629mg; Total Carbs 8.6g; Fiber 2.6g; Sugars 13.8g; Protein 4.3g

Spicy Bacon Cheeseburger Soup

Prep time: 10 minutes. | Cooking time: 15 minutes. | Serves: 6

1 pound 85% lean ground beef	1 teaspoon salt
½ medium onion, sliced	½ teaspoon pepper
½ (14.5-ounce) can fire-roasted tomatoes	½ teaspoon garlic powder
	2 teaspoons Worcestershire sauce
3 cups beef broth	4 ounces cream cheese
¼ cup cooked crumbled bacon	1 cup sharp cheddar cheese
1 tablespoon chopped pickled jalapeños	1 pickle spear, diced

1. Hit the sauté button on the Instant Pot and add ground beef. Brown beef halfway and add onion. Continue cooking beef until no pink remains. Hit the cancel button. Add tomatoes, broth, bacon, jalapeños, salt, pepper, garlic powder, and Worcestershire sauce, and stir. Place cream cheese on top in middle. 2. Turn the pot's lid to close. Hit the soup button and adjust time for almost 15 minutes. When the pot beeps, quick-release the pressure. Top with diced pickles. Feel free to add additional cheese and bacon.
Per Serving: Calories 120; Total Fat 2.3g; Sodium 2mg; Total Carbs 4.1g; Fiber 2.3g; Sugars 10g; Protein 3.6g

Chicken and Cauliflower Rice Soup

Prep time: 10 minutes. | Cooking time: 20 minutes. | Serves: 4

4 tablespoons butter	¼ teaspoon dried parsley
¼ cup diced onion	1 bay leaf
2 stalks celery, chopped	2 cups chicken broth
½ cup fresh spinach	2 cups diced cooked chicken
½ teaspoon salt	¾ cup uncooked cauliflower rice
¼ teaspoon pepper	½ teaspoon xanthan gum
¼ teaspoon dried thyme	

1. Hit the sauté button on the Instant Pot and add butter to Instant Pot. Add onions and sauté until translucent. Place celery and spinach into Instant Pot and sauté for almost 2–3 minutes until spinach is wilted. Hit the cancel button. 2. Sprinkle seasoning into Instant Pot and add bay leaf, broth, and cooked chicken. Turn the pot's lid to close. Hit the soup button and adjust time for almost 10 minutes. 3. When the pot beeps, quick-release the pressure and stir in cauliflower rice. Leave Instant Pot on keep warm setting to finish cooking cauliflower rice additional 10 minutes. Serve warm.
Per Serving: Calories 139; Total Fat 11.9g; Sodium 60mg; Total Carbs 5.4g; Fiber 3.1g; Sugars 1g; Protein 5g

Broccoli Cheddar Soup

Prep time: 10 minutes. | Cooking time: 10 minutes. | Serves: 4

2 tablespoons butter	1 cup broccoli, chopped
⅛ cup onion, diced	1 tablespoon cream cheese, softened
½ teaspoon garlic powder	
½ teaspoon salt	¼ cup heavy cream
¼ teaspoon pepper	1 cup shredded cheddar cheese
2 cups chicken broth	

1. Hit the sauté button on the Instant Pot and add butter to Instant Pot. Add onion and sauté until translucent. Hit the cancel button and add garlic powder, salt, pepper, broth, and broccoli to pot. 2. Turn the pot's lid to close. Hit the soup button and set time for almost 5 minutes. When the pot beeps, stir in heavy cream, cream cheese, and cheddar.
Per Serving: Calories 666; Total Fat 3.5g; Sodium 198mg; Total Carbs 8.5g; Fiber 44.1g; Sugars 15.4g; Protein 39g

Loaded Taco Soup

Prep time: 10 minutes. | Cooking time: 10 minutes. | Serves: 4

1 pound 85% lean ground beef	3 cups beef broth
½ medium onion, diced	⅓ cup heavy cream
1 (7-ounce) can diced tomatoes and chilies	¼ teaspoon xanthan gum
	1 avocado, diced
1 teaspoon salt	½ cup sour cream
1 tablespoon chili powder	1 cup shredded cheddar cheese
2 teaspoons cumin	¼ cup chopped cilantro

1. Hit the sauté button on the Instant Pot and brown ground beef in Instant Pot. When halfway done, add onion. Once beef is completely cooked, add diced tomatoes with chilies, seasoning, and broth. 2. Turn the pot's lid to close. Hit the soup button and adjust time for almost 10 minutes. When the pot beeps, quick-release the pressure. Stir in cream and xanthan gum. Serve warm and top with diced avocado, sour cream, cheddar, and cilantro.
Per Serving: Calories 110; Total Fat 3.4g; Sodium 1446mg; Total Carbs 3.9g; Fiber 5.4g; Sugars 3.8g; Protein 8.2g

Balsamic Beef Stew

Prep time: 10 minutes. | Cooking time: 6 hours. | Serves: 6

1 pound sirloin steak, cubed	1 cup beef broth
1 red onion, sliced	¼ cup parsley, freshly chopped
3 cloves garlic, chopped	1 teaspoon salt
2 carrots, chopped	¼ teaspoon black pepper
¼ cup balsamic vinegar	¼ cup sour cream, for serving

1. Add the sirloin steak to the base of a slow cooker and cook for almost 10 minutes. 2. Add in the remaining ingredients and cook on low for almost 6 hours. 3. Serve with a dollop of sour cream per serving.
Per Serving: Calories 164; Total Fat 1.8g; Sodium 469mg; Total Carbs 9.2g; Fiber 12.6g; Sugars 8.2g; Protein 14g

Mac & Cheese Stew

Prep time: 10 minutes| Cooking time: 4 hours| Serves: 6

1 pound lean ground beef	2 cups shredded cheddar cheese
1 cup butternut squash, cubed	1 cup broccoli florets, chopped
1 yellow onion, chopped	1 teaspoon dried thyme
3 cloves garlic, chopped	Salt & black pepper, to taste

1. Add all the recipe ingredients minus the salt and black pepper to the base of a slow cooker and cook on high for almost 4 hours. 2. Season with salt and black pepper and serve.
Per Serving: Calories 529; Total Fat 7.7g; Sodium 743mg; Total Carbs 1g; Fiber 19g; Sugars 9.5g; Protein 28g

Creamy Tuscan Soup

Prep time: 10 minutes. | Cooking time: 17 minutes. | Serves: 4

4 slices bacon	4 ounces cream cheese
1 pound ground Italian sausage	2 cups kale, chopped
4 tablespoons butter	½ cup heavy cream
½ medium onion, diced	1 teaspoon salt
2 cloves garlic, finely minced	½ teaspoon pepper
3 cups store-bought chicken broth	

1. Hit the sauté button on the Instant Pot and fry bacon until crispy. Remove bacon and chop into pieces, then keep it aside. Add Italian sausage to Instant Pot and sauté until no pink remains. Add butter and onion to Instant Pot. Sauté until onions are translucent. Add garlic and sauté for almost 30 seconds. Hit the cancel button. 2. Add broth and cream cheese to pot. Turn the pot's lid to close. Hit the soup button and adjust time for almost 7 minutes. 3. When the pot beeps, quick-release the pressure and add remaining ingredients to pot. Leave Instant Pot on keep warm setting and allow to cook additional 10 minutes, stirring occasionally until kale is wilted. Serve warm.
Per Serving: Calories 122; Total Fat 10.1g; Sodium 143mg; Total Carbs 4.9g; Fiber 1.2g; Sugars 1.1g; Protein 3.6g

Pumpkin Kale Vegetarian Stew

Prep time: 10 minutes. | Cooking time: 40 minutes. | Serves: 6

4 cups vegetable broth
1 cup pumpkin, cubed
2 carrots, chopped
1 yellow onion, chopped

2 cloves garlic, chopped
1 cup kale, chopped
Salt & black pepper, to taste

1. Add all the recipe ingredients minus the salt and black pepper to a stockpot and cook to a boil. Reduce its heat to a simmer and cook for almost 40 minutes. 2. Season with salt and black pepper and serve.
Per Serving: Calories 100; Total Fat 1.1g; Sodium 741mg; Total Carbs 9.4g; Fiber 5.2g; Sugars 6.2g; Protein 4.3g

Herbed Broccoli Stew

Prep time: 10 minutes. | Cooking time: 4 hours. | Serves: 6

6 cups vegetable broth
1 cup full-fat coconut milk
2 cups broccoli florets
1 cup canned diced tomatoes (no sugar added)
1 yellow onion, chopped

2 cloves garlic, chopped
1 teaspoon dried sage
1 teaspoon dried oregano
1 teaspoon dried rosemary
Salt & black pepper to taste

1. Add all the recipe ingredients minus the salt, black pepper, and coconut milk to a slow cooker and cook on high for almost 4 hours. 2. Stir in the coconut milk and season with salt and black pepper.
Per Serving: Calories 390; Total Fat 15.3g; Sodium 1086mg; Total Carbs 5g; Fiber 17.3g; Sugars 6.6g; Protein 18.2g

Creamy Mixed Vegetable Stew

Prep time: 10 minutes. | Cooking time: 4 hours. | Serves: 6

4 cups vegetable broth
1 cup heavy cream
1 cup shredded parmesan cheese
1 cup broccoli florets, chopped

1 cup canned diced tomatoes
1 yellow onion, chopped
Salt & black pepper, to taste

1. Add all the recipe ingredients minus the heavy cream, salt and black pepper to the base of a slow cooker. Cook on high for almost 4 hours. 2. Once cooked, warm the cream, and then stir into the stew. 3. Season with salt and black pepper and serve.
Per Serving: Calories 562; Total Fat 2.1g; Sodium 238mg; Total Carbs 1.8g; Fiber 19g; Sugars 5.3g; Protein 28.6g

Autumn Harvest Stew

Prep time: 10 minutes. | Cooking time: 4 hours. | Serves: 6

1 pound beef chuck, cubed
¼ cup beef broth
¼ cup balsamic vinegar
1 cup butternut squash, cubed
1 carrot, chopped
1 yellow onion, chopped

3 cloves garlic, chopped
1 cup kale, chopped
1 teaspoon dried thyme
1 teaspoon dried oregano
1 teaspoon dried sage
Salt & black pepper, to taste

1. Add all the recipe ingredients minus the salt and black pepper to the base of a slow cooker and cook on high for almost 4 hours. 2. Season with salt and black pepper and serve.
Per Serving: Calories 425; Total Fat 8.8g; Sodium 284mg; Total Carbs 8.6g; Fiber 15.2g; Sugars 3.1g; Protein 20.6g

Turkey, Onion & Sage Stew

Prep time: 10 minutes. | Cooking time: 4 hours. | Serves: 6

1 pound ground turkey
1 yellow onion, chopped
3 cloves garlic, chopped
2 cups shredded mozzarella cheese

3 cups fresh spinach
2 teaspoons dried sage
1 teaspoon dried oregano
Salt & black pepper, to taste
Water

1. Add all the recipe ingredients minus the salt and black pepper to the base of a slow cooker and cover with about ¼ cup of water. Cook on high for almost 4 hours. 2. Season with salt and black pepper and serve.
Per Serving: Calories 300; Total Fat 4.3g; Sodium 1377mg; Total Carbs 5.2g; Fiber 7.7g; Sugars 6.2g; Protein 21.6g

Hamburger Beef Stew

Prep time: 10 minutes. | Cooking time: 4 hours. | Serves: 6

1 pound lean ground beef
¼ cup beef broth
½ cup tomato paste
½ cup canned diced tomatoes

1 yellow onion, chopped
2 cups shredded cheddar cheese
1 teaspoon Italian seasoning
Salt & black pepper, to taste

1. Add all the recipe ingredients minus the salt and black pepper to the base of a slow cooker and cook on high for almost 4 hours. 2. Season with salt and black pepper and serve.
Per Serving: Calories 557; Total Fat 10g; Sodium 2706mg; Total Carbs 7.6g; Fiber 17.8g; Sugars 5.6g; Protein 29.2g

Delicious Sausage-Sauerkraut Soup

Prep time: 15 minutes| Cook time: 6 hours| Serves: 6

1 tablespoon extra-virgin olive oil
6 cups beef broth
1 pound organic sausage, cooked and sliced
2 cups sauerkraut
2 celery stalks, chopped
1 sweet onion, chopped

2 teaspoons minced garlic
2 tablespoons butter
1 tablespoon hot mustard
½ teaspoon caraway seeds
½ cup sour cream
2 tablespoons chopped fresh parsley for garnish

1. Lightly oil the slow cooker with olive oil. 2. Place the broth, sausage, sauerkraut, celery, onion, garlic, butter, mustard, and caraway seeds in the insert. 3. Cover it and cook on low temp setting for 6 hours. 4. Stir in the sour cream. 5. Serve topped with the parsley.
Per Serving: Calories 332; Fat 28g; Sodium 69mg; Carbs 6g; Fiber 2g; Sugar 2g; Protein 15g

No Bean Chili

Prep time: 10 minutes. | Cooking time: 40 minutes. | Serves: 6

4 cups vegetable broth
4 ounces tomato paste
¼ cup balsamic vinegar
1 yellow onion, chopped
1 green bell pepper, seeded and

chopped
2 cloves garlic, chopped
2 teaspoons chili powder
Salt & black pepper, to taste

1. Add all the recipe ingredients minus the salt and black pepper to a stockpot and cook to a boil. Reduce its heat to a simmer and cook for almost 40 minutes. 2. Season with salt and black pepper and serve.
Per Serving: Calories 300; Total Fat 4g; Sodium 429mg; Total Carbs 6.8g; Fiber 22.7g; Sugars 11.3g; Protein 19.7g

Asparagus & Mushroom Nutmeg Stew

Prep time: 10 minutes. | Cooking time: 4 hours. | Serves: 6

6 cups vegetable broth
1 cup heavy cream
1 cup asparagus, chopped
1 cup cremini mushrooms

2 cloves garlic, chopped
1 yellow onion, chopped
½ teaspoon nutmeg
Salt & black pepper, to taste

1. Add all the recipe ingredients minus the heavy cream, salt, and black pepper to a slow cooker and cook on high for almost 4 hours. 2. Once cooked, warm the heavy cream, and then stir into the stew. 3. Season with salt and black pepper and serve.
Per Serving: Calories 276; Total Fat 11.8g; Sodium 888mg; Total Carbs 3.1g; Fiber 6.2g; Sugars 2.6g; Protein 14.4g

Balsamic Tofu Stew

Prep time: 10 minutes. | Cooking time: 20 minutes. | Serves: 4

2 cups vegetable broth
¼ cup balsamic vinegar
1½ cups firm tofu, cubed
1 green bell pepper, seeded and chopped

1 yellow onion, chopped
1 teaspoon garlic powder
1 tablespoon coconut oil, for cooking
Salt & black pepper, to taste

1. Add the coconut oil to a suitable skillet over medium heat and sauté the tofu, bell pepper, and onion for almost 10 minutes. 2. Add the vegetable broth, balsamic and garlic powder and bring to a simmer. 3. Cook for 10 minutes more or until the stew begins to thicken. 4. Season with salt and black pepper and serve.
Per Serving: Calories 589; Total Fat 22.7g; Sodium 266mg; Total Carbs 6.5g; Fiber 23.9g; Sugars 5.1g; Protein 25.5g

Chapter 3 Beef, Pork, and Lambs

Cheese Stuffed Meatballs

Prep time: 30 minutes| Cook time: 5-6 hours| Serves: 6

3 tablespoons extra-virgin olive oil, divided
1½ pounds ground beef
1 egg
¼ cup grated parmesan cheese
2 teaspoons minced garlic
2 teaspoons dried basil
½ teaspoon salt
¼ teaspoon freshly ground black pepper
6 ounces mozzarella, cut into 16 small cubes
4 cups marinara sauce

1. Lightly grease the slow cooker with 1 tablespoon of olive oil. 2. In large bowl, combine the beef, egg, Parmesan, garlic, basil, salt, and pepper until well mixed. Shape the mixture into 16 meatballs and press a mozzarella piece into the center of each, making sure to thoroughly enclose the cheese thoroughly. 3. In a pan heat 2 tablespoons of the olive oil. Add the meatballs and sear all over, about 10 minutes. 4. Transfer the meatballs to the insert and add the marinara sauce. 5. Cover it and cook on low temp setting for 5 to 6 hours. Serve warm.
Per Serving: Calories 508; Fat 36g; Sodium 643mg; Carbs 6g; Fiber 2g; Sugar 3g; Protein 39g

Delicious Beef Goulash

Prep time: 15 minutes| Cook time: 9-10 hours| Serves: 6

1 tablespoon extra-virgin olive oil
1½ pounds beef, cut into 1-inch pieces
½ sweet onion, chopped
1 carrot, cut into ½-inch-thick slices
1 red bell pepper, diced
2 teaspoons minced garlic
1 cup beef broth
¼ cup tomato paste
1 tablespoon Hungarian paprika
1 bay leaf
1 cup sour cream
2 tablespoons chopped fresh parsley, for garnish

1. Lightly oil the slow cooker with olive oil. 2. Add the beef, onion, carrot, red bell pepper, garlic, broth, tomato paste, paprika, and bay leaf to the insert. 3. Cover it and cook on low temperature setting for 9 to 10 hours. 4. Remove the bay leaf and stir in the sour cream. 5. Serve topped with the parsley.
Per Serving: Calories 548; Fat 42g; Sodium 234mg; Carbs 8g; Fiber 2g; Sugar 2g; Protein 32g

Spiced Braised Beef Short Ribs

Prep time: 10 minutes| Cook time: 7-8 hours| Serves: 8

1 tablespoon extra-virgin olive oil
2 pounds beef short ribs
1 sweet onion, sliced
2 cups beef broth
2 tablespoons granulated
erythritol
2 tablespoons balsamic vinegar
2 teaspoons dried thyme
1 teaspoon hot sauce

1. Lightly oil the slow cooker with olive oil. 2. Place the ribs, onion, broth, erythritol, balsamic vinegar, thyme, and hot sauce in the insert. 3. Cover it and cook on low temperature setting for 7 to 8 hours. 4. Serve warm.
Per Serving: Calories 473; Fat 43g; Sodium 850mg; Carbs 2g; Fiber 0g; Sugar 1g; Protein 18g

Balsamic Beef Roast

Prep time: 15 minutes| Cook time: 7-8 hours| Serves: 8

3 tablespoons of extra-virgin olive oil, divided
2 pounds boneless beef chuck roast
1 cup beef broth
½ cup balsamic vinegar
1 tablespoon minced garlic
1 tablespoon granulated erythritol
½ teaspoon red pepper flakes
1 tablespoon chopped fresh thyme

1. Lightly grease the slow cooker with 1 tablespoon of olive oil. 2. In a large pan over medium-high heat, heat the remaining 2 tablespoons of the olive oil. Sear the meat on all sides, sear about 7 minutes in total. Transfer to the instant pot. In a small bowl, whisk the broth, balsamic vinegar, garlic, erythritol, red pepper flakes, and thyme until blended. 3. Pour the sauce over the beef. Cover it and cook on low temperature setting for 7 to 8 hours. Serve warm.
Per Serving: Calories 476; Fat 39g; Sodium 157mg; Carbs 1g; Fiber 0g; Sugar 0g; Protein 28g

Curry Beef

Prep time: 10 minutes| Cook time: 7 to 8 hours| Serves: 6

1 tablespoon extra-virgin olive oil
1 pound beef chuck roast, cut into 2-inch pieces
1 sweet onion, chopped
1 red bell pepper, diced
2 cups coconut milk
2 tablespoons hot curry powder
1 tablespoon coconut aminos
2 teaspoons grated fresh ginger
2 teaspoons minced garlic
1 cup shredded baby bok choy

1. Lightly oil the slow cooker with olive oil. 2. Add the beef, onion, and bell pepper to the insert. 3. Whisk together the coconut milk, curry, coconut aminos, ginger, and garlic in a medium bowl. Pour the sauce into the insert and stir to combine. 4. Cover it and cook on low temperature setting for 7 to 8 hours. Stir in the bok choy and let stand for 15 minutes. Serve warm.
Per Serving: Calories 504; Fat 42g; Sodium 780mg; Carbs 7g; Fiber 3g; Sugar 2g; Protein 23g

Burger in a Lettuce Bun

Prep time: 10 minutes| Cook time: 15 minutes| Serves: 4

1 pound ground beef, formed into 4 burger patties
½ teaspoon onion powder
½ teaspoon garlic powder
½ teaspoon salt
¼ teaspoon freshly ground black
pepper
4 bacon slices
8 large lettuce leaves
4 cheddar cheese slices
4 eggs

1. Sprinkle the beef patties generously with the onion powder, garlic powder, salt, and pepper. Make dimple with thumb into the middle of each cake, which will help them keep a flat shape as they cook. Heat a pan and cook the bacon for 5-7 minutes until crisp over medium heat. Transfer to a paper towel, leaving the bacon grease in the pan. 2. Cook the burger patties in the bacon grease in the pan, covered, over medium-high heat for 2-4 minutes on each side. Add cheese to each burger patty, cover the pan, and let cook for another 30 seconds until the cheese is melted. Remove the burgers from the pan. 3. Cook the eggs over medium-high heat for 30 seconds for soft sunny-side-up doneness. Don't flip them! 4. Place lettuce leaf on a serving plate, topped by a burger patty, 1 slice of bacon, and 1 egg—season with salt and pepper. 5. Top with 1 more lettuce leaf and serve immediately.
Per Serving: Calories 492; Fat 38g; Sodium 904mg; Carbs 3.5g; Fiber 1.5g; Sugar 2g; Protein 34g

Delicious Beef Stroganoff

Prep time: 10 minutes| Cook time: 35 minutes| Serves: 6

1 tablespoon lard
1½ pounds beef sirloin, cut against the grain into thin strips
½ teaspoon sea salt, plus additional
¼ teaspoon freshly ground black pepper, plus additional
2 tablespoons butter or ghee
½ cup chopped onion
3 garlic cloves, minced
3 cups sliced mushrooms (about 8
ounces)
1 teaspoon dried oregano
⅛ teaspoon cayenne pepper
1 cup bone broth
½ cup heavy (whipping) cream
½ cup sour cream
½ to 1 teaspoon xanthan or guar gum, for thickening
½ teaspoon garlic powder
½ teaspoon onion powder
Chopped fresh parsley, for garnish

1. Heat the lard in a cooking pot. 2. Spice the beef strips with the salt and pepper and add the beef to the pot and cook for 1-2 minutes, just until browned. Once all the beef is browned and removed to the bowl, reduce the heat to medium and add the butter to the pan along with the onion, garlic, and mushrooms. Season with the oregano and cayenne (if using). Add more salt and pepper. Cook the onions and mushrooms for 7 to 10 minutes, occasionally stirring, until tender. Remove the onion, mushrooms, and garlic to the bowl with the beef. 3. Add the bone broth to the pan and bring to a boil. Once boiling, lower the heat to low and slowly whisk in the cream, sour cream, xanthan or guar gum, garlic powder, and onion powder. Stir for 3 to 5 minutes until the broth starts to thicken. 4. Return the cooked beef and veggies mixture to the pot. Cook on low heat for another 5-10 minutes until the beef is cooked through and the sauce is thickened. Garnish with parsley and serve.
Per Serving: Calories 326; Fat 22g; Sodium 784mg; Carbs 5g; Fiber 1g; Sugar 3g; Protein 27g

Cabbage Rolls

Prep time: 15 minutes| Cook time: 7-8 hours| Serves: 4

3 tablespoons extra-virgin olive oil, divided
1 pound ground beef
1 sweet onion, chopped
2 cups finely chopped cauliflower
2 teaspoons minced garlic
1 teaspoon dried thyme
¼ teaspoon salt
¼ teaspoon freshly ground black pepper
4 cups shredded cabbage
2 cups marinara sauce
½ cup cream cheese

1. Lightly grease the slow cooker with 1 tablespoon of olive oil. 2. Press the ground beef along the bottom of the insert. 3. Heat 2 tablespoons of olive oil. Add the onion, cauliflower, garlic, thyme, salt, and pepper, and sauté until the onion is softened about 3 minutes. 4. Add the cabbage and sauté for an additional 5 minutes. 5. Transfer the cabbage mixture to the insert, pour the marinara sauce over the cabbage, and top with the cream cheese. Cover it and cook on low temperature setting for 7 to 8 hours. 6. Stir before serving.
Per Serving: Calories 547; Fat 42g; Sodium 133mg; Carbs 6g; Fiber 4g; Sugar 2g; Protein 34g

Savory Peppers

Prep time: 25 minutes| Cook time: 6 hours| Serves: 4

3 tablespoons extra-virgin olive oil, divided
1 pound ground beef
½ cup finely chopped cauliflower
1 tomato, diced
½ sweet onion, chopped
2 teaspoons minced garlic
2 teaspoons dried oregano
1 teaspoon dried basil
4 bell peppers, deseeded1 cup shredded cheddar cheese
½ cup chicken broth
1 tablespoon basil, sliced into thin strips, for garnish

1. Lightly grease the slow cooker with 1 tablespoon of olive oil. 2. Heat the oil. Add the beef and sauté until it is cooked through about 10 minutes. 3. Add the cauliflower, tomato, onion, garlic, oregano, and basil. Sauté for an additional 5 minutes. 4. Spoon the meat-veggie mixture into the peppers and top with the cheese. Place the peppers in the slow cooker and add the broth to the bottom. 5. Cover it and cook on low temperature setting for 6 hours. Cover the pot and cook. Serve warm and top with the basil.
Per Serving: Calories 571; Fat 41g; Sodium 371mg; Carbs 12g; Fiber 3g; Sugar 2g; Protein 38g

Beef with Broccoli

Prep time: 10 minutes| Cook time: 20 minutes| Serves: 4

For the marinade
3 tablespoons coconut aminos
2 tablespoons coconut oil, melted
2 tablespoons toasted sesame oil
2 tablespoons fish sauce
1 tablespoon apple cider vinegar
1 teaspoon onion powder
1 teaspoon garlic powder
½ teaspoon ground ginger
¼ teaspoon red pepper flakes
For the beef and broccoli
1 pound beef sirloin or flank, sliced thinly across the grain
2 cups broccoli florets
1 tablespoon coconut oil
2 garlic cloves, minced
½ teaspoon sea salt
¼ teaspoon freshly ground black pepper
1 tablespoon toasted sesame seeds

To make the marinade: In a medium bowl, add the coconut aminos along coconut oil, sesame oil, vinegar, onion powder, fish sauce, garlic powder, ginger, and red pepper flakes and mix well with the whisk.
To make the beef and broccoli: 1 In a large plastic bag pour one-third of the marinade mix over the beef. Let marinate in the refrigerator for a few hours or overnight. Use the remaining marinade for the sauce for the sauce. 2. In a large pot, steam the broccoli until just tender. 3. Transfer the broccoli to cold water to stop the cooking. Drain and set aside. Heat the coconut oil over high heat in a large pan or wok. Add the marinated meat to the pan. Let brown the meat for 4 to 5 minutes. 4. Add the garlic, salt, and pepper and stir to combine. 5. Add the cooked broccoli florets and the reserved marinade. 6. Stir well and let simmer low heat for 5-10 minutes or until the sauce thickens and the meat is cooked through. Top with sesame seeds.
Per Serving: Calories 365; Fat 24g; Sodium 804mg; Carbs 6g; Fiber 1.5g; Sugar 2g; Protein 29g

Skirt Steak with Fresh Herb Butter

Prep time: 20 minutes| Cook time: 10 minutes| Serves: 4

For the butter
1½ cups butter
1 tablespoon minced garlic
½ cup finely chopped basil
1 tablespoon chopped parsley
1 tablespoon minced chives
1½ teaspoons sea salt
For the steak
1 pound skirt steak, cut into 4 separate steaks
1 teaspoon garlic powder
1 teaspoon sea salt
½ teaspoon freshly ground pepper
1 tablespoon coconut oil

To make the butter: 1. Combine the butter with the garlic, basil, parsley, chives, and salt, and stir until the mixture is well combined and smooth. Set aside ¼ cup of the mixture for the steak, refrigerate the rest in an airtight container or rolled into a log wrapped in parchment paper. 2. Store the butter in the refrigerator for up to 1 week or in the freezer for 3 months.
To make the steak: 1. Season the steak generously with garlic powder, salt, and pepper, then sit at room temperature for 10 to 15 minutes. 2. Oil a cast-iron pan and heat it over medium-high heat. 3. Cook each steak in the pan for 2 to 6 minutes on each side, depending on how you like your steak. 4. Serve hot; each steak topped with 1 tablespoon of butter. Let the butter melt, then enjoy!
Per Serving: Calories 376; Fat 32g; Sodium 999mg; Carbs 1g; Fiber 0g; Sugar 0.2g; Protein 21g

Veggies Beef Stir-Fry

Prep time: 10 minutes| Cook time: 12 minutes| Serves: 4

2 tablespoons toasted sesame oil
3 tablespoons canola oil
1 pound boneless sirloin, cut in paper-thin slices
Sea salt
Freshly ground black pepper
2 tablespoons minced ginger
2 teaspoons minced garlic
Pinch red pepper flakes
1 broccoli, diced
¼ cup low-sodium soy sauce
2 tablespoons dry sherry

1. Heat the both sesame oil and canola oil in a wok over medium-high heat until very hot. 2. Season the sirloin generously with salt and pepper. Stir-fry the sirloin until just cooked through, about 5 minutes. 3. Cook the ginger, garlic, and red pepper flakes for 1 minute until fragrant. Transfer the beef to a separate dish with a slotted spoon. 4. Add the broccoli to the pan and stir-fry for 5 minutes until bright green and crisp-tender. 5. Return the beef with accumulated juices to the pan, and add the soy sauce and sherry. 6. Simmer for 2 minutes until the liquid has reduced, and the beef and broccoli are coated in the sauce.
Per Serving: Calories 472; Fat 29g; Sodium 784mg; Carbs 12g; Fiber 5g; Sugar 3g; Protein 41g

Steak with Broccoli Noodles

Prep time: 15 minutes| Cook time: 15 minutes| Serves: 4

1 tablespoon vegetable oil
1 Thai chili, seeded and very finely chopped
1 pound thinly sliced steak
½ white onion, spiralized
2 garlic cloves, minced
2 teaspoons fish sauce
4 heads broccoli, florets removed,
stems peeled and spiralized
2 scallions, cut into 1- to 2-inch pieces
Salt
¼ cup soy sauce
2 tablespoons oyster sauce
Freshly ground black pepper
½ cup Thai basil leaves

1. Heat the vegetable oil. Add the onion noodles and sauté for 2 to 3 minutes. 2. Add in the chili and garlic, cook for just under 1 minute. Then add the beef in the pan and stir-fry for 4 to 5 minutes. Add the fish sauce, broccoli florets, and broccoli noodles. Cook, for 3-4 minutes. Whisk the soy sauce and oyster sauce to combine. Whisk the soy sauce and oyster sauce to combine. 4. Pour the sauce and add the scallions in the pan. Toss to combine—cook for 1 to 2 minutes. Season with salt and pepper, as needed. 5. Add the basil, tossing until slightly wilted from the heat and remove from heat. Serve immediately.
Per Serving: Calories 355; Fat 17g; Sodium 796mg; Carbs 21g; Fiber 7g; Sugar 7g; Protein 33g

Roast Beef

Prep time: 10 minutes. | Cooking time: 60 minutes. | Serves: 6

1 (2-pound) top round beef roast
1 teaspoon salt
½ teaspoon ground black pepper
1 teaspoon dried rosemary
½ teaspoon garlic powder
1 tablespoon coconut oil, melted

1. Sprinkle all sides of roast with salt, pepper, rosemary, and garlic powder. Drizzle with coconut oil. 2. Place roast into ungreased air fryer basket, fatty side down. Set the temperature to 375°F/191°C and set the timer for almost 60 minutes, turning the roast halfway through cooking. Roast will be done when no pink remains and internal temperature is at least 180°F/82°C. Serve warm.
Per Serving: Calories 231; Total Fat 2.1g; Sodium 816mg; Total Carbs 8.1g; Fiber 14.4g; Sugars 4.5g; Protein 16.6g

Gingery Pork Meatballs

Prep time: 10 minutes| Cook time: 15 minutes| Serves: 4

1 large egg, whisked
¼ cup almond flour
1 teaspoon minced fresh ginger
1 teaspoon minced garlic
½ teaspoon sea salt
¼ teaspoon freshly ground black
pepper
¼ cup minced cilantro
1 cup roughly chopped spinach
1 scallion, thinly sliced
1 pound ground pork
2 tablespoons coconut oil

1. Whisk the egg, almond flour, ginger, garlic, salt, and pepper in a large bowl. Stir in the cilantro, spinach, and scallion. 2. Add the pork and mix the ingredients until combined. Shape the pork mixture into 8 to 12 meatballs. 3. Heat a large pan over medium-high heat. Melt the coconut oil. Sear the meatballs until well brown and cooked through to an internal temperature of 160°F/71°C, for about 15 minutes.
Per Serving: Calories 460; Fat 35g; Sodium 1040mg; Carbs 3g; Fiber 1g; Sugar 0.26g; Protein 33g

Regular Beef Fajitas

Prep time: 20 minutes| Cook time: 22 minutes| Serves: 4

¼ cup olive oil, divided
1 tablespoon freshly squeezed lime juice
1 teaspoon ground cumin
1 teaspoon chili powder
1 teaspoon paprika
¼ teaspoon cayenne pepper
Pinch sea salt
Pinch freshly ground black pepper
1 pound boneless rib eye steak
1 red onion, thinly sliced
1 red bell pepper, thinly sliced
1 green bell pepper, thinly sliced
2 tablespoons chopped fresh cilantro
½ cup sour cream

1. In a resealable plastic bag, add oil, the lime juice, cumin, chili powder, paprika, cayenne, salt, and black pepper and shake to combine. 2. Pierce the steak well all over with a knife or a fork and place the meat in the bag with the marinade. 3. Marinate the steak for 1 hour in the refrigerator, turning the bag over once. 4. Heat the remaining oil in a large pan over medium-high heat. Pan sear the steak until medium-rare, turning 6 to 7 minutes per side. 5. Remove the cooked steak and let rest for 10 minutes. While the meat rests, sauté the onion and peppers until they are lightly caramelized, about 5 minutes. 6. Remove the cooked vegetables from the heat and stir in the cilantro. 7. Slice the steak thinly on a bias across the grain and serve the meat topped with the vegetable mixture and sour cream.
Per Serving: Calories 435; Fat 32g; Sodium 632mg; Carbs 11g; Fiber 2g; Sugar 2g; Protein 24g

Southwest-Style Beef Fajita Bowls

Prep time: 15 minutes| Cook time: 25 minutes| Serves: 6

For the marinade
⅓ cup olive oil
½ cup freshly squeezed lime juice
2 garlic cloves, minced
1 teaspoon salt
1 teaspoon chili powder
½ teaspoon onion powder
½ teaspoon garlic powder
½ teaspoon freshly ground black pepper
½ teaspoon red pepper flakes
½ teaspoon dried oregano
½ teaspoon ground cumin
1 or 2 dashes hot sauce
For the cauliflower rice
1 pound frozen riced cauliflower
1 tablespoon olive oil
2 tablespoons lime juice
¼ cup chopped fresh cilantro
1 teaspoon salt
½ teaspoon ground cumin
For the fajitas
2 pounds stir-fry beef or thinly sliced sirloin
3 bell peppers (red or green), sliced
1 medium white onion, halved and sliced
For the garnish
Lime wedges
1 avocado, sliced
Sour cream
2 or 3 scallions, sliced

1. Combine all the ingredients in a bowl. 2. Reserve half of the marinade. In a large bowl, combine the steak slices and half the marinade. Toss to coat the steak well and allow to sit, covered, for 15 to 20 minutes while you prepare the rice. 3. In a pan, sauté the cauliflower in the oil for about 8 minutes or until the cauliflower is the texture of rice over medium heat. Remove from the heat and add the lime juice, cilantro, salt, and cumin. Mix well. 4. Transfer to a bowl and set aside. Wipe out the pan and heat it over medium-high heat. When the pan is hot, put the marinated steak and any marinade left in the bowl into the pan. Cook, for 6-8 minutes until the steak is cooked through. 5. Transfer to a bowl and set aside. In the same pan, combine the peppers and onion with 2 tablespoons of the reserved marinade. 6. Sauté for about 6 minutes or until the peppers are soft and the onion is translucent. To assemble, divide the cauliflower rice among 6 wide bowls or plates. 7. Top the rice with the steak and vegetables. Spoon

a bit of reserved marinade on top. 8. Garnish with lime wedges for squeezing avocado, a dollop of sour cream, and scallions.
Per Serving: Calories 499; Fat 34g; Sodium 1020mg; Carbs 16g; Fiber 6g; Sugar 6g; Protein 34g

Garlic Steak

Prep time: 5 minutes| Cook time: 15 minutes| Serves: 2

1 tablespoon beef tallow
1 pound boneless chuck steak, cut into 1-inch cubes
Pink Himalayan sea salt
Freshly ground black pepper
3 tablespoons butter
2 garlic cloves, minced
½ teaspoon dried rosemary

1. In a large pan, melt the fat over medium-high heat. Season the steak cubes with salt and pepper on all sides. 2. Add the steak cubes to the pan. Cook on all sides, turning and stirring, for 30 seconds to 1 minute per side. Transfer the meat to a bowl; leave the drippings in the pan. Add the butter, garlic, and rosemary to the drippings. 3. Cook it for 2-3 minutes, until the garlic, starts to sear on medium heat. Return the steak to the pan, and cook, occasionally stirring, for 5 to 10 minutes, until the pieces reach your desired doneness.
Per Serving: Calories 730; Fat 62g; Sodium 695mg; Carbs 1g; Fiber 0g; Sugar 0g; Protein 43g

Soy-Ginger Steak Roll-Ups

Prep time: 15 minutes| Cook time: 35 minutes| Serves: 4

3 tablespoons olive oil, divided
½ red onion, spiralized
2 garlic cloves, minced, divided
1 bell pepper, any color, spiralized
1 large zucchini, spiralized
Salt
Freshly ground black pepper
1 teaspoon minced peeled fresh ginger
¼ cup soy sauce
1 pound flank steak

1. Preheat the oven to 350°F/177°C. 2. In an ovenproof pan over medium-high heat pan, heat 1 tablespoon of olive oil. Add the red onion and sauté for 2 to 3 minutes. 3. Add 1 clove of garlic and cook for 1 minute more, then add the bell pepper and zucchini. 4. Season with salt and pepper to taste. Cook for 4 to 5 minutes, then transfer to a bowl and let cool slightly. Return the pan to the heat and add 1 tablespoon of olive oil and the remaining 1 clove of garlic. 5. Sauté for 1 to 2 minutes, and stir in the ginger and the soy sauce. Bring the sauce to a simmer. While the sauce simmers, place the flank steak on a work surface and season with salt and pepper. 6. Spread the veggie noodle mixture over the steak and, starting from one side, roll it tightly, using toothpicks to secure the roll. 7. Pour the soy-ginger sauce into a ramekin and set aside. Return the pan to the stovetop and turn the heat to high. Add the remaining olive oil to heat. 8. Carefully transfer the steak roll-ups to the pan and sear for 1 minute per side, brushing the soy-ginger sauce over the steak as you sear it. 9. Put the pan to the oven and bake for 10 to 15 minutes, until the roll-ups are browned and cooked through when cut into. 10. When cooked, remove and let rest for about 5 minutes before slicing and serving.
Per Serving: Calories 319; Fat 20g; Sodium 547mg; Carbs 8g; Fiber 2g; Sugar 1g; Protein 27g

Hanger Steak with Herb Cream Sauce

Prep time: 5 minutes| Cook time: 1 hour| Serves: 4

1 head garlic
1 pint heavy (whipping) cream
2 to 4 fresh herb sprigs (e.g., tarragon, rosemary)
2 teaspoons salt, divided
1½ pounds hanger steak
1 teaspoon freshly ground black pepper
2 tablespoons olive oil
2 tablespoons unsalted butter

1. Separate the garlic cloves and crush them with a knife. 2. In a small saucepan, combine the garlic, cream, herbs, and 1 teaspoon salt. Simmer on low heat, uncovered for about 1 hour, stirring occasionally. Strain to remove the herbs and garlic. While the sauce is simmering, allow the steak to come to room temperature. 3. Cook the steak when the cream sauce is almost ready. Heat a heavy pan over medium-high heat. Spiced the steak with the pepper and the remaining 1 teaspoon of salt. Pour the oil into the hot pan, then add the steak. 4. Cook it for 4 minutes without lifting or moving it. Turn the steak and add the butter to the pan. 5. Cook the steak for 4 minutes while continuously spooning the melted butter over the top. Transfer to a plate when a thermometer reads 125°F/52°C (for medium-rare) in the thickest part of the steak. 6. Cover and allow the steak to rest for 8 to 10 minutes. Thinly slice the steak against the grain. Spoon the cream sauce over the sliced steak.
Per Serving: Calories 884; Fat 80g; Sodium 1564mg; Carbs 5g; Fiber 0g; Sugar 0g; Protein 37g

Flank Steak with Chimichurri

Prep time: 15 minutes| Cook time: 12 minutes| Serves: 4

½ cup olive oil
½ cup finely chopped kale
2 tablespoons finely chopped fresh parsley
2 tablespoons freshly squeezed lime juice
1 tablespoon minced garlic

1 tablespoon finely chopped chili pepper
½ teaspoon salt, plus more for seasoning
½ teaspoon black pepper, plus more for seasoning
1 pound flank steak

1. Stir the olive oil, kale, parsley, lime juice, garlic, chili pepper, salt, and pepper in a medium bowl until well combined. Set aside. Preheat the barbecue to medium-high heat. Lightly spiced the steak with salt and pepper. Grill the steak 5 to 6 minutes per side for medium-rare. 2. If you do not have a barbecue, preheat the oven to broil and broil the steak until it is the desired doneness, 5 to 6 minutes per side for medium-rare. 3. Let the steak rest for 10 minutes before slicing it thinly across the grain. Serve with the chimichurri.
Per Serving: Calories 426; Fat 35g; Sodium 896mg; Carbs 2g; Fiber 0g; Sugar 0g; Protein 25g

Delicious Flank Steak with Orange-Herb Pistou

Prep time: 10 minutes| Cook time: 20 minutes| Serves: 4

1 pound flank steak
½ cup extra-virgin olive oil, divided
2 teaspoons salt, divided
1 teaspoon freshly ground black pepper, divided
½ cup chopped fresh flat-leaf

Italian parsley
¼ cup chopped fresh mint leaves
2 garlic cloves, roughly chopped
Zest and juice of 1 orange
1 teaspoon red pepper flakes
1 tablespoon red wine vinegar

1. Heat the grill to medium-high heat or, if using an oven, preheat to 400°F/204°C. 2. Rub the steak with 2 tablespoons of olive oil and sprinkle with 1 teaspoon salt and ½ teaspoon pepper. 3. In a blender, combine the parsley, mint, garlic, orange zest, and juice, remaining 1 teaspoon salt, red pepper flakes and remaining ½ teaspoon pepper. 4. Pulse until finely chopped. With the processor running, stream in the red wine vinegar and remaining 6 tablespoons of olive oil until well combined. This pistou will be more oil-based than traditional basil pesto. 5. Cook the steak on the grill, for 6 to 8 minutes per side. Remove from the grill and allow to rest for 10 minutes on a cutting board. 6. If cooking in the oven, heat cast iron. Add the steak and brown for 1 to 2 minutes per side until browned. 7. Place the cast iron pan to the oven and cook for 10 to 12 minutes, or until the steak reaches your desired temperature. To serve, slice the steak and drizzle with the pistou.
Per Serving: Calories 441; Fat 36g; Sodium 986mg; Carbs 3g; Fiber 0g; Sugar 1g; Protein 25g

Steak Fingers with Gravy

Prep time: 15 minutes| Cook time: 20 minutes| Serves: 6

For the chicken-fried steak
1 cup almond flour
1 cup crushed pork rinds
⅓ cup grated Parmesan cheese
1 teaspoon paprika
1 teaspoon salt, plus more for seasoning
½ teaspoon garlic powder
½ teaspoon black pepper, plus more for seasoning
2 large eggs, lightly beaten
2 tablespoons unsweetened

almond milk
1½ pounds (about 4 steaks) cubed beef steak, cut into 1½-inch strips
Lard or tallow, for frying
For the gravy
2 tablespoons pan drippings
2 tablespoons finely diced onion
4 ounces cream cheese
1 cup unsweetened almond milk
1¼ cups heavy (whipping) cream
Kosher salt
Freshly ground black pepper

1. Make the chicken-fried steak. Stir the almond flour, pork rinds, Parmesan cheese, paprika, salt, garlic powder, and pepper in a shallow dish. 2. Whisk the eggs along with almond milk well in a shallow dish. Place the steak strips on a layer of paper towels and pat dry. 3. Lightly season with salt and pepper. Dip the strips into the egg-milk mixture, one at time. 4. Then dredge the strips in the almond flour mixture. In a large sauté pan or pan over medium heat, melt the lard and heat it to 375°F/191°C. This will take 3 to 5 minutes. 5. You need about 1½ inches of fat in the pan—fry the steak strips for 2 to 3 minutes per side, or until golden brown. 6. Drain on paper towels, reserving 2 tablespoons of pan drippings. Serve with gravy or sugar-free ketchup. 7. Combine the reserved pan drippings and onion in a medium sauté pan or pan over medium heat. Sauté for 2 to 3 minutes. 8. Add the

cream cheese and almond milk and cook, stirring, until smooth and the cream cheese is melted. 9. Add the heavy cream and stir well than simmer the gravy for 3 to 5 minutes, or until thick. Spice the sauce with salt and pepper, and serve immediately.
Per Serving: Calories 643; Fat 51g; Sodium 1248mg; Carbs 4g; Fiber 2g; Sugar 1g; Protein 40g

Spicy Tandoori Beef Fajitas

Prep time: 10 minutes plus 2 to 24 hours to marinate| Cook time: 15 minutes| Serves: 2

½ cup sugar-free Greek yogurt
2 tablespoons avocado oil
½ teaspoon garlic powder
½ teaspoon ground cumin
½ teaspoon paprika
½ teaspoon ground coriander
¼ teaspoon ground cinnamon
¼ teaspoon ground turmeric
¼ teaspoon cayenne pepper
¼ teaspoon ground ginger
¼ teaspoon erythritol "brown sugar"
Salt
1 pound steak, sliced into strips
1 tablespoon butter or butter-

flavored coconut oil
2 medium bell peppers (any color), sliced
1 medium red onion, sliced
4 ounces button mushrooms, sliced
8 asparagus spears, trimmed and chopped
2 to 4 coconut or almond flour wraps or grain-free chips
1 cup shredded romaine lettuce
Sugar-free salsa, sour cream, guacamole, and shredded cheese, for serving

1. Combine the Greek yogurt, avocado oil, garlic powder, cumin, paprika, coriander, cinnamon, turmeric, cayenne, ginger, erythritol, and salt in resealable bag. Add the steak, seal the bag tightly, and massage the marinade into the meat. Marinate in the refrigerator for at least 2 hours or 24 hours. 2. In a pan over medium-high heat pan, melt the butter. Sauté the bell peppers, onion, mushrooms, and asparagus for 5 to 8 minutes, or until the onion is translucent. 3. Add the beef strips and marinade to the pan and stir-fry for 5 to 8 minutes, or until the meat is cooked through. 4. Be sure the marinade boils for at least 1 full minute to kill any harmful bacteria. Place the wraps or chips on plates and top with shredded lettuce. 5. Top with the beef fajita mixture, then salsa, sour cream, guacamole, and cheese.
Per Serving: Calories 655; Fat 43g; Sodium 875mg; Carbs 16g; Fiber 4g; Sugar 6g; Protein 51g

Delicious Mediterranean Meatloaf

Prep time: 15 minutes| Cook time: 7 to 8 hours| Serves: 8

3 tablespoons extra-virgin olive oil, divided
½ sweet onion, chopped
2 teaspoons minced garlic
1 pound ground beef
1 pound ground pork
½ cup almond flour
½ cup heavy (whipping) cream

2 eggs
2 teaspoons dried oregano
1 teaspoon dried basil
¼ teaspoon salt
¼ teaspoon freshly ground black pepper
¾ cup tomato purée
1 cup goat cheese

1. Lightly grease the slow cooker with 1 tablespoon of olive oil. 2. In a medium pan over medium-high heat, heat the remaining 2 tablespoons of olive oil. Sauté garlic and onion until softened about 3 minutes. In a large bowl, mix the onion mixture, beef, pork, almond flour, heavy cream, eggs, oregano, basil, salt, and pepper until well combined. 3. Transfer the meat mixture to the insert and form into a loaf with about a ½-inch gap on the sides. Spread the tomato purée on top of the meatloaf and sprinkle with goat cheese. 4. Cover it and cook on low temperature setting for 7 to 8 hours. Serve warm.
Per Serving: Calories 410; Fat 29g; Sodium 158mg; Carbs 4g; Fiber 1g; Sugar 1g; Protein 32g

Quick Bratwurst

Prep time: 10 minutes. | Cooking time: 8 minutes. | Serves: 4

1 cup water
4 (4-ounce) bratwursts

1 tablespoon coconut oil

1. Pour water into Instant Pot and place steam rack in bottom of pot. Put brats on steam rack and turn the pot's lid to close. Adjust time for almost 10 minutes. When the pot beeps, quick-release the pressure. Remove brats and pour out water. 2. Replace inner pot and hit the sauté button. Place brats and coconut oil into Instant Pot. Brown for almost 2–4 minutes or until golden. Remove brats with tongs when golden. Serve alone or with buttered cabbage.
Per Serving: Calories 323; Total Fat 17.9g; Sodium 838mg; Total Carbs 4.3g; Fiber 1.5g; Sugars 1g; Protein 35.5g

Beef Eggplant Lasagna

Prep time: 10 minutes. | Cooking time: 60 minutes. | Serves: 8

½ cup olive oil, extra-virgin
2 eggs, beaten
2 teaspoons salt
1 cup shredded parmesan cheese
2½ cups mozzarella cheese
2 small eggplants, unpeeled, trimmed and cut into ¼-inch

rounds
1 pound ground beef, preferably grass-fed
2 cups whole-milk ricotta cheese
2 teaspoons dried basil or oregano
¼ teaspoon black pepper
3 cups basic marinara

1. At 425°F/218°C, preheat your oven. 2. Layer a suitable baking sheet with foil sheet and coat with 2 tablespoons of olive oil. 3. In a suitable, shallow bowl, mix the beaten eggs and 1 teaspoon of salt. 4. In a second bowl, mix ½ cup of parmesan cheese and ½ cup of mozzarella cheese. 5. One at a time, dredge each eggplant round first in the egg mixture and then in the cheese mixture, coating each side. 6. Place the coated eggplant rounds on the prepared baking sheet and drizzle with 2 tablespoons of olive oil. 7. Bake until golden brown and eggplant is softened, for 18 to 20 minutes. 8. While the eggplant bakes, prepare the filling. 9. Heat 2 tablespoons oil in a suitable skillet over medium heat. 10. Add the ground beef and cook, breaking it apart, until browned and cooked through, for 5 to 6 minutes. 11. To the skillet with the beef, stir in the ricotta cheese, basil, remaining 1 teaspoon of salt, and the pepper. Remove it from the heat and keep it aside. 12. In a suitable bowl, mix the marinara sauce with the remaining 2 tablespoons of olive oil and whisk until smooth. 13. In a suitable bowl, mix the remaining 2 cups of mozzarella and ½ cup of parmesan. 14. Once the eggplant is cooked, assemble the lasagna. 15. Spoon one-third of the sauce mixture into a 9-by-13-inch glass baking dish and spread evenly to coat the bottom. Place half of the eggplant rounds in one layer to fully cover the sauce. 16. Add half of the beef and ricotta mixture on top of the eggplant, spreading evenly. 17. Top with half of the cheese mixture. Repeat another layer with sauce, eggplant, beef and ricotta, and cheese, topping with the final third of the sauce mixture. 18. Bake until the cheese is bubbly and melted, 30 to 35 minutes. 19. Turn the broiler to low and broil until the top is golden brown. for almost 5 minutes. 20. Remove it from your oven and allow to cool slightly before slicing.
Per Serving: Calories 448; Total Fat 32.9g; Sodium 71mg; Total Carbs 8.1g; Fiber 9.4g; Sugars 6.3g; Protein 14.6g

Mozzarella-Stuffed Meatloaf

Prep time: 10 minutes. | Cooking time: 30 minutes. | Serves: 6

1 pound 80/20 ground beef
½ medium green bell pepper, seeded and chopped
¼ medium yellow onion, peeled and chopped

½ teaspoon salt
¼ teaspoon ground black pepper
2 ounces mozzarella cheese, sliced into ¼"-thick slices
¼ cup low-carb ketchup

1. In a suitable bowl, mix ground beef, bell pepper, onion, salt, and black pepper. Cut a piece of parchment to fit air fryer basket. Place half beef mixture on ungreased parchment and form a 9" × 4" loaf. for almost ½" thick. 2. Center mozzarella slices on beef loaf, leaving at least ¼" around each edge. 3. Press remaining beef into a second 9" × 4" loaf and place on top of mozzarella, pressing edges of loaves to seal. 4. Place parchment with meatloaf into air fryer basket. Set the temperature to 350°F/177°C and set the timer for almost 30 minutes, carefully turning loaf and brushing top with ketchup halfway through cooking. Loaf will be browned and have an internal temperature of at least 180°F/82°C when done. Slice and serve warm.
Per Serving: Calories 542; Total Fat 17.8g; Sodium 801mg; Total Carbs 9g; Fiber 10.7g; Sugars 3.9g; Protein 19.2g

Cheesy Southwestern Meat Loaf

Prep time: 10 minutes. | Cooking time: 60 minutes. | Serves: 8

½ cup avocado oil or olive oil, extra-virgin
2 cups shredded (not spiralized) zucchini, from 2 small or 1 large zucchini
1½ teaspoons salt
1 pound ground beef, preferably grass-fed
1 pound ground pork chorizo
½ cup chopped cilantro
¼ cup chopped scallions, green

and white parts
1 large egg, beaten
1 tablespoon chopped chipotle pepper with adobo sauce
1 teaspoon garlic powder
¼ cup almond flour
2 cups shredded Mexican cheese blend or cheddar cheese
1 tablespoon tomato paste (no sugar added)

1. At 375°F/191°C, preheat your oven. Coat a loaf pan with 2 tablespoons of avocado oil. 2. Layer a colander with a layer of paper towels and add the shredded zucchini. Sprinkle with ½ teaspoon of salt, tossing to coat. Let sit for almost 10 minutes, then press down with another layer of paper towels to release some of the excess moisture. 3. While the zucchini drains, in a suitable bowl, mix the ground beef, chorizo, cilantro, scallions, ¼ cup of oil, egg, chipotle with adobo, garlic powder, and remaining 1 teaspoon of salt. Mix well with a fork. 4. Add the almond flour to the drained zucchini and toss to coat. Add the zucchini to the meat mixture and mix until well combined. Add half of the prepared mixture to the prepared pan and spread evenly. 5. Top with 1 cup of shredded cheese, spreading evenly. Top with the remaining half of the prepared mixture and spread evenly. 6. In a suitable bowl, beat the tomato paste and remaining 2 tablespoons of oil and spread evenly on top of the meat mixture. Sprinkle with the remaining 1 cup of cheese. Bake for almost 50 to 55 minutes, or until cooked through. Let sit for almost 10 minutes before cutting.
Per Serving: Calories 589; Total Fat 18.2g; Sodium 513mg; Total Carbs 5.6g; Fiber 24.5g; Sugars 13.2g; Protein 26g

Shepherd's Pie

Prep time: 10 minutes. | Cooking time: 70 minutes. | Serves: 6

4 tablespoons olive oil, extra-virgin
2 cups cauliflower florets (from about half a head of cauliflower)
2 tablespoons unsalted butter
½ cup heavy cream
1 cup shredded cheddar cheese
2 teaspoons salt
2 teaspoons dried thyme
½ teaspoon black pepper, divided
1 pound ground beef, preferably grass-fed

½ small yellow onion, diced
1 cup chopped cabbage
1 carrot, peeled and diced
2 ribs celery, diced
4 ounces mushrooms, sliced
4 cloves garlic, minced
1 (14½-ounce) can diced tomatoes, with juices
2 tablespoons tomato paste
½ cup beef stock
8 ounces cream cheese, room temperature

1. At 375°F/191°C, preheat your oven. 2. Heat 2 tablespoons oil in a suitable saucepan over medium-low heat. Add the cauliflower and sauté until just tender, 6 to 8 minutes. Add the butter and heavy cream, cover, reduce heat to low, and cook until cauliflower is very tender, another 6 to 8 minutes. Remove it from the heat and allow to cool slightly. 3. Add the cheese, 1 teaspoon of salt, 1 teaspoon of thyme, and ¼ teaspoon of pepper to the cauliflower. 4. Using an immersion blender or hand mixer, puree until very smooth. Keep it aside. 5. In a suitable saucepan or skillet, heat the remaining 2 tablespoons of olive oil over medium heat. 6. Add the ground beef and sauté for almost 5 minutes, breaking it apart. 7. Add the onion, cabbage, carrot, celery, and mushrooms and sauté for another 5 to 6 minutes, or until the vegetables are just tender and the meat is browned. 8. Add the garlic, remaining 1 teaspoon of salt, remaining 1 teaspoon of thyme, and remaining ¼ teaspoon of pepper and sauté, stirring, for another 30 seconds. 9. Stir in the tomatoes with their juices and the tomato paste. 10. Bring to a simmer, reduce heat to low, cover, and simmer for almost 8 to 10 minutes, or until the vegetables are very tender and sauce has thickened. 11. In a suitable microwave-safe bowl, mix the stock and cream cheese and microwave on high for almost 1 minute or until cheese is melted. Whisk until creamy. 12. Add the cream cheese mixture to the meat and vegetables and stir to mix well. Place the prepared mixture in an 8-inch square glass baking dish or pie pan. Spread the pureed cauliflower over the meat mixture and bake until golden, 25 to 30 minutes.
Per Serving: Calories 687; Total Fat 17.1g; Sodium 495mg; Total Carbs 2.7g; Fiber 27.3g; Sugars 12.9g; Protein 26g

Marinated Steak Kebabs

Prep time: 10 minutes. | Cooking time: 5 minutes. | Serves: 4

1 pound strip steak, fat trimmed, cut into 1" cubes
½ cup soy sauce
¼ cup olive oil
1 tablespoon granular brown

erythritol
½ teaspoon salt
¼ teaspoon ground black pepper
1 medium green bell pepper, seeded and chopped into 1" cubes

1. Place steak into a suitable sealable bowl or bag and pour in soy sauce and olive oil. Add erythritol, then stir to coat steak. Marinate at room temperature 30 minutes. 2. Remove streak from marinade and sprinkle with salt and black pepper. 3. Place meat and vegetables onto 6" skewer sticks, alternating between steak and bell pepper. 4. Place kebabs into ungreased air fryer basket. Set the temperature to 400°F/204°C and set the timer for almost 5 minutes. Steak will be done when crispy at the edges and peppers are tender. Serve warm.
Per Serving: Calories 499; Total Fat 9.4g; Sodium 422mg; Total Carbs 3.4g; Fiber 17.2g; Sugars 1.6g; Protein 26.9g

Beef and Broccoli Foil Packs

Prep time: 10 minutes. | Cooking time: 10 minutes. | Serves: 4

¼ cup beef stock
¼ cup low-sodium soy sauce
¼ cup sesame oil
¼ cup plus 2 tablespoons olive oil, extra-virgin
4 cloves garlic, minced
2 tablespoons chopped fresh

ginger
1 pound flank steak, sliced
2 cups broccoli florets, cut into bite-size pieces
¼ cup minced scallion, green and white parts
2 tablespoons sesame seeds

1. In a suitable bowl, beat the stock, soy sauce, sesame oil, ¼ cup of olive oil, the garlic, and ginger. Pour half of the prepared mixture into a suitable zip-top plastic bag and add the steak slices. 2. Marinate in the refrigerator for 1 hour, or up to 24 hours. 3. Heat the remaining 2 tablespoons oil in a suitable skillet over high heat. Remove the steak from its marinade. Sear the steak for almost 2 to 3 minutes, until just browned per side, but not cooked through. 4. Lay four 8-inch squares of foil sheet on the counter. Place ½ cup of broccoli and a quarter of the seared steak in the middle of each piece of foil. Pour a quarter of the remaining soy sauce mixture over each steak and broccoli pile, garnish with the scallions and sesame seeds, and cover with a second 8-inch foil square. Fold the foil up to about 1 inch from the prepared mixture per side. Fold in each corner once to secure and seal the foil pack. 5. Preheat the grill on medium-high heat. Place the prepared foil packs in a single layer on the grill and grill for almost 8 minutes.
Per Serving: Calories 483; Total Fat 6g; Sodium 184mg; Total Carbs 7.2g; Fiber 31.2g; Sugars 6g; Protein 30.4g

Weeknight Chili

Prep time: 10 minutes. | Cooking time: 35 minutes. | Serves: 6

¼ cup olive oil, extra-virgin
1 small yellow onion, diced
1 green bell pepper, diced
1 pound ground beef, preferably grass-fed
½ pound ground Italian sausage (hot or sweet)
1 tablespoon chili powder
2 teaspoons ground cumin

1½ teaspoons salt
6 cloves garlic, minced
1 (14½-ounce) can diced tomatoes, with juices
1 (6-ounce) can tomato paste
2 cups water
2 ripe avocados, pitted, peeled, and chopped
1 cup sour cream

1. Preheat the olive oil in a suitable pot over medium heat. Add the onion and bell pepper and sauté for almost 5 minutes, or until just tender. 2. Stir in the ground beef and sausage and cook until meat is browned, 5 to 6 minutes, stirring to break into small pieces. Add the chili powder, cumin, salt, and garlic and sauté, stirring frequently, for almost 1 minute, until fragrant. 3. Add the tomatoes and their juices, tomato paste, and water, stirring to mix well. Bring the prepared mixture to a boil, reduce heat to low, cover, and simmer for almost 15 to 20 minutes, stirring occasionally. Add additional water for a thinner chili if desired. 4. Serve hot, garnished with chopped avocado and sour cream.
Per Serving: Calories 396; Total Fat 8.6g; Sodium 596mg; Total Carbs 5.9g; Fiber 3.4g; Sugars 3.8g; Protein 12.1g

Slow Cooker Herb-and-Garlic Short Rib Stew

Prep time: 10 minutes. | Cooking time: 6 hours. | Serves: 4

1 pound boneless beef short ribs
1 teaspoon salt
½ teaspoon garlic powder
¼ teaspoon black pepper
4 tablespoons olive oil, extra-virgin
½ small yellow onion, diced
1 carrot, peeled and diced
2 ribs celery, diced
4 ounces sliced mushrooms

6 cloves garlic, minced
2 teaspoons dried thyme
2 teaspoons dried rosemary (or 2 tablespoons fresh)
1 teaspoon dried oregano
3 cups beef stock
1 (14½-ounce) can diced tomatoes, with juices
½ cup dry red wine (such as merlot)

1. Season the short ribs with the salt, garlic powder, and pepper. 2. Preheat 2 tablespoons oil in a suitable skillet over high heat. Add the short ribs and brown until dark in color, 2 to 3 minutes per side. Transfer to the bowl of a slow cooker. 3. Add the rest of the 2 tablespoons of oil to the skillet and reduce heat to medium. Add the onion, carrot, celery, and mushrooms and sauté until just tender but not fully cooked, 3 to 4 minutes. Add the garlic and sauté, stirring, for an additional 30 seconds. Transfer the contents of the skillet to the slow cooker with the ribs. 4. Add the thyme, rosemary, oregano, stock, tomatoes with their juices, and wine, and cook on low for almost 4 to 6 hours, or until meat is very tender. 5. Remove the ribs from the stew and shred using two forks. Return the shredded meat to the stew and stir to mix well. Serve warm.

Per Serving: Calories 426; Total Fat 8.6g; Sodium 588mg; Total Carbs 7g; Fiber 16.4g; Sugars 2.4g; Protein 23.2g

Steak with Blue Cheese Butter

Prep time: 10 minutes. | Cooking time: 10 minutes. | Serves: 4

4 (4-ounce) filet mignon or New York strip steaks
1 teaspoon salt
1 teaspoon garlic powder
¼ teaspoon black pepper
¼ cup unsalted butter, room

temperature
¼ cup crumbled blue cheese
½ teaspoon dried thyme
2 tablespoons olive oil, extra-virgin

1. At 450°F/232°C, preheat your oven. Rub the steaks with the salt, ½ teaspoon of garlic powder, and the pepper. Let sit at room temperature for almost 15 to 30 minutes. 2. To make the blue cheese butter, in a suitable bowl, mix the butter, blue cheese, remaining ½ teaspoon of garlic powder, and thyme and whisk until well combined and smooth. Keep it aside. 3. Heat the olive oil in a suitable, oven-proof skillet over high heat. When the oil is very hot, add the steaks and sear for almost 1 minute per side. Transfer the skillet to your oven and roast to desired doneness. 4. For almost 1-inch-thick steaks, it will take 3 to 6 minutes for rare (130 to 135 degrees F), 6 to 8 minutes for medium-rare (140 to 155 degrees F), and 8 to 10 minutes for well-done (150 to 155 degrees F). For almost 1½-inch-thick steaks, cook 4 to 6 minutes for rare and 8 to 10 minutes for well-done. 5. Remove the prepared steaks from the skillet and place each on a separate plate. Top each with 2 tablespoons of blue cheese butter and allow the steak to rest and butter to melt for almost 5 minutes before serving.
Per Serving: Calories 336; Total Fat 9.9g; Sodium 1672mg; Total Carbs 2.6g; Fiber 1.7g; Sugars 2.1g; Protein 12.3g

Slow Cooker Swedish Meatballs

Prep time: 10 minutes. | Cooking time: 4 hrs. | Serves: 8

1 pound ground Italian pork sausage
1 pound ground beef, preferably grass-fed
½ small yellow onion, minced
¼ cup almond flour
1 large egg, beaten
3 teaspoons Worcestershire sauce
2 teaspoons salt
1 teaspoon ground allspice

½ teaspoon ground nutmeg
½ teaspoon ground ginger
½ teaspoon black pepper
1½ cups beef stock or broth
1 cup heavy cream
1 tablespoon Dijon mustard
4 ounces cream cheese, room temperature
1 cup sour cream, room temperature

1. In a suitable bowl, mix the pork, beef, onion, almond flour, egg, 1 teaspoon of Worcestershire, 1 teaspoon of salt, the allspice, nutmeg, ginger, and ¼ teaspoon of pepper and mix well with a fork. 2. Form the meat mixture into small 1-inch meatballs, and place on a suitable baking sheet or cutting board. 3. In the bowl of a 5- or 6-quart slow cooker, beat the stock, heavy cream, mustard, remaining 2 teaspoons of Worcestershire sauce, remaining 1 teaspoon of salt, and remaining ¼ teaspoon of pepper until smooth and creamy. Place the meatballs in the sauce, trying to not overcrowd. Set the slow cooker to low and cook for almost 4 hours. 4. After 4 hours of cooking, beat the cream cheese and sour cream and add to the warm mixture, gently stirring to incorporate well. 5. Serve the meatballs in their sauce with toothpicks, or over spiralized zucchini for a complete meal. Leftover meatballs and sauce can be frozen for up to 3 months.
Per Serving: Calories 371; Total Fat 4.9g; Sodium 1207mg; Total Carbs 7.5g; Fiber 25g; Sugars 7g; Protein 25.6g

Cheese-Stuffed Steak Burgers

Prep time: 10 minutes. | Cooking time: 10 minutes. | Serves: 4

1 pound 80/20 ground sirloin
4 ounces mild cheddar cheese, cubed

½ teaspoon salt
¼ teaspoon ground black pepper

1. Form ground sirloin into four equal balls, then separate each ball in half and flatten into two thin patties, for eight total patties. Place 1 ounce cheddar into center of one patty, then top with a second patty and press edges to seal burger closed. Repeat with remaining patties and cheddar to create four burgers. 2. Sprinkle black pepper and salt over both sides of burgers and carefully place burgers into ungreased air fryer basket. Set the temperature to 350°F/177°C and set the timer for almost 10 minutes. Burgers will be done when browned on the edges and top. Serve warm.
Per Serving: Calories 499; Total Fat 9.4g; Sodium 422mg; Total Carbs 3.4g; Fiber 17.2g; Sugars 1.6g; Protein 26.9g

Corn Dogs

Prep time: 10 minutes. | Cooking time: 8 minutes. | Serves: 4

1½ cups shredded mozzarella cheese
1 ounce cream cheese
½ cup blanched finely ground almond flour
4 beef hot dogs

1. Place mozzarella, cream cheese, and flour in a suitable microwave-safe bowl. Microwave on high 45 seconds, then stir with a fork until a soft ball of dough forms. 2. Press dough out into a 12" × 6" rectangle, then use a knife to separate into four smaller rectangles. 3. Wrap each hot dog in one rectangle of dough and place into ungreased air fryer basket. Set the temperature to 400°F/204°C and set the timer for almost 8 minutes, turning corn dogs halfway through cooking. Corn dogs will be golden brown when done. Serve warm.
Per Serving: Calories 161; Total Fat 12.4g; Sodium 375mg; Total Carbs 9.8g; Fiber 1.5g; Sugars 2.6g; Protein 3.8g

Marinated Rib Eye

Prep time: 10 minutes. | Cooking time: 10 minutes. | Serves: 4

1 pound rib eye steak
¼ cup soy sauce
1 tablespoon Worcestershire sauce
1 tablespoon granular brown
erythritol
2 tablespoons olive oil
½ teaspoon salt
¼ teaspoon ground black pepper

1. Place rib eye in a suitable sealable bowl or bag and pour in soy sauce, Worcestershire sauce, erythritol, and olive oil. Seal and let marinate 30 minutes in the refrigerator. 2. Remove rib eye from marinade, pat dry, and sprinkle on all sides with black pepper and salt. Place rib eye into ungreased air fryer basket. 3. Set the temperature to 400°F/204°C and set the timer for almost 10 minutes. Steak will be done when browned at the edges and has an internal temperature of 150°F/66°C for medium or 180°F/82°C for well-done. Serve warm.
Per Serving: Calories 339; Total Fat 14g; Sodium 556mg; Total Carbs 4.6g; Fiber 6.4g; Sugars 3.8g; Protein 10.5g

Mexican-Style Shredded Beef

Prep time: 10 minutes. | Cooking time: 35 minutes. | Serves: 6

1 (2-pound) beef chuck roast, cut into 2" cubes
1 teaspoon salt
½ teaspoon ground black pepper
½ cup no-sugar-added chipotle sauce

1. In a suitable bowl, sprinkle beef cubes with black pepper and salt and toss to coat. 2. Place beef into ungreased air fryer basket. Set the temperature to 400°F/204°C and set the timer for almost 30 minutes, shaking the basket halfway through cooking. Beef will be done when internal temperature is at least 160°F/71°C. 3. Place cooked beef into a suitable bowl and shred with two forks. Pour in chipotle sauce and toss to coat. 4. Return beef to air fryer basket for an additional 5 minutes at 400°F/204°C to crisp with sauce. Serve warm.
Per Serving: Calories 373; Total Fat 3.1g; Sodium 687mg; Total Carbs 9.2g; Fiber 9.6g; Sugars 3.4g; Protein 17.8g

Bacon and Blue Cheese Burgers

Prep time: 10 minutes. | Cooking time: 15 minutes. | Serves: 4

1 pound 70/30 ground beef
6 slices cooked sugar-free bacon, finely chopped
½ cup crumbled blue cheese
¼ cup peeled and chopped yellow onion
½ teaspoon salt
¼ teaspoon ground black pepper

1. In a suitable bowl, mix ground beef, bacon, blue cheese, and onion. Separate into four sections and shape each section into a patty. Sprinkle with black pepper and salt. 2. Place patties into ungreased air fryer basket. Set the temperature to 350°F/177°C and set the timer for almost 15 minutes, turning patties halfway through cooking. Burgers will be done when internal temperature is at least 150°F/66°C for medium and 180°F/82°C for well. Serve warm.
Per Serving: Calories 254; Total Fat 2.6g; Sodium 482mg; Total Carbs 9.1g; Fiber 4.8g; Sugars 0.2g; Protein 7.8g

Blackened Steak Nuggets

Prep time: 10 minutes. | Cooking time: 7 minutes. | Serves: 2

1 pound rib eye steak, cut into 1" cubes
2 tablespoons salted butter,
melted
½ teaspoon paprika
½ teaspoon salt

¼ teaspoon garlic powder
¼ teaspoon onion powder
¼ teaspoon ground black pepper
⅛ teaspoon cayenne pepper

1. Place steak into a suitable bowl and pour in butter. Toss to coat. Sprinkle with remaining ingredients. 2. Place bites into ungreased air fryer basket. Set the temperature to 400°F/204°C and set the timer for almost 7 minutes, shaking the basket three times during cooking. Steak will be crispy on the outside and browned when done and internal temperature is at least 150°F/66°C for medium and 180°F/82°C for well-done. Serve warm.
Per Serving: Calories 244; Total Fat 9.1g; Sodium 1399mg; Total Carbs 4.3g; Fiber 8.7g; Sugars 15.7g; Protein 8.3g

Spinach and Provolone Steak Rolls

Prep time: 10 minutes. | Cooking time: 12 minutes. | Serves: 8

1 (1-pound) flank steak, butterflied
8 (1-ounce, ¼"-thick) deli slices provolone cheese
1 cup fresh spinach leaves
½ teaspoon salt
¼ teaspoon ground black pepper

1. Place steak on a suitable plate. Place provolone slices to cover steak, leaving 1" at the edges. Lay spinach leaves over cheese. 2. Gently roll steak and tie with kitchen twine or secure with toothpicks. Carefully slice into eight pieces. Sprinkle each with black pepper and salt. 3. Place rolls into ungreased air fryer basket, cut side up. Set the temperature to 400°F/204°C and set the timer for almost 12 minutes. Steak rolls will be browned and cheese will be melted when done and have an internal temperature of at least 150°F/66°C for medium steak and 180°F/82°C for well-done steak. Serve warm.
Per Serving: Calories 669; Total Fat 53.8g; Sodium 905mg; Total Carbs 1.7g; Fiber 8.6g; Sugars 12.3g; Protein 14g

Spicy Brisket

Prep time: 10 minutes. | Cooking time: 110 minutes. | Serves: 6

3 teaspoons salt
2 teaspoons pepper
1 teaspoon garlic powder
1 teaspoon dried thyme
½ teaspoon dried rosemary
1 (4- to 5-pound) beef brisket
1 tablespoon avocado oil
1 cup beef broth
½ cup pickled jalapeño juice
½ cup pickled jalapeños
½ medium onion, chopped

1. In a suitable bowl mix salt, pepper, garlic powder, thyme, and rosemary. Sprinkle over brisket; keep it aside. 2. Hit the sauté button on the Instant Pot and add avocado oil to Instant Pot. Sear each side of brisket for almost 5 minutes. 3. Add beef broth, jalapeño juice, jalapeños, and onions to Instant Pot. Hit the cancel button and click to close lid. 4. Hit the manual button and adjust time to 100 minutes. When the pot beeps, allow pot to naturally release, for almost 30–40 minutes. Don't do a quick release; it will result in tougher meat. 5. Remove brisket, slice, and pour all the strained broth over meat for additional flavor.
Per Serving: Calories 541; Total Fat 12.4g; Sodium 250mg; Total Carbs 5.4g; Fiber 21.3g; Sugars 6.1g; Protein 26.5g

Buttery Pot Roast

Prep time: 10 minutes. | Cooking time: 90 minutes. | Serves: 4

4 teaspoons onion powder
2 teaspoons dried parsley
1 teaspoon salt
1 teaspoon garlic powder
½ teaspoon dried oregano
½ teaspoon pepper
1 (2-pound) chuck roast
1 tablespoon coconut oil
1 cup store-bought beef broth
½ packet dry ranch seasoning
1 stick butter
10 pepperoncini

1. Hit the sauté button on the Instant Pot and allow to heat. In suitable bowl, mix onion powder, parsley, salt, garlic powder, oregano, and pepper. Rub seasoning onto roast. Add coconut oil to preheat. Place roast in pot and sear for almost 5 minutes each side; remove roast and keep it aside. 2. Hit the cancel button. Add broth to Instant Pot. Using rubber spatula or wooden spoon, scrape bottom to loosen any stuck-on seasoning or meat. 3. Place roast back into Instant Pot and sprinkle dry ranch powder on top. Place stick of butter on roast and add pepperoncini. Turn the pot's lid to close. Hit the manual button and adjust time for almost 90 minutes. 4. When the pot beeps, allow a natural release to retain meat tenderness. When pressure indicator drops, remove lid and remove cooked roast. Slice or shred and top with broth from pot.
Per Serving: Calories 344; Total Fat 3g; Sodium 603mg; Total Carbs 3.8g; Fiber 11.5g; Sugars 8.6g; Protein 9.4g

Steak Bites and Roasted Garlic Dipping Sauce

Prep time: 10 minutes. | Cooking time: 10 minutes. | Serves: 4

Steak bites
1 pound sirloin steak
1 teaspoon salt
¼ teaspoon pepper
4 tablespoons butter

Dipping sauce
½ cup mayo
1 teaspoon lemon juice
1 roasted garlic clove, mashed
⅛ teaspoon red pepper flakes

1. Cut steak into 1-inch cubes. Sprinkle with black pepper and salt. Hit the sauté button on the Instant Pot and add butter to Instant Pot. When butter is melted, add steak and sear each side until desired doneness, for almost 10 minutes. Hit the cancel button and place steak bites into dish. 2. In suitable bowl, mix mayo, lemon juice, roasted garlic, and red pepper flakes. 3. Serve steak bites with dipping sauce.
Per Serving: Calories 357; Total Fat 16.1g; Sodium 80mg; Total Carbs 6g; Fiber 7.3g; Sugars 9.2g; Protein 29.4g

Sausage Stuffing with Veggies

Prep time: 15 minutes| Cook time: 45 minutes| Serves: 4

4 cups cauliflower florets, broken or chopped into ½-inch pieces
½ cup extra-virgin olive oil, divided
1 teaspoon salt, divided
8 ounces bulk pork sausage
½ small onion, diced small
4 ribs celery, diced small
¼ cup chopped carrot
4 ounces chopped mushrooms

1 tablespoon fresh sage, finely chopped
1 teaspoon dried thyme
¼ teaspoon freshly ground black pepper
4 cloves garlic, minced
1 cup chicken or vegetable stock
¼ cup dry white wine
2 tablespoons fresh parsley, chopped

1. Preheat the oven to 425°F/218°C. 2. Prepare a rimmed baking tray with aluminum foil. 3. In a large bowl, toss the cauliflower with ¼ cup of olive oil and ½ teaspoon of salt. Spread the cauliflower on the baking sheet, reserving the bowl. 4. Cook the cauliflower until golden brown and crispy but not soft, for 10 to 12 minutes. Remove from the oven, reduce temperature to 375°F/191°C, and allow the cauliflower to cool slightly before transferring back to the reserved bowl. 5. Heat the olive oil over medium-high heat. Add the sausage and sear for 10 minutes, breaking it into small pieces. Do not drain the rendered fat. 6. To the pan along with sausage, add onion, celery, carrot, mushrooms, sage, thyme, remaining ½ teaspoon of salt, and pepper, and sauté well until the vegetables begin to soften, 5 to 7 minutes. Add the garlic and sauté, stirring, for another 30 seconds. 7. Add the stock and white wine, increase heat to high, and sauté, continuously stirring, until half the liquid evaporates. 8. Transfer the sausage-and-vegetable mixture to the bowl with the cauliflower and stir in the parsley. Transfer the mixture to an 8-inch square glass baking dish. 9. Bake uncovered until the top is browned and crispy, for 15 to 20 minutes. Allow resting for 10 minutes before serving.
Per Serving: Calories 496; Fat 45g; Sodium 784mg; Carbs 10g; Fiber 3g; Sugar 6g; Protein 12g

Creamy Mushroom Pot Roast

Prep time: 10 minutes. | Cooking time: 90 minutes. | Serves: 6

1 cup sliced button mushrooms
½ medium onion, sliced
1 tablespoon coconut oil
2 teaspoons dried minced onion
2 teaspoons dried parsley
1 teaspoon pepper
1 teaspoon garlic powder

½ teaspoon dried oregano
1 teaspoon salt
1 (2–3-pound) chuck roast
1 cup beef broth
4 tablespoons butter
2 ounces cream cheese
¼ cup heavy cream

1. Hit the sauté button on the Instant Pot and add mushrooms, onion, and coconut oil to Instant Pot. Stir-fry for almost 5 minutes or until onions turn translucent. While stir-frying, mix dried minced onion, parsley, pepper, garlic, oregano, and salt in suitable bowl. Rub into chuck roast. Hit the cancel button. 2. Add beef broth and roast into pot. Place butter and cream cheese on top. Turn the pot's lid to close. Hit the meat button and hit the adjust button to set heat to more. Set time to 90 minutes. 3. When the pot beeps allow a full natural release to retain moisture in meat. When pressure valve drops, stir in heavy cream. Remove roast carefully; it will be fall-apart tender. Hit the sauté button on the Instant Pot and reduce sauce in Instant Pot for almost 10 minutes, stirring occasionally. Hit the cancel button and spoon over roast to serve.
Per Serving: Calories 459; Total Fat 3.6g; Sodium 1614mg; Total Carbs 2g; Fiber 11.5g; Sugars 8.3g; Protein 25.9g

Crispy Baked Pork Chops with Veggie Gravy

Prep time: 10 minutes| Cook time: 25 minutes| Serves: 4

4 tablespoons extra-virgin olive oil, divided
½ cup almond flour
2 teaspoons dried sage, divided
1½ teaspoons salt, divided
½ teaspoon freshly ground black pepper, divided
1 large egg
¼ cup flax meal
¼ cup walnuts, very finely

chopped
4 (4-ounce) boneless pork chops
1 tablespoon unsalted butter
4 ounces chopped mushrooms
2 cloves garlic, minced
1 teaspoon dried thyme
8 ounces cream cheese, room temperature
½ cup heavy cream
¼ cup chicken stock

1. Preheat the oven to 400°F/204°C. Prepare a baking tray with aluminum foil lining and grease with 1 tablespoon of olive oil. 2. In a shallow bowl, Mix almond flour with 1 teaspoon of sage, ½ teaspoon of salt, and ¼ teaspoon of pepper. 3. In another bowl, whisk the egg. In another shallow bowl, stir the flax meal and walnuts. 4. Dredge each pork chop first in the flour mixture, then in the egg, then in the flax-and-walnut mixture to thoroughly coat all sides. Place the prepared baking sheet and drizzle the pork chops evenly with 1 tablespoon of olive oil. 5. Bake until cooked through and golden brown, for 18 to 25 minutes, depending on the thickness of the pork. 6. While the pork is baking, prepare the gravy. Heat the olive oil and the butter in a medium saucepan. Add the mushrooms and sauté until very tender, for 4 to 6 minutes. Add the garlic, remaining 1 teaspoon of sage and 1 teaspoon of salt, thyme, and remaining ¼ teaspoon of pepper, and sauté for an additional 30 seconds. 7. Add the cream cheese to the mushrooms, reduce heat to low, and stir until melted and creamy, for 2 to 3 minutes. Whisk in the cream and stock until smooth. Cook over low heat, frequently whisking, until the mixture is thick and creamy, another 3 to 4 minutes. 8. Serve each pork chop covered with a quarter of the mushroom gravy.
Per Serving: Calories 799; Fat 69g; Sodium 654mg; Carbs 11g; Fiber 4g; Sugar 4g; Protein 36g

Herb Pork Tenderloin

Prep time: 5 minutes| Cook time: 20 minutes| Serves: 6

¼ cup mayonnaise
2 tablespoons Dijon mustard
½ teaspoon dried thyme
¼ teaspoon dried rosemary

1 (1-pound) pork tenderloin
½ teaspoon salt
¼ teaspoon ground black pepper

1. Mix mayonnaise, mustard, thyme, and rosemary in a small bowl. Brush tenderloin with the mixture on all sides, then sprinkle with salt and pepper on all sides. 2. Place tenderloin into an ungreased air fryer basket. Set the temp setting to 400°F/204°C and the timer for 20 minutes, turning the tenderloin halfway through cooking. Tenderloin will be golden and have an internal temperature of at least 145°F/63°C when done. Serve warm.
Per Serving: Calories 158; Fat 9g; Sodium 557mg; Carbs 1g; Fiber 0g; Sugar 0g; Protein 16g

Chops with Kalamata Tapenade

Prep time: 15 minutes| Cook time: 25 minutes| Serves: 4

For the tapenade
1 cup pitted Kalamata olives
2 tablespoons chopped fresh parsley
2 tablespoons extra-virgin olive oil
2 teaspoons minced garlic
2 teaspoons freshly squeezed

lemon juice
For the lamb chops
2 (1-pound) racks French-cut lamb chops (8 bones each)
Sea salt
Freshly ground black pepper
1 tablespoon olive oil

To make the tapenade: 1. Place the olives, parsley, olive oil, garlic, and lemon juice in a food processor and process until the mixture is puréed but still slightly chunky. 2. Transfer the tapenade to a container and store sealed in the refrigerator until needed
To make the lamb chops: 1. Preheat the oven to 450°F/232°C. 2. Spice the lamb racks with salt and pepper. Place a large ovenproof pan over medium-high heat and add the olive oil. 3. Sear the lamb racks brown, about 5 minutes. 4. Arrange the racks upright in the pan, with the bones interlaced, and roast them in the oven about 20 minutes for medium-rare or until the internal temperature reaches 125°F/52°C. 5. Let the roasted lamb rest for 10 minutes, and then cut the lamb racks into chops. Arrange 4 chops per person on the plate and top with the Kalamata tapenade.
Per Serving: Calories 348; Fat 28g; Sodium 987mg; Carbs 2g; Fiber 1g; Sugar 1g; Protein 21g

Wrapped Pork Tenderloin

Prep time: 20 minutes| Cook time: 10 minutes| Serves: 6

1 (1-pound) pork tenderloin
½ teaspoon salt
½ teaspoon garlic powder
¼ teaspoon ground black pepper
8 slices sugar-free bacon

1. Sprinkle tenderloin with salt, garlic powder, and pepper. Wrap bacon around the tenderloin and secure it with toothpicks. 2. Place tenderloin into an ungreased air fryer basket. Set the temperature setting to 400°F/204°C and the timer for 20 minutes, turning the tenderloin after 15 minutes. When done, bacon will be crispy, and tenderloin will have an internal temperature of at least 145°F/63°C. 3. Cut the tenderloin into six even portions, transfer each to a medium plate, and serve warm.
Per Serving: Calories 144; Fat 6g; Sodium 590mg; Carbs 0g; Fiber 0g; Sugar 0g; Protein 20g

Parmesan Pork Chops

Prep time: 5 minutes| Cook time: 12 minutes| Serves: 4

1 large egg
½ cup grated Parmesan cheese
4 (4-ounce) boneless pork chops
½ teaspoon salt
¼ teaspoon ground black pepper

1. Whisk egg in a medium bowl and place Parmesan in a separate medium bowl. 2. Sprinkle pork chops on both sides with salt and pepper. Dip pork chop into the egg, then press both sides into Parmesan. 3. Place pork chops into an ungreased air fryer basket. Set the temperature setting to 400°F/204°C and the timer for 12 minutes, turning chops halfway through cooking. When done, pork chops will be golden and have an internal temperature of at least 145°F/63°C. Serve warm.
Per Serving: Calories 298; Fat 17g; Sodium 626mg; Carbs 2g; Fiber 0g; Sugar 0g; Protein 29g

Crispy Pork

Prep time: 40 minutes| Cook time: 20 minutes| Serves: 4

1 pound pork belly, cut into 1" chunks
¼ cup soy sauce
1 tablespoon Worcestershire sauce
2 teaspoons sriracha hot chili sauce
½ teaspoon salt
¼ teaspoon ground black pepper

1. Place pork belly into a medium sealable bowl or bag and pour in soy sauce, Worcestershire sauce, and sriracha. Seal and let marinate for 30 minutes in the refrigerator. 2. Remove pork from marinade, pat dry with a paper towel, and sprinkle with salt and pepper. 3. Place pork in an ungreased air fryer basket. Set the temperature setting to 360°F/182°C and the timer for 20 minutes, shaking the basket halfway through cooking. Pork belly will be done with an internal temperature of at least 145°F/63°C and is golden brown. 4. Let pork belly rest on a large plate for 10 minutes. Serve warm.
Per Serving: Calories 588; Fat 56g; Sodium 423mg; Carbs 0g; Fiber 0g; Sugar 0g; Protein 11g

Pork Ribs

Prep time: 10 minutes| Cook time: 30 minutes| Serves: 4

1 (4-pound) rack pork spare ribs
1 teaspoon ground cumin
2 teaspoons salt
1 teaspoon ground black pepper
1 teaspoon garlic powder
½ teaspoon dry ground mustard
½ cup low-carb barbecue sauce

1. Place ribs on an ungreased aluminum foil sheet. Sprinkle meat evenly with cumin, salt, pepper, garlic powder, and ground mustard. 2. Cut the rack into portions that will fit in your air fryer, and wrap each piece in aluminum foil, working in batches if needed. 3. Place ribs into an ungreased air fryer basket. 4. Set the temperature setting to 400°F/204°C and the timer for 25 minutes. 5. When the timer beeps, carefully remove ribs from the foil and brush them with barbecue sauce. Return ribs back to the air fryer and cook at 400°F/204°C for an additional 5 minutes to brown. Serve warm.
Per Serving: Calories 192; Fat 12g; Sodium 1374mg; Carbs 3g; Fiber 0g; Sugar 0g; Protein 13g

Silky Pork Chops

Prep time: 5 minutes| Cook time: 12 minutes| Serves: 4

4 (4-ounce) boneless pork chops
½ teaspoon salt

¼ teaspoon ground black pepper
2 tablespoons salted butter,
softened

1. Sprinkle pork chops on all sides with salt and pepper. Place chops into an ungreased air fryer basket in a single layer. 2. Set the temperature setting to 400°F/204°C and the timer for 12 minutes. When done, pork chops will be golden and have an internal temperature of at least 145°F/63°C. 3. Use tongs to remove cooked pork chops from the air fryer and place them onto a large plate. Top each chop with ½ tablespoon butter and let sit 2 minutes to melt. Serve warm.
Per Serving: Calories 278; Fat 19g; Sodium 428mg; Carbs 0g; Fiber 0g; Sugar 0g; Protein 24g

Sweet and Spicy Ribs

Prep time: 10 minutes| Cook time: 30 minutes| Serves: 6

¼ cup granular brown erythritol
2 teaspoons paprika
2 teaspoons chili powder
1 teaspoon garlic powder
½ teaspoon cayenne pepper
2 teaspoons salt
1 teaspoon ground black pepper
1 (4-pound) rack pork spare ribs

1. Mix erythritol, paprika, chili powder, garlic powder, cayenne pepper, salt, and black pepper in a small bowl. Rub spice mix over ribs on both sides. Place ribs on an ungreased aluminum foil sheet and wrap to cover. 2. Place ribs into an ungreased air fryer basket. Set the temp setting to 400°F/204°C and the timer for 25 minutes. 3. When the timer beeps, remove ribs from the foil, then place them back into the air fryer basket to cook for an additional 5 minutes, turning halfway through cooking. Ribs will be browned and have an internal temperature of at least 180°F/82°C when done. Serve warm.
Per Serving: Calories 474; Fat 32g; Sodium 898mg; Carbs 9g; Fiber 1g; Sugar 0g; Protein 35g

London Broil

Prep time: 10 minutes. | Cooking time: 12 minutes. | Serves: 4

1 pound top round steak
1 tablespoon Worcestershire sauce
¼ cup soy sauce
2 cloves garlic, peeled and finely minced
½ teaspoon ground black pepper
½ teaspoon salt
2 tablespoons salted butter, melted

1. Place steak in a suitable sealable bowl or bag. Pour in Worcestershire sauce and soy sauce, then add garlic, pepper, and salt. Toss to coat. Seal and place into refrigerator to let marinate 2 hours. 2. Remove steak from marinade and pat dry. Drizzle top side with butter, then place into ungreased air fryer basket. Set the temperature to 375°F/191°C and set the timer for almost 12 minutes, turning steak halfway through cooking. Steak will be done when browned at the edges and it has an internal temperature of 150°F/66°C for medium or 180°F/82°C for well-done. 3. Let steak rest on a suitable plate 10 minutes before slicing into thin pieces. Serve warm.
Per Serving: Calories 283; Total Fat 3.6g; Sodium 381mg; Total Carbs 5.4g; Fiber 8.1g; Sugars 3.1g; Protein 8.7g

Pork Chops in Mushroom Gravy

Prep time: 10 minutes. | Cooking time: 15 minutes. | Serves: 4

4 (5-ounce) pork chops
1 teaspoon salt
½ teaspoon pepper
2 tablespoons avocado oil
1 cup chopped button mushrooms
½ medium onion, sliced
1 clove garlic, minced
1 cup chicken broth
¼ cup heavy cream
4 tablespoons butter
¼ teaspoon xanthan gum
1 tablespoon chopped fresh parsley

1. Sprinkle pork chops with black pepper and salt. Place avocado oil and mushrooms in Instant Pot and hit the sauté button. Sauté for 3–5 minutes until mushrooms begin to soften. Add onions and pork chops. Sauté additional 3 minutes until pork chops reach a golden brown. 2. Add garlic and broth to Instant Pot. Turn the pot's lid to close. Hit the manual button and adjust time for almost 15 minutes. When the pot beeps, allow a 10-minute natural release. Quick-release the remaining pressure. 3. Remove lid and place pork chops on plate. Hit the sauté button on the Instant Pot and add heavy cream, butter, and xanthan gum. Reduce for almost 5–10 minutes or until sauce begins to thicken. 4. Add pork chops back into pot. Serve warm topped with mushroom sauce and parsley.
Per Serving: Calories 609; Total Fat 19.5g; Sodium 132mg; Total Carbs 9g; Fiber 6g; Sugars 13.3g; Protein 57.5g

Delicious Pork Meatballs

1 pound ground pork
1 large egg, whisked
½ teaspoon garlic powder
½ teaspoon salt
½ teaspoon ground ginger

¼ teaspoon crushed red pepper flakes
1 medium scallion, trimmed and sliced

1. Combine all ingredients in a large bowl. Spoon out 2 tablespoons of mixture and roll into a ball. Repeat to form eighteen meatballs total. 2. Place meatballs into an ungreased air fryer basket. Set the temperature setting to 400°F/204°C and the timer for 12 minutes, shaking the basket three times throughout the cooking. 3. When done, meatballs will be browned and have an internal temperature of at least 145°F/63°C when done. Serve warm.
Per Serving: Calories 164; Fat 10g; Sodium 252mg; Carbs 1g; Fiber 0g; Sugar 0g; Protein 15g

Spiced Pork Loin

1 teaspoon paprika
½ teaspoon ground cumin
½ teaspoon chili powder
½ teaspoon garlic powder

2 tablespoons coconut oil
1 (1½-pound) boneless pork loin
½ teaspoon salt
¼ teaspoon ground black pepper

1. Combine paprika, ground cumin, chili powder, and garlic powder in a small bowl. Drizzle coconut oil over pork. Spice pork loin with salt and pepper, then rub the spice mixture evenly on all sides. 2. Place pork loin into an ungreased air fryer basket. Set the temperature setting to 400°F/204°C and the timer for 20 minutes, turning the pork halfway through cooking. When done, pork loin will be browned and have an internal temperature of at least 145°F/63°C when done. Serve warm.
Per Serving: Calories 249; Fat 16g; Sodium 278mg; Carbs 1g; Fiber 0g; Sugar 0g; Protein 24g

Cabbage Egg Roll

1 pound 84% lean ground pork
2 tablespoons soy sauce
½ teaspoon salt
½ cup diced onion

1 clove garlic, minced
2 stalks green onion, sliced
8 cabbage leaves
1 cup water

1. Hit the sauté button on the Instant Pot and add ground pork, soy sauce, and salt to Instant Pot. Brown pork until no pink remains. Carefully drain grease. 2. Add diced onion and continue cooking until translucent, 2–4 minutes. Add garlic and cook for additional 30 seconds. Hit the cancel button. 3. Pour mixture into suitable bowl; keep it aside. Mix green onions into pork. Rinse pot and replace. Add water and steam rack. 4. Take 2–3 tablespoons of pork mixture and spoon it into cabbage leaf in rectangle shape, off to one side of the leaf. Fold the short ends of the leaf toward the middle. Complete the roll by starting at the filled edge and rolling toward the empty side, as you would get a burrito. 5. Place rolls onto steam rack. Turn the pot's lid to close. Hit the manual button and adjust time for almost 1 minute. When the pot beeps, quick-release the steam. Serve warm.
Per Serving: Calories 570; Total Fat 29.3g; Sodium 845mg; Total Carbs 5.8g; Fiber 1.6g; Sugars 2.7g; Protein 68.6g

Italian-Spiced Pork Tenderloin

1 teaspoon dried oregano
1 onion, peeled and diced
1 slice gluten-free bread (use ½ cup of almond flour for a paleo version)
1 garlic clove, peeled and minced
1 large egg white, beaten

½ pound pork tenderloin, trimmed of excess fat
Essentials
Salt and ground black pepper, to taste
Cooking spray (use coconut oil for a paleo version)

1. At 400°F/204°C, preheat your oven. Spray a broiler pan with cooking oil spray. 2. Mix the oregano, onion, garlic, and bread in a food processor and process until finely ground. You should have about ⅓ cup breadcrumbs. 3. Transfer the breadcrumbs to a plate. 4. Season the pork with salt and black pepper. 5. Dip the meat into the beaten egg white, and then roll in the bread crumb mixture until coated evenly. 6. Place the pork on the broiler pan and roast for almost 20 minutes. Remove from your oven and let rest for almost 5 minutes. 7.

Cut the pork into ¼-inch thick slices and serve.
Per Serving: Calories 494; Total Fat 27.1g; Sodium 106mg; Total Carbs 23.4g; Fiber 7.5g; Sugars 10.5g; Protein 42.7g

Nut-stuffed pork chops

3 ounces goat cheese
½ cup chopped walnuts
¼ cup toasted chopped almonds
1 teaspoon chopped fresh thyme
4 center-cut pork chops,

butterflied
Sea salt
Black pepper
2 tablespoons olive oil

1. At 400°F/204°C, preheat your oven. 2. In a suitable bowl, make the filling by stirring the goat cheese, walnuts, almonds, and thyme until well mixed. 3. Rub the pork chops inside and outside with black pepper and salt. 4. Stuff each pork chop, pushing the filling to the bottom of the cut section. Secure the stuffing with toothpicks through the meat. 5. Place a suitable skillet over medium-high heat and add the olive oil. 6. Pan-sear the pork chops until they're browned per side, for almost 10 minutes in total. 7. Transfer the prepared pork chops to a baking dish and roast the chops in your oven until cooked through. for almost 20 minutes. 8. Serve after removing the toothpicks.
Per Serving: Calories 414; Total Fat 20.8g; Sodium 156mg; Total Carbs 4.5g; Fiber 0.4g; Sugars 1.6g; Protein 49.8g

Lamb Dogs with Tzatziki

For the tzatziki
½ medium cucumber, peeled and grated on the large holes of a box grater
1 cup full-fat plain Greek yogurt
1 tablespoon olive oil, extra-virgin
1 tablespoon chopped fresh dill (or ½ teaspoon dried dill weed)
1 teaspoon freshly squeezed lemon juice
1 garlic clove, minced (or ½ teaspoon garlic powder)
½ teaspoon sea salt

¼ teaspoon black pepper
For the lamb dogs
Oil or cooking spray, for greasing
2 pounds ground lamb
2 eggs
2 tablespoons Italian seasoning
2 tablespoons olive oil
2 scallions, finely chopped
¼ cup chopped fresh mint
2 teaspoons lemon-pepper seasoning
1 teaspoon garlic powder
1 teaspoon sea salt
½ teaspoon black pepper

1. Wrap the cucumber shreds in a clean dishtowel and squeeze out as much liquid as possible. 2. In a suitable bowl, beat the cucumber, yogurt, oil, lemon juice, dill, garlic, salt, and pepper. Cover and keep it in the refrigerator while you prepare the lamb dogs. 3. At 350°F/177°C, preheat your oven. 3. Layer a suitable baking sheet with foil sheet and a baking rack. 4. Grease or spray the rack with oil to prevent the lamb from sticking. 5. In a suitable bowl, mix the ground meat, eggs, Italian seasoning, oil, scallions, mint (if using), lemon-pepper seasoning, garlic powder, salt, and pepper. 6. Divide the meat mixture into 10 equal portions. 7. Form the prepared mixture into one large, flat rectangle. 8. Score it with your hand down the middle lengthwise and then score it 4 more times in the opposite direction so that you end up with 10 squares. 9. Form each portion into a log (or hot dog shape) and place on the prepared baking rack. 10. Bake for almost 20 to 25 minutes until browned and cooked through. 11. Serve the lamb dogs topped with the sauce.
Per Serving: Calories 397; Total Fat 19.1g; Sodium 431mg; Total Carbs 6.8g; Fiber 5.3g; Sugars 6.4g; Protein 39.4g

Cheese-Stuffed Tenderloin

½ pound pork tenderloin
2 tablespoons grated pecorino cheese
2 tablespoons crumbled feta cheese
1 green onion, chopped

1 tablespoon cashews, finely crushed
½ teaspoon onion, diced
Essentials
Salt and ground black pepper, to taste

1. Preheat grill. 2. Using a sharp knife, cut a pocket, running lengthwise, into the pork tenderloin. 3. Place the green onion, onions, crushed cashews, pecorino cheese, and feta cheese in a suitable bowl and mix well to combine. 4. Spoon the prepared mixture into the pocket and secure the pocket with a skewer or wrap in butcher's twine. 5. Sprinkle the pork with salt and freshly ground pepper and grill until golden brown and juices run clear.
Per Serving: Calories 347; Total Fat 17.7g; Sodium 1655mg; Total Carbs 6.8g; Fiber 1.2g; Sugars 2.8g; Protein 33.3g

Herbed Lamb Chops

Prep time: 10 minutes| Cook time: 25 minutes| Serves: 2

4 lamb chops
2 teaspoons fresh rosemary
1 tablespoon extra-virgin olive oil
1 tablespoon butter (use extra olive oil for a paleo version),

optional
Fresh garlic, to taste
Salt and ground black pepper, to taste

1. Add the butter along with olive oil to a pan and place over medium-high heat. Place the lamb chops in the hot pan, cook for 2-3 minutes, and flip. 2. Sprinkle the top side with ¾ of the fresh rosemary, cook for 7-8 minutes, and flip to sear the other side. 3. Once the chops are golden brown, reduce the heat to low and cook for another 4-5 minutes until they are cooked through. 4. Place the chops on a serving plate, garnish with the remaining rosemary and serve.
Per Serving: Calories 198; Fat 15g; Sodium 865mg; Carbs 0g; Fiber 0g; Sugar 0g; Protein 16g

Cheesy Bacon Stuffed Pork Chops

Prep time: 10 minutes| Cook time: 12 minutes| Serves: 4

½ ounce plain pork rinds, finely crushed
½ cup shredded sharp cheddar cheese
4 slices of cooked sugar-free

bacon, crumbled
4 (4-ounce) boneless pork chops
½ teaspoon salt
¼ teaspoon ground black pepper

1. In a small bowl, mix pork rinds, cheddar, and bacon. 2. Make a 3" slit in the side of each pork chop and stuff with ¼ pork rind mixture. Sprinkle pork chops with salt and pepper. Place pork chops into an ungreased air fryer basket, stuffed side up. Set the temperature setting to 400°F/204°C and the timer for 12 minutes. When done, pork chops will be browned and have an internal temperature of at least 145°F/63°C. Serve warm.
Per Serving: Calories 348; Fat 22g; Sodium 694mg; Carbs 0g; Fiber 0g; Sugar 0g; Protein 33g

Lamb Kebabs with Mint Pesto

Prep time: 15 minutes plus 1 hour to marinate| Cook time: 15 minutes| Serves: 4

1½ cups fresh mint leaves
¼ cup shelled pistachios
2 cloves garlic, chopped
Zest and juice of 1 orange
¼ cup sesame oil
1 teaspoon salt

¼ teaspoon freshly ground black pepper
¼ cup extra-virgin olive oil
½ cup apple cider vinegar
1 pound leg of lamb, boneless, cut into 1-inch cubes

1. In a food processor, combine the mint, pistachios, and garlic in a bowl and process until very finely chopped. Add the orange zest and juice, sesame oil, salt, and pepper, and pulse until smooth. With the processor running, stream in the olive oil until soft. 2. Place ¼ cup of the mint pesto in a small bowl, add the vinegar, and whisk to form a marinade. Place the lamb cubes in the marinade and toss to coat. Cover and refrigerate for at least 1 hour, up to 24 hours. 3. While the lamb is marinating, soak four wooden skewers in water for 30 to 60 minutes—Preheat the oven to 450°F/232°C. 4. Thread the lamb cubes onto the soaked skewers, dividing evenly among the four. Place the skewers on a broiler pan or rimmed baking sheet lined with foil. 5. Cook until browned and cooked through, for 12 to 15 minutes, flipping halfway through cooking time. 6. Serve the skewers drizzled with the remaining mint pesto.
Per Serving: Calories 592; Fat 52g; Sodium 1745mg; Carbs 5g; Fiber 1g; Sugar 1g; Protein 22g

Keto Crusted Lamb Chops

Prep time: 10 minutes| Cook time: 75 minutes| Serves: 2

2 lamb chops, 1-inch thick
2 teaspoons Dijon mustard
½ cup ground almonds
10 asparagus spears, trimmed

4 cherry tomatoes
Salt and ground black pepper to taste

1. Preheat the oven to 350°F/177°C. 2. Spice the lamb chops with salt and pepper. Coat the chops with mustard and sprinkle with ground almonds until covered. Reserve a bit of the almond for the vegetables. 3. Arrange the lamb chops in a roasting pan and roast for about 50-60 minutes until they acquire a golden crust. 4. Coat the asparagus and cherry tomatoes with oil, and then sprinkle the remaining ground almonds over the vegetables—roast next to the chops for about 15 minutes. Serve hot.
Per Serving: Calories 219; Fat 14g; Sodium 1714mg; Carbs 6g; Fiber 4g; Sugar 2g; Protein 15g

Shepherd's Pie with Cauliflower Mash

Prep time: 10 minutes. | Cooking time: 30 minutes. | Serves: 8

6 cups fresh or frozen cauliflower florets or rice
2 pounds ground beef or lamb
1 tablespoon butter or ghee, plus ¼ cup, melted
½ cup chopped onion
3 garlic cloves, minced
2 tablespoons Italian seasoning
1 tablespoon tomato paste

2 cups chopped mushrooms
2 teaspoons sea salt
1 teaspoon black pepper
4 ounces cream cheese, at room temperature
1 tablespoon Italian seasoning
1 teaspoon garlic powder
½ cup grated parmesan or white cheddar cheese

1. Preheat your oven to 375°F/191°C. 2. Place the cauliflower in a microwave-safe dish and cook on high for almost 6 to 8 minutes if using frozen (10 to 15 minutes if using fresh), until tender. Transfer to a colander to drain. 3. Meanwhile, in a suitable skillet over medium heat, cook the ground meat until browned, for 5 to 7 minutes. Drain the excess liquid and transfer the meat to a bowl. 4. In the same skillet, melt 1 tablespoon of butter and add the onion. Cook for almost 3 minutes over medium-high heat. 5. Add the garlic, Italian seasoning, tomato paste, mushrooms, 1 teaspoon of salt, and ½ teaspoon of pepper and cook for another 5 to 8 minutes until the mushrooms are cooked down. 6. While the mushrooms are cooking, strain off any excess liquid from the cauliflower and add it to your high-speed blender or food processor with the remaining ¼ cup of melted butter, cream cheese, Italian seasoning, garlic powder, remaining 1 teaspoon of salt, and remaining ½ teaspoon of pepper. Blend until smooth. Taste and set the seasoning. 7. Return the meat to the skillet with the mushrooms and onions and stir well. 8. Transfer the meat mixture to a 9-by-13-inch baking dish. Spoon the cauliflower mixture over the top and smooth it into an even layer. Sprinkle with the cheese and bake for almost 20 minutes. 9. Let cool and cut into 8 squares.
Per Serving: Calories 681; Total Fat 30.7g; Sodium 1245mg; Total Carbs 4.9g; Fiber 9.9g; Sugars 5g; Protein 42.5g

Herb-Braised Pork Chops

Prep time: 10 minutes. | Cooking time: 8 hours. | Serves: 6

¼ cup olive oil
1½ pounds pork loin chops
Salt, for seasoning
Black pepper, for seasoning
1 cup chicken broth
½ sweet onion, chopped

2 teaspoons minced garlic
1 teaspoon dried thyme
1 teaspoon dried oregano
1 cup heavy (whipping) cream
1 tablespoon chopped fresh basil, for garnish

1. Lightly grease the insert of the slow cooker with 1 tablespoon of the olive oil. 2. In a suitable skillet over medium-high heat, heat the remaining 3 tablespoons of the olive oil. 3. Rub the pork with black pepper and salt. Add the pork to the skillet and brown for almost 5 minutes. Transfer the chops to the insert. 4. In a suitable bowl, stir the broth, onion, garlic, thyme, and oregano. 5. Add the broth mixture to the chops. 5. Cover and cook on low for almost 7 to 8 hours. 6. Stir in the heavy cream. 7. Serve topped with the basil.
Per Serving: Calories 404; Total Fat 19.4g; Sodium 187mg; Total Carbs 5g; Fiber 1.1g; Sugars 0.8g; Protein 52g

Pork-and-Sauerkraut Casserole

Prep time: 10 minutes. | Cooking time: 10 hours. | Serves: 6

3 tablespoons olive oil, extra-virgin
2 tablespoons butter
2 pounds pork shoulder roast
1 (28-ounce) jar sauerkraut,

drained
1 cup chicken broth
½ sweet onion, sliced
¼ cup granulated erythritol

1. Lightly grease the insert of the slow cooker with 1 tablespoon of the olive oil. 2. In a suitable skillet over medium-high heat, heat the remaining 2 tablespoons of the olive oil and the butter. 3. Add the pork to the skillet and brown on all sides for almost 10 minutes. 4. Transfer to the insert and add the sauerkraut, broth, onion, and erythritol. 5. Cover and cook on low for almost 9 to 10 hours. Serve warm.
Per Serving: Calories 636; Total Fat 25g; Sodium 259mg; Total Carbs 0.9g; Fiber 0.5g; Sugars 0g; Protein 95.6g

Herb-Crusted Lamb Chops

Prep time: 10 minutes. | Cooking time: 15 minutes. | Serves: 3

1 pound lamb chops	4 garlic cloves, minced
2 tablespoons Dijon mustard	1 teaspoon onion powder
4 fresh rosemary sprigs, chopped	¼ teaspoon salt
4 fresh thyme sprigs, chopped	¼ teaspoon black pepper
3 tablespoons almond flour	¼ cup olive oil

1. At 350°F/177°C, preheat your oven. 2. Coat the lamb chops with the mustard. Keep it aside. 3. To your high-speed blender or food processor, add the rosemary, thyme, almond flour, garlic, onion powder, salt, and pepper. Pulse until finely chopped. 4. Slowly add about 2 tablespoons of olive oil to form a thick paste. 5. Hit the herb paste firmly around the edges of the mustard-coated chops, creating a crust. In a suitable oven-safe skillet over medium heat, heat the remaining 2 tablespoons of olive oil for almost 2 minutes. 6. Add the chops to the skillet on their sides to brown. 7. Cook, undisturbed, for almost 2 to 3 minutes so the crust adheres properly to the meat. Turn and cook on the opposite edge for almost 2 to 3 minutes more. 8. Transfer the chops to a suitable baking sheet. Place the sheet in the preheated oven. 9. Cook for almost 7 to 8 minutes, for medium. Remove the sheet from your oven. Serve immediately.
Per Serving: Calories 348; Total Fat 11.1g; Sodium 139mg; Total Carbs 7.9g; Fiber 3g; Sugars 1.6g; Protein 52.8g

Dijon Pork Chops

Prep time: 10 minutes. | Cooking time: 8 hours. | Serves: 4

1 tablespoon olive oil, extra-virgin	1 teaspoon maple extract
1 cup chicken broth	4 (4-ounce) boneless pork chops
1 sweet onion, chopped	1 cup heavy (whipping) cream
¼ cup Dijon mustard	1 teaspoon chopped fresh thyme, for garnish
1 teaspoon minced garlic	

1. Lightly grease the insert of the slow cooker with the olive oil. 2. Add the broth, onion, Dijon mustard, garlic, and maple extract to the insert, and stir to combine. Add the pork chops. 3. Cover and cook on low for almost 8 hours. 4. Stir in the heavy cream. 5. Serve topped with the thyme. (Make it paleo: replace the heavy cream with coconut milk to create a lovely sauce with very little change in flavor. Dijon mustard is strong enough to mask the coconut taste, especially when it is reduced in a slow cooker.)
Per Serving: Calories 305; Total Fat 16.7g; Sodium 148mg; Total Carbs 2.5g; Fiber 1.1g; Sugars 0.1g; Protein 36.5g

Pancetta-And-Brie-Stuffed Pork Tenderloin

Prep time: 10 minutes. | Cooking time: 8 hours. | Serves: 4

1 tablespoon olive oil	4 ounces triple-cream brie
2 (½-pound) pork tenderloins	1 teaspoon minced garlic
4 ounces pancetta, cooked crispy and chopped	1 teaspoon chopped fresh basil
	⅛ teaspoon black pepper

1. Lightly grease the insert of the slow cooker with the olive oil. 2. Place the pork on a cutting board and make a lengthwise cut, holding the knife parallel to the board, through the center of the meat without cutting right through. Open the meat up like a book and cover it with plastic wrap. 3. Pound the meat with a mallet or rolling pin until each piece is about ½ inch thick. Lay the butterflied pork on a clean work surface. 4. In a suitable bowl, stir this pancetta, brie, garlic, basil, and pepper. 5. Divide the cheese mixture between the tenderloins and spread it evenly over the meat leaving about 1 inch around the edges. 6. Roll the tenderloin up and secure with toothpicks. 7. Place the pork in the insert, cover, and cook on low for almost 8 hours. Remove the toothpicks and serve.
Per Serving: Calories 315; Total Fat 15g; Sodium 91mg; Total Carbs 0g; Fiber 0g; Sugars 0g; Protein 42.3g

Tender Lamb Roast

Prep time: 10 minutes. | Cooking time: 7 to 8 hours. | Serves: 6

1 tablespoon olive oil, extra-virgin	2 teaspoons minced garlic
2 pounds lamb shoulder roast	1 teaspoon paprika
Salt, for seasoning	1 teaspoon chili powder
Black pepper, for seasoning	1 cup sour cream
1 (14.5-ounce) can diced tomatoes	2 teaspoons chopped fresh parsley, for garnish
1 tablespoon cumin	

1. Lightly grease the insert of the slow cooker with the olive oil. 2. Lightly season the lamb with black pepper and salt. 3. Place the lamb in the insert and add the tomatoes, cumin, garlic, paprika, and chili powder. 4. Cover and cook on low for almost 7 to 8 hours. 5. Stir in the sour cream. Serve topped with the parsley.
Per Serving: Calories 392; Total Fat 23.4g; Sodium 88mg; Total Carbs 1.4g; Fiber 1.9g; Sugars 3.7g; Protein 34.5g

Tangy Pulled Pork

Prep time: 5 minutes| Cook time: 30 minutes| Serves: 4

1 tablespoon chili adobo sauce	1 (2½–3 pound) cubed pork butt
1 tablespoon chili powder	1 tablespoon coconut oil
2 teaspoons salt	2 cups beef broth
1 teaspoon garlic powder	1 lime, cut into wedges
1 teaspoon cumin	¼ cup chopped cilantro
½ teaspoon pepper	

1. Mix adobo sauce, chili powder, salt, garlic powder, cumin, and pepper in a small bowl. 2. Press the Sauté button on Instant Pot and add coconut oil to the pot. Rub spice mixture onto the cubed pork butt. Place pork into pot and sear for 3–5 minutes per side. Add broth. 3. Press the Cancel button—lock Lid. Press the Manual setting of the pot and set the time to 30 minutes. When the timer beeps, let the pressure naturally release until the float valve drops and unlock the lid. 4. Shred pork with a fork. Pork should easily fall apart. For extra-crispy pork, place a single layer in a pan on the stove over medium heat. Cook pork for 10–15 minutes or until water has cooked out and meat becomes brown and crisp. Serve warm with fresh lime wedges and cilantro garnish.
Per Serving: Calories 570; Fat 35g; Sodium 1725mg; Carbs 3.2g; Fiber 1.1g; Sugar 0.4g; Protein 55g

Cranberry Pork Roast

Prep time: 10 minutes. | Cooking time: 8 hours 10 minutes. | Serves: 6

3 tablespoons olive oil, extra-virgin	ground
2 tablespoons butter	½ cup cranberries
2 pounds pork shoulder roast	½ cup chicken broth
1 teaspoon ground cinnamon	½ cup granulated erythritol
¼ teaspoon allspice	2 tablespoons Dijon mustard
¼ teaspoon salt	Juice and zest of ½ orange
⅛ teaspoon black pepper, freshly	1 scallion, white and green parts, chopped, for garnish

1. Lightly grease the insert of the slow cooker with 1 tablespoon of the olive oil. 2. In a suitable skillet over medium-high heat, heat the remaining 2 tablespoons of the olive oil and the butter. 3. Lightly season the pork with cinnamon, allspice, salt, and pepper. Add the pork to the skillet and brown on all sides for almost 10 minutes. Transfer to the insert. 4. In a suitable bowl, stir the cranberries, broth, erythritol, mustard, and orange juice and zest, and add the prepared mixture to the pork. 5. Cover and cook on low for almost 7 to 8 hours. Serve topped with the scallion.
Per Serving: Calories 367; Total Fat 22.9g; Sodium 101mg; Total Carbs 8g; Fiber 1.9g; Sugars 3g; Protein 31.8g

Carnitas

Prep time: 10 minutes. | Cooking time: 10 hours 10 minutes. | Serves: 8

3 tablespoons olive oil, extra-virgin	1 teaspoon ground coriander
2 pounds pork shoulder, cut into 2-inch cubes	1 teaspoon ground cumin
2 cups diced tomatoes	½ teaspoon salt
2 cups chicken broth	1 avocado, peeled, pitted, and diced, for garnish
½ sweet onion, chopped	1 cup sour cream, for garnish
2 fresh chipotle peppers, chopped	2 tablespoons chopped cilantro, for garnish
Juice of 1 lime	

1. Lightly grease the insert of the slow cooker with 1 tablespoon of the olive oil. 2. In a suitable skillet over medium-high heat, heat the remaining 2 tablespoons of the olive oil. 3. Add the pork meat and brown on all sides for almost 10 minutes. 4. Transfer to the insert and add the tomatoes, broth, onion, peppers, lime juice, coriander, cumin, and salt. 5. Cover and cook on low for almost 9 to 10 hours. 6. Shred the cooked pork with a fork and mix the meat into the sauce. 7. Serve topped with the avocado, sour cream, and cilantro.
Per Serving: Calories 278; Total Fat 15.4g; Sodium 321mg; Total Carbs 1.3g; Fiber 0.5g; Sugars 0.1g; Protein 32.1g

Herbed Lamb Racks

Prep time: 1 hour 10 minutes| Cook time: 25 minutes| Serves: 4

4 tablespoons extra-virgin olive oil	2 teaspoons minced garlic
2 tablespoons finely chopped fresh rosemary	Pinch sea salt
	2 (1-pound) racks French-cut lamb chops (8 bones each)

1. Whisk the olive oil, rosemary, garlic, and salt in a small bowl. Place the racks in a sealable freezer bag and pour the olive oil mixture into the bag. Massage the meat through the bag so it is coated with the marinade. Press the air out of the bag and seal it. 2. Marinate the lamb racks in the refrigerator for 1 to 2 hours. 3. Preheat the oven to 450°F/232°C. 4. Place a large ovenproof pan over medium-high heat. Take the lamb racks out of the bag and sear them in the pan on all sides, about 5 minutes. 5. Arrange the racks upright in the pan, with the bones interlaced, and roast for about 20 minutes for medium-rare. 6. Let the roasted lamb rest for 10 minutes, and then cut the racks into chops. 7. Serve 4 chops per person.
Per Serving: Calories 354; Fat 30g; Sodium 687mg; Carbs 0g; Fiber 0g; Sugar 0g; Protein 21g

Lamb Shanks with Mushrooms

Prep time: 15 minutes| Cook time: 7-8 hours| Serves: 6

3 tablespoons extra-virgin olive oil, divided	1 tablespoon minced garlic
2 pounds lamb shanks	1 (15-ounce) can crushed tomatoes
½ pound wild mushrooms, sliced	½ cup beef broth
1 leek, thoroughly cleaned and chopped	2 tablespoons apple cider vinegar
2 celery stalks, chopped	1 teaspoon dried rosemary
1 carrot, diced	½ cup sour cream, for garnish

1. Lightly grease the slow cooker with 1 tablespoon of olive oil. 2. In a large pan over medium-high heat, heat the remaining 2 tablespoons of the olive oil. Add the lamb; sear for 6 minutes, turning once; and transfer to the insert. In the pan, sauté the mushrooms, leek, celery, carrot, and garlic for 5 minutes. 3. Transfer the vegetables to the insert and the tomatoes, broth, apple cider vinegar, and rosemary. 4. Cover it and cook on low temperature setting for 7 to 8 hours. 5. Serve topped with sour cream.
Per Serving: Calories 475; Fat 36g; Sodium 666mg; Carbs 11g; Fiber 5g; Sugar 6g; Protein 31g

Spiced Curried Lamb

Prep time: 15 minutes| Cook time: 7-8 hours| Serves: 6

3 tablespoons extra-virgin olive oil, divided	½ sweet onion, sliced
1½ pounds lamb shoulder chops	¼ cup curry powder
Salt, for seasoning	1 tablespoon grated fresh ginger
Freshly ground black pepper, for seasoning	2 teaspoons minced garlic
3 cups coconut milk	1 carrot, diced
	2 tablespoons chopped cilantro for garnish

1. Lightly grease the slow cooker with 1 tablespoon of olive oil. 2. In a large pan over medium-high heat, heat the remaining 2 tablespoons of the olive oil. 3. Season the lamb with salt and pepper. Season the lamb with salt and pepper. Sear it for 6 minutes, turning once. Transfer to the insert. Stir together the coconut milk, onion, curry, ginger, and garlic in a medium bowl. 4. Add the mixture to the lamb along with the carrot. 5. Cover it and cook on low temperature setting for 7 to 8 hours. 6. Serve topped with cilantro.
Per Serving: Calories 490; Fat 41g; Sodium 500mg; Carbs 10g; Fiber 5g; Sugar 2g; Protein 26g

Rack of Lamb with Kalamata Tapenade

Prep time: 10 minutes. | Cooking time: 25 minutes. | Serves: 4

For the tapenade	lemon juice
1 cup pitted Kalamata olives	For the lamb chops
2 tablespoons chopped fresh parsley	2 (1-pound) racks French-cut lamb chops (8 bones each)
2 tablespoons olive oil, extra-virgin	Sea salt
2 teaspoons minced garlic	Black pepper
2 teaspoons freshly squeezed	1 tablespoon olive oil

1. Place the olives, parsley, olive oil, garlic, and lemon juice in a food processor and process until the prepared mixture is puréed but still slightly chunky. 2. Transfer the tapenade to a container and store sealed in the refrigerator until needed. At 450°F/232°C, preheat your oven.
Rub the lamb racks with black pepper and salt. Place a suitable ovenproof skillet over medium-high heat and add the olive oil. 3. Pan sear the lamb racks on all sides until browned. for almost 5 minutes in total. 4. Arrange the racks upright in the skillet, with the bones interlaced, and roast them in your oven until they reach your desired doneness. For almost 20 minutes for medium-rare or until the internal temperature reaches 125°F/52°C. 5. Let the lamb rest for almost 10 minutes and then cut the lamb racks into chops. 6. Top with the Kalamata tapenade.
Per Serving: Calories 841; Fat 65.7g; Sodium 1153mg; Carbs 2.9g; Fiber 1.2g; Sugar 0.1g; Protein 57g

Broiled Lamb Chops with Mint Gremolata and Pan-Fried Zucchini

Prep time: 10 minutes. | Cooking time: 20 minutes. | Serves: 4

8 (4-ounce) bone-in lamb chops	½-inch-thick coins
Salt	½ cup fresh mint leaves
Black pepper	Grated zest of 1 lemon
2 tablespoons olive oil	2 teaspoons minced garlic
4 medium zucchini, sliced into	

1. Preheat the broiler to high. Season the lamb chops on both sides with black pepper and salt and place on a suitable baking sheet. Broil for almost 4 minutes per side for rare, 5 minutes per side for medium-rare, 7 minutes per side for medium, and 9 minutes per side for well-done. Let rest for almost 5 minutes. 2. Meanwhile, in a suitable skillet, heat the oil over medium heat. 3. Add the zucchini and cook, stirring frequently, for almost 10 minutes, or to desired tenderness. 4. Finely chop the mint and place in a suitable bowl. Add the lemon zest and garlic and mix well.
Per Serving: Calories 396; Total Fat 11.4g; Sodium 448mg; Total Carbs 0.7g; Fiber 3.7g; Sugars 0.8g; Protein 40.2g

Rosemary Mint Marinated Lamb Chops

Prep time: 10 minutes. | Cooking time: 10 minutes. | Serves: 4

3 tablespoons olive oil, extra-virgin, plus more for greasing	1 tablespoon chopped mint leaves
½ teaspoon sea salt	½ teaspoon garlic salt
1 tablespoon fresh rosemary leaves (from about 4 sprigs), plus more sprigs for garnish	4 (4-ounce) lamb chops (about ½-inch thick)
	Black pepper

1. In your high-speed blender, mix the olive oil, salt, rosemary, mint, and garlic salt and blend until smooth. Rub the prepared mixture all over the lamb chops and let them marinate in an airtight container in the refrigerator for almost 30 minutes or up to 4 hours. 2. Oil a suitable skillet over medium-high heat. Add the lamb chops and cook for almost 3 minutes per side (for medium-rare), or to desired doneness. 3. Plate the chops and let them rest for almost 3 minutes. 4. Pour the leftover extra juices over the lamb chops and garnish with rosemary sprigs and pepper.
Per Serving: Calories 348; Total Fat 11.1g; Sodium 139mg; Total Carbs 7.9g; Fiber 3g; Sugars 1.6g; Protein 52.8g

Sweet-and-Sour Pork Chops

Prep time: 10 minutes. | Cooking time: 6 hours. | Serves: 4

3 tablespoons olive oil, extra-virgin	2 tablespoons coconut aminos
1 pound boneless pork chops	2 tablespoons red chili paste
½ cup granulated erythritol	2 teaspoons minced garlic
¼ cup chicken broth	¼ teaspoon salt
¼ cup tomato paste	¼ teaspoon black pepper

1. Lightly grease the insert of the slow cooker with 1 tablespoon of the olive oil. 2. In a suitable skillet over medium-high heat, heat the remaining 2 tablespoons of the olive oil. Add the pork chops, brown for almost 5 minutes, and transfer to the insert. 3. In a suitable bowl, stir the erythritol, broth, tomato paste, coconut aminos, chili paste, garlic, salt, and pepper. Add the sauce to the chops. 4. Cover and cook on low for almost 6 hours. Serve warm.
Per Serving: Calories 340; Total Fat 27.7g; Sodium 109mg; Total Carbs 2.6g; Fiber 0.3g; Sugars 3g; Protein 15.7g

Lamb Leg with Red Pesto

Prep time: 15 minutes| Cook time: 70 minutes| Serves: 8

For the pesto	2 teaspoons minced garlic
1 cup sun-dried tomatoes packed in oil	For the lamb leg
¼ cup pine nuts	1 (2-pound) lamb leg
2 tablespoons extra-virgin olive oil	Sea salt
	Freshly ground black pepper
2 tablespoons chopped fresh basil	2 tablespoons olive oil

To make the pesto: Place the sun-dried tomatoes, pine nuts, olive oil, basil, and garlic in a blender or food processor; process until smooth. Set aside until needed.
To make the lamb leg: 1. Preheat the oven to 400°F/204°C. Season the lamb leg all over with salt and pepper. 2. Place a large ovenproof pan over medium-high heat and add the olive oil. 3. Sear the lamb on all sides until nicely browned, about 6 minutes. 4. Spread the sun-dried tomato pesto all over the lamb and place the lamb on a baking sheet. 5. Roast for about 1 hour for medium. 6. Let the roasted lamb rest for 10 minutes before slicing and serving.
Per Serving: Calories 352; Fat 29g; Sodium 1024mg; Carbs 5g; Fiber 2g; Sugar 3g; Protein 17g

Lamb-Vegetable

Prep time: 10 minutes| Cook time: 6 hours| Serves: 4

¼ cup extra-virgin olive oil, divided	½ sweet onion, sliced
	½ fennel bulb, cut into 2-inch chunks
1 pound boneless lamb chops, about ½-inch thick	1 zucchini, cut into 1-inch chunks
Salt, for seasoning	¼ cup chicken broth
Freshly ground black pepper, for seasoning	2 tablespoons chopped fresh basil for garnish

1. Lightly grease the slow cooker with 1 tablespoon of olive oil. 2. Spiced the lamb with salt and pepper. 3. In a medium bowl, toss the onion along with fennel, and zucchini with the olive oil, and then place half of the vegetables in the cooker. 4. Place the lamb on the vegetables, cover with the remaining vegetables, and add the broth. 5. Cover it and cook on low temperature setting for 6 hours. Cover the pot and cook. 6. Serve topped with the basil.
Per Serving: Calories 431; Fat 37g; Sodium 972mg; Carbs 5g; Fiber 2g; Sugar 2g; Protein 21g

Tunisian Lamb Ragout

Prep time: 10 minutes. | Cooking time: 8 hours. | Serves: 6

¼ cup olive oil	2 carrots, diced
1½ pounds lamb shoulder, cut into 1-inch chunks	1 (14.5-ounce) can diced tomatoes
1 sweet onion, chopped	3 cups beef broth
1 tablespoon minced garlic	2 tablespoons Ras el Hanout
4 cups pumpkin, cut into 1-inch pieces	1 teaspoon hot chili powder
	1 teaspoon salt
	1 cup Greek yogurt

1. Lightly grease the slow cooker insert with 1 tablespoon olive oil. 2. Place a suitable skillet over medium–high heat and add the remaining oil. 3. Brown the lamb for almost 6 minutes, then add the onion and garlic. 4. Sauté for 3 minutes more, then transfer the lamb and vegetables to the insert. 5. Add the pumpkin, carrots, tomatoes, broth, Ras el Hanout, chili powder, and salt to the insert and stir to combine. 6. Cover and cook on low for almost 8 hours. Serve topped with yogurt.
Per Serving: Calories 423; Total Fat 18.4g; Sodium 137mg; Total Carbs 4.6g; Fiber 1.9g; Sugars 0.8g; Protein 56.2g

Lemon Pork

Prep time: 10 minutes. | Cooking time: 8 hours 10 minutes. | Serves: 6

3 tablespoons olive oil	¼ cup chicken broth
1 tablespoon butter	Juice and zest of 1 lemon
2 pounds pork loin roast	1 tablespoon minced garlic
½ teaspoon salt	½ cup heavy (whipping) cream
¼ teaspoon black pepper	

1. Lightly grease the insert of the slow cooker with 1 tablespoon of the olive oil. 2. In a suitable skillet over medium-high heat, heat the remaining 2 tablespoons of the olive oil and the butter. 3. Rub the pork with black pepper and salt. 4. Add the pork to the skillet and brown the roast on all sides for almost 10 minutes. Transfer it to the insert. 5. In a suitable bowl, stir the broth, lemon juice and zest, and garlic. 6. Add the broth mixture to the roast. 7. Cover, and cook on low for almost 7 to 8 hours. 8. Stir in the heavy cream and serve.
Per Serving: Calories 786; Total Fat 24.2g; Sodium 252mg; Total Carbs 1.6g; Fiber 3.9g; Sugars 22.8g; Protein 106.9g

Rosemary Lamb Chops

Prep time: 10 minutes. | Cooking time: 6 hours. | Serves: 4

3 tablespoons olive oil, extra-virgin	½ cup chicken broth
	1 sweet onion, sliced
1½ pounds lamb shoulder chops	2 teaspoons minced garlic
Salt, for seasoning	2 teaspoons dried rosemary
Black pepper, for seasoning	1 teaspoon dried thyme

1. Lightly grease the insert of the slow cooker with 1 tablespoon of the olive oil. 2. In a suitable skillet over medium-high heat, heat the remaining 2 tablespoons of the olive oil. 3. Season the lamb with black pepper and salt. Add the lamb to the skillet and brown for almost 6 minutes, turning once. 4. Transfer the lamb to the insert, and add the broth, onion, garlic, rosemary, and thyme. 5. Cover and cook on low for almost 6 hours. Serve warm.
Per Serving: Calories 443; Total Fat 16.3g; Sodium 305mg; Total Carbs 7.4g; Fiber 7.8g; Sugars 11.4g; Protein 38.5g

Chipotle Pork Chops

Prep time: 10 minutes. | Cooking time: 15 minutes. | Serves: 4

2 tablespoons coconut oil	½ medium onion, chopped
3 chipotle chilies	2 bay leaves
2 tablespoons adobo sauce	1 cup chicken broth
2 teaspoons cumin	½ (7-ounce) can fire-roasted diced tomatoes
1 teaspoon dried thyme	
1 teaspoon salt	⅓ cup chopped cilantro
4 (5-ounce) boneless pork chops	

1. Hit the sauté button on the Instant Pot and add coconut oil to preheat. While it heats, add chilies, adobo sauce, cumin, thyme, and salt to food processor. Pulse to make paste. Rub paste into pork chops. Place in Instant Pot and sear each side 5 minutes or until browned. 2. Hit the cancel button and add onion, bay leaves, broth, tomatoes, and cilantro to Instant Pot. Turn the pot's lid to close. Hit the manual button and adjust time for almost 15 minutes. When the pot beeps, allow a 10-minute natural release, then quick-release the remaining pressure. Serve warm with additional cilantro as garnish if desired.
Per Serving: Calories 419; Total Fat 15.8g; Sodium 3342mg; Total Carbs 0.4g; Fiber 0.2g; Sugars 0g; Protein 65.4g

Roasted Pork Loin with Grainy Mustard Sauce

Prep time: 10 minutes. | Cooking time: 70 minutes. | Serves: 8

1 (2-pound) boneless pork loin roast	3 tablespoons olive oil
	1½ cups heavy (whipping) cream
Sea salt	3 tablespoons grainy mustard
Black pepper	

1. At 375°F/191°C, preheat your oven. 2. Season the pork roast all over with sea black pepper and salt. 3. Place a suitable skillet over medium-high heat and add the olive oil. 4. Brown the roast on all sides in the skillet. for almost 6 minutes in total, and place the roast in a baking dish. Roast until a meat thermometer inserted in the thickest part of the roast reads 155 degrees F, for almost 1 hour. 5. When there is approximately 15 minutes of roasting time left, place a suitable saucepan over medium heat and add the heavy cream and mustard. 6. Mix the sauce until it simmers, then reduce its heat to low. Simmer the sauce until it is very rich and thick, for almost 5 minutes. Remove this pan from the heat and keep it aside. 7. Let the pork rest for almost 10 minutes before slicing and serve with the sauce.
Per Serving: Calories 506; Total Fat 23.9g; Sodium 197mg; Total Carbs 3.6g; Fiber 0.7g; Sugars 1.2g; Protein 66.1g

Chicken Burgers

Prep time: 10 minutes| Cook time: 25 minutes| Serves: 6

1 pound ground chicken	Pinch freshly ground black pepper
8 bacon slices, chopped	2 tablespoons coconut oil
¼ cup ground almonds	4 large lettuce leaves
1 teaspoon chopped fresh basil	1 avocado, peeled, pitted, and
¼ teaspoon sea salt	sliced

1. Preheat the oven to 350°F/177°C. 2. Add the chicken, bacon, ground almonds, basil, salt, and pepper in a medium bowl and combined until well mixed. Form the mixture into 6 equal patties. 3. Place a pan and add the coconut oil over medium heat. Pan sear the chicken patties until brown on both sides, about 6 minutes. 4. Place the browned patties on the baking sheet and bake until thoroughly cooked through about 15 minutes. 5. Serve on the lettuce leaves, topped with the avocado slices.
Per Serving: Calories 374; Fat 33g; Sodium 421mg; Carbs 3g; Fiber 2g; Sugar 1g; Protein 18g

Spicy Paprika Chicken

Prep time: 10 minutes| Cook time: 25 minutes| Serves: 4

4 (4-ounce) chicken breasts, skin-on	½ cup heavy (whipping) cream
Sea salt	2 teaspoons smoked paprika
Freshly ground black pepper	½ cup sour cream
1 tablespoon olive oil	2 tablespoons chopped fresh
½ cup chopped sweet onion	parsley

1. Lightly spiced the chicken with salt and pepper. Place a large pan over medium-high heat and add the olive oil. 2. Sear the chicken on both sides until almost cooked through, about 15 minutes. Remove the chicken to a plate. 3. Sauté the onion to the pan until tender, about 4 minutes. Stir in the cream and paprika and bring the liquid to a simmer. 4. Return the chicken with accumulated juices to the pan and simmer the chicken for 5 minutes until thoroughly cooked. 5. Stir in the sour cream and remove the pan from the heat. 6. Serve topped with the parsley.
Per Serving: Calories 389; Fat 30g; Sodium 475mg; Carbs 4g; Fiber 0g; Sugar 0g; Protein 25g

Chicken Breasts with Mushrooms

Prep time: 30 minutes| Cook time: 30 minutes| Serves: 4

1 tablespoon butter	2 tablespoons chopped fresh basil
¼ cup chopped sweet onion	4 (5-ounce) chicken breasts, skin-on
½ cup goat cheese, at room temperature	2 tablespoons extra-virgin olive oil
¼ cup Kalamata olives, chopped	
¼ cup chopped roasted red pepper	

1. Preheat the oven to 400°F/204°C. 2. Melt the butter. Sauté the onion in butter until tender in a small pan over medium heat. In a medium bowl transfer the onion and add the cheese, olives, red pepper, and basil. Stir until well blended, then refrigerate for about 30 minutes. 3. Cut horizontal pockets into each chicken breast, and stuff them evenly with the filling. Secure the two sides of each breast with toothpicks. 4. Place a large ovenproof pan over medium-high heat and add the olive oil. 5. Sear the chicken on both sides, about 10 minutes in total. 6. Place the pan in the oven and roast until the chicken is just cooked through, about 15 minutes. Remove the toothpicks and serve.
Per Serving: Calories 389; Fat 30g; Sodium 724mg; Carbs 3g; Fiber 0g; Sugar 0g; Protein 25g

Tropical Chicken

Prep time: 15 minutes| Cook time: 25 minutes| Serves: 4

2 tablespoons olive oil	1 tablespoon curry powder
4 (4-ounce) chicken breasts, cut into 2-inch chunks	1 teaspoon ground cumin
½ cup chopped sweet onion	1 teaspoon ground coriander
1 cup coconut milk	¼ cup chopped fresh cilantro

1. In a pan heat olive oil over medium-high heat. Sauté the chicken until almost cooked through, for about 10 minutes. 2. Add the onion and sauté for an additional 3 minutes. 3. Whisk together the coconut milk, curry powder, cumin, and coriander in a medium bowl. 4. Pour the sauce into the cooking pan with the cooked chicken and boil the liquid. Simmer on low heat until the chicken is tender and the sauce has thickened for about 10 minutes. 5. Serve the chicken with the sauce, top with cilantro.
Per Serving: Calories 382; Fat 31g; Sodium 632mg; Carbs 5g; Fiber 1g; Sugar 2g; Protein 23g

Creamy Tangy Chicken

Prep time: 10 minutes| Cook time: 7 to 8 hours| Serves: 6

3 tablespoons extra-virgin olive oil	½ teaspoon salt
2 tablespoons butter	⅛ teaspoon pepper, depending on taste
1½ pounds boneless chicken thighs	1½ cups chicken broth
½ sweet onion, diced	Juice and zest of 1 lemon
2 teaspoons minced garlic	1 tablespoon Dijon mustard
2 teaspoons dried oregano	1 cup heavy (whipping) cream

1. Lightly grease the slow cooker with 1 tablespoon of olive oil. 2. Heat the remaining 2 tablespoons of the olive oil and the butter in a large pan over medium-high heat. Sear the chicken for 5 minutes, turning once. Transfer the chicken to the insert and add the onion, garlic, oregano, salt, and pepper. 3. Whisk together the broth, lemon juice, zest, and mustard in a small bowl. Pour the mixture over the chicken. 4. Cover it and cook on low temperature setting for 7 to 8 hours. 5. Remove from the heat, stir in the heavy cream, and serve.
Per Serving: Calories 558; Fat 44g; Sodium 1416mg; Carbs 20g; Fiber 0g; Sugar 2g; Protein 22g

Crispy Bacon-Mushroom Chicken

Prep time: 15 minutes| Cook time: 7 to 8 hours| Serves: 8

3 tablespoons coconut oil, divided	1 sweet onion, diced
¼ pound bacon, diced	1 tablespoon minced garlic
2 pounds chicken (breasts, thighs, drumsticks)	½ cup chicken broth
2 cups quartered button mushrooms	2 teaspoons chopped thyme
	1 cup coconut cream

1. Lightly grease the slow cooker with 1 tablespoon of coconut oil. 2. In a large pan over medium-high heat, heat the remaining 2 tablespoons of coconut oil and cook the bacon till crispy. Transfer the bacon to a plate and set it aside. 3. Sear the chicken to the pan with the bacon fat for 5 minutes, turning once. 4. Transfer the chicken and bacon to the insert and add the mushrooms, onion, garlic, broth, and thyme. 5. Cover it and cook on low temperature setting for 7 to 8 hours. 6. Stir in the coconut cream and serve.
Per Serving: Calories 406; Fat 34g; Sodium 870mg; Carbs 5g; Fiber 2g; Sugar 1g; Protein 22g

Chicken Mole with Black Pepper

Prep time: 15 minutes| Cook time: 7 to 8 hours| Serves: 6

3 tablespoons ghee, divided	water for 2 hours and chopped
2 pounds boneless chicken thighs and breasts	3 ounces dark chocolate, chopped
Salt, for seasoning	¼ cup natural peanut butter
Freshly ground black pepper, for seasoning	1½ teaspoons ground cumin
1 sweet onion, chopped	¾ teaspoon ground cinnamon
1 tablespoon minced garlic	½ teaspoon chili powder
1 (28-ounce) can diced tomatoes	½ cup coconut cream
4 dried chili peppers, soaked in	2 tablespoons chopped cilantro, for garnish

1. Lightly grease the slow cooker with 1 tablespoon of ghee. 2. In a large pan over medium-high heat, heat the remaining 2 tablespoons of the ghee. 3. Lightly spiced the chicken with salt and pepper, add to the pan, and sear for about 5 minutes. 4. Sauté the onion and garlic for an additional 3 minutes. 5. Transfer the chicken, onion, and garlic to the slow cooker, and stir in the tomatoes, chiles, chocolate, peanut butter, cumin, cinnamon, and chili powder. 6. Cover it and cook on low temperature setting for 7 to 8 hours. 7. Stir in the coconut cream, and serve hot, topped with the cilantro.
Per Serving: Calories 501; Fat 28g; Sodium 310mg; Carbs 22.5g; Fiber 6g; Sugar 11g; Protein 41g

Braised Chicken Thighs

Prep time: 15 minutes| Cook time: 7 to 8 hours| Serves: 4

¼ cup extra-virgin olive oil, divided
1½ pounds boneless chicken thighs
1 teaspoon paprika
salt, for seasoning
freshly ground black pepper, for

seasoning
1 sweet onion, chopped
4 garlic cloves, thinly sliced
½ cup chicken broth
2 tablespoons freshly squeezed lemon juice
½ cup Greek yogurt

1. Lightly grease the slow cooker with 1 tablespoon of olive oil. 2. Season the thighs with paprika, salt, and pepper. 3. Heat the remaining olive oil. Sear the chicken for 5 minutes, turning once. Transfer the chicken to the insert and add the onion, garlic, broth, and lemon juice. 4. Cover it and cook on low temperature setting for 7 to 8 hours. 5. Stir in the yogurt and serve.
Per Serving: Calories 434; Fat 36g; Sodium 1080mg; Carbs 5g; Fiber 1g; Sugar 1g; Protein 22g

Tropical-Chicken Curry

Prep time: 15 minutes| Cook time: 7 to 8 hours | Serves: 6

3 tablespoons extra-virgin olive oil, divided
1½ pounds boneless chicken breasts
½ sweet onion, chopped
1 cup quartered baby bok choy
1 red bell pepper, diced
2 cups coconut milk
2 tablespoons almond butter

1 tablespoon red Thai curry paste
1 tablespoon coconut aminos
2 teaspoons grated fresh ginger
Pinch red pepper flakes
¼ cup chopped peanuts, for garnish
2 tablespoons chopped cilantro, for garnish

1. Lightly grease the slow cooker with 1 tablespoon of olive oil. 2. In a large pan over medium-high heat, heat the remaining 2 tablespoons of the olive oil. Add the chicken and sear for about 7 minutes. 3. Transfer the chicken to the slow cooker and add the onion, baby bok choy, and bell pepper. 4. In a bowl whisk the coconut milk, almond butter, curry paste, coconut aminos, ginger, and red pepper flakes, until well blended. 5. Pour the coconut sauce over the cooked chicken and vegetables, and mix to coat. Cover it and cook on low temperature setting for 7 to 8 hours. 5. Serve topped with peanuts and cilantro.
Per Serving: Calories 543; Fat 42g; Sodium 1001mg; Carbs 10g; Fiber 5g; Sugar 2g; Protein 35g

Regular Buffalo Chicken

Prep time: 10 minutes| Cook time: 6 hours| Serves: 4

3 tablespoons olive oil, divided
1 pound boneless chicken breasts
1 cup hot sauce
½ sweet onion, finely chopped
⅓ cup coconut oil, melted

¼ cup water
1 teaspoon minced garlic
2 tablespoons chopped fresh parsley, for garnish

1. Lightly grease the slow cooker with 1 tablespoon of olive oil. 2. In a large pan over medium-high heat, heat the remaining 2 tablespoons of the olive oil. Sear the chicken for 5 minutes, turning once. Transfer the chicken to the insert and arrange in one layer on the bottom. 3. Whisk together the hot sauce, onion, coconut oil, water, and garlic in a small bowl. Pour the mixture over the chicken. 4. Cover it and cook on low temperature setting for 6 hours. 5. Serve topped with the parsley.
Per Serving: Calories 473; Fat 39g; Sodium 535mg; Carbs 8g; Fiber 2g; Sugar 4.7g; Protein 25g

Traditional Hungarian Chicken

Prep time: 10 minutes| Cook time: 7 to 8 hours| Serves: 4

1 tablespoon extra-virgin olive oil
2 pounds boneless chicken thighs
½ cup chicken broth
Juice and zest of 1 lemon
2 teaspoons minced garlic

2 teaspoons paprika
¼ teaspoon salt
1 cup sour cream
1 tablespoon chopped parsley, for garnish

1. Lightly oil the slow cooker with olive oil. 2. Place the chicken thighs in the insert. 3. Stir together the broth, lemon juice and zest, garlic, paprika, and salt in a small bowl. Pour the broth mixture over the chicken. 4. Cover it and cook on low temperature setting for 7 to 8 hours. 5. Turn off the heat and stir in the sour cream. 6. Serve topped with the parsley.
Per Serving: Calories 404; Fat 32g; Sodium 121mg; Carbs 4g; Fiber 0g; Sugar 0g; Protein 23g

Roasted Chicken

Prep time: 15 minutes| Cook time: 7 to 8 hours| Serves: 8

¼ cup extra-virgin olive oil, divided
1 (3-pound) whole chicken, washed and patted dry
Salt, for seasoning
Freshly ground black pepper, for

seasoning
1 lemon, quartered
6 thyme sprigs
4 garlic cloves, crushed
3 bay leaves
1 sweet onion, quartered

1. Lightly grease the slow cooker with 1 tablespoon of olive oil. 2. Rub the remaining olive oil all over the chicken and season with salt and pepper. Stuff the lemon quarters, thyme, garlic, and bay leaves into the chicken cavity. 3. Spread the onion quarters on the bottom of the slow cooker and place the chicken on top so it does not touch the base of the insert. 4. Cover it and cook on low temp setting for 7 to 8 hours, or until the internal temperature reaches 165°F/74°C on an instant-read thermometer. 5. Serve warm.
Per Serving: Calories 427; Fat 34g; Sodium 689mg; Carbs 2g; Fiber 0g; Sugar 0g; Protein 29g

Delicious Turkey Meatloaf

Prep time: 10 minutes| Cook time: 35 minutes| Serves: 6

1 tablespoon olive oil
½ sweet onion, chopped
1½ pounds ground turkey
⅓ cup heavy (whipping) cream
¼ cup freshly grated Parmesan

cheese
1 tablespoon chopped fresh parsley
Pinch sea salt
Pinch freshly ground black pepper

1. Heat the oven to 450°F/232°C. 2. Heat the olive oil over medium heat. Sauté the onion until it is tender, about 4 minutes. 3. Transfer the cooked onion to a bowl and add the turkey, heavy cream, Parmesan cheese, parsley, salt, and pepper. 4. Stir until the ingredients are combined and held together. Press the mixture into a loaf pan. Bake until cooked through, about 30 minutes. 5. Rest the meatloaf for 10 minutes and serve.
Per Serving: Calories 216; Fat 19g; Sodium 774mg; Carbs 1g; Fiber 0g; Sugar 0g; Protein 19g

Cheesy Turkey Rissoles

Prep time: 10 minutes| Cook time: 25 minutes| Serves: 4

1 pound ground turkey
1 scallion, finely chopped
1 teaspoon minced garlic
Pinch sea salt

Pinch freshly ground black pepper
1 cup ground almonds
2 tablespoons olive oil

1. Preheat the oven to 350°F/177°C. Arrange a baking sheet with aluminum foil and set it aside. 2. In a medium bowl, mix the turkey, scallion, garlic, salt, and pepper until well combined. 3. Shape the turkey mixture into 8 patties and flatten them out. 4. Place the ground almonds in a shallow bowl and dredge the turkey patties in the ground almonds to coat. 5. Heat olive oil over medium heat. Sear the turkey patties on both sides, about 10 minutes in total. 6. Transfer the browned patties to the baking sheet and bake them until cooked through, flipping them once, for about 15 minutes.
Per Serving: Calories 440; Fat 34g; Sodium 965mg; Carbs 7g; Fiber 4g; Sugar 3g; Protein 27g

Delicious Jerk Chicken

Prep time: 15 minutes| Cook time: 7 to 8 hours| Serves: 6

½ cup extra-virgin olive oil, divided
2 pounds boneless chicken (breast and thighs)
1 sweet onion, quartered
4 garlic cloves
2 scallions, coarsely chopped
2 habanero chiles, stemmed and seeded

2 tablespoons granulated erythritol
1 tablespoon grated fresh ginger
2 teaspoons allspice
1 teaspoon dried thyme
½ teaspoon cardamom
½ teaspoon salt
2 tablespoons chopped cilantro, for garnish

1. Lightly grease the slow cooker with 1 tablespoon of olive oil. 2. Arrange the chicken pieces in the bottom of the insert. 3. In a blender, pulse the remaining olive oil, onion, garlic, scallions, chiles, erythritol, ginger, allspice, thyme, cardamom, and salt until a thick, uniform sauce forms. 4. Pour the sauce over the chicken, turning the pieces to coat. 5. Cover it and cook on low temperature setting for 7 to 8 hours. 6. Serve topped with cilantro.
Per Serving: Calories 457; Fat 30g; Sodium 464mg; Carbs 9g; Fiber 1g; Sugar 4g; Protein 37g

Chicken Cacciatore with Mushroom

Prep time: 15 minutes| Cook time: 8 hours| Serves: 6

3 tablespoons extra-virgin olive oil, divided	1 cup quartered button mushrooms
2 pounds boneless chicken thighs	½ sweet onion, chopped
Salt, for seasoning	1 tablespoon minced garlic
Freshly ground black pepper, for seasoning	1 tablespoon dried oregano
	1 teaspoon dried basil
1 (14-ounce) can stewed tomatoes	Pinch red pepper flakes
2 cups chicken broth	

1. Lightly grease the slow cooker with 1 tablespoon of olive oil. 2. Lightly season the chicken thighs with salt and pepper. 3. Heat remaining olive oil in a pan over medium heat and add the chicken thighs and sear for about 8 minutes, turning once. 4. Transfer the chicken to the pot and add the tomatoes, broth, mushrooms, onion, garlic, oregano, basil, and red pepper flakes. 5. Cover it and cook on low temperature setting for 8 hours. Serve warm.
Per Serving: Calories 425; Fat 32g; Sodium 128mg; Carbs 8g; Fiber 1g; Sugar 4g; Protein 27g

Turkey Ragout with Pumpkin

Prep time: 15 minutes| Cook time: 8 hours| Serves: 6

1 tablespoon extra-virgin olive oil	1½ cups chicken broth
1 pound boneless turkey thighs, cut into 1½-inch chunks	1½ cups coconut milk
3 cups cubed pumpkin, cut into 1-inch chunks	2 teaspoons chopped fresh thyme
	½ cup coconut cream
1 red bell pepper, diced	Salt, for seasoning
½ sweet onion, cut in half and sliced	Freshly ground black pepper, for seasoning
1 tablespoon minced garlic	12 slices cooked bacon, chopped, for garnish

1. Lightly oil the slow cooker with olive oil. 2. Add the turkey, pumpkin, red bell pepper, onion, garlic, broth, coconut milk, and thyme. 3. Cover it and cook on low temperature setting for 8 hours. 4. Stir in the coconut cream and season with salt and pepper. 5. Serve topped with the bacon.
Per Serving: Calories 418; Fat 34g; Sodium 665mg; Carbs 6g; Fiber 1g; Sugar 1g; Protein 25g

Herbed Turkey Legs

Prep time: 15 minutes| Cook time: 7 to 8 hours| Serves: 6

3 tablespoons extra-virgin olive oil, divided	1 tablespoon dried thyme
2 pounds boneless turkey legs	2 teaspoons poultry seasoning
Salt, for seasoning	½ cup chicken broth
Freshly ground black pepper, for seasoning	2 tablespoons chopped fresh parsley, for garnish

1. Lightly grease the slow cooker with 1 tablespoon of olive oil. 2. In a large pan over medium-high heat, heat the remaining 2 tablespoons of the olive oil. 3. Spiced the turkey with salt and pepper. Sprinkle with thyme and poultry seasoning. Add the turkey to the pan and sear for about 7 minutes, turning once. 4. Transfer the turkey to the slow cooker and add the broth. 5. Cover it and cook on low temperature setting for 7 to 8 hours. 6. Serve topped with the parsley.
Per Serving: Calories 363; Fat 29g; Sodium 1001mg; Carbs 1g; Fiber 0g; Sugar 0g; Protein 28g

Spice -Infused Turkey Breast

Prep time: 15 minutes| Cook time: 7 to 8 hours| Serves: 6

3 tablespoons extra-virgin olive oil, divided	2 teaspoons minced garlic
1½ pounds boneless turkey breasts	2 teaspoons dried thyme
	1 teaspoon dried oregano
Salt, for seasoning	1 avocado, peeled, pitted, and chopped
Freshly ground black pepper, for seasoning	1 tomato, diced
1 cup coconut milk	½ jalapeño pepper, diced
	1 tablespoon chopped cilantro

1. Lightly grease the slow cooker with 1 tablespoon of olive oil. 2. In a large pan over medium-high heat, heat the remaining 2 tablespoons of the olive oil. 3. Lightly spice the turkey with salt and pepper. Add the turkey to the pan and sear for about 7 minutes, turning once. 4. Transfer the turkey to the insert and add the coconut milk, garlic, thyme, and oregano. 5. Cover it and cook on low temperature setting for 7 to 8 hours. 6. Stir

together the avocado, tomato, jalapeño pepper, and cilantro in a small bowl. 7. Serve the turkey topped with avocado salsa.
Per Serving: Calories 347; Fat 27g; Sodium 701mg; Carbs 5g; Fiber 3g; Sugar 2g; Protein 25g

Crispy Chicken Thighs

Prep time: 10 minutes| Cook time: 50 minutes| Serves: 4

Coconut or olive oil, for greasing	⅛ teaspoon cayenne pepper
¼ teaspoon paprika	4 skin-on, bone-in chicken thighs
¼ teaspoon onion powder	1 yellow onion, quartered
¼ teaspoon garlic powder	8 garlic cloves, peeled and left whole
⅛ teaspoon dried oregano	
⅛ teaspoon dried basil	¼ cup extra-virgin olive oil
⅛ teaspoon dried thyme	1 tablespoon freshly squeezed lemon juice
⅛ teaspoon dried rosemary	
⅛ teaspoon dried parsley	

1. Preheat the oven to 350°F/177°C. Grease a cast iron pan with oil. 2. Stir the paprika, onion powder, garlic powder, oregano, basil, thyme, rosemary, parsley, and cayenne in a large bowl. Add the chicken and toss to coat. 3. Place the chicken in the prepared pan, skin-side up along with the quartered onion, and sprinkle the whole garlic in the pan, preferably to touch the bottom. 4. Drizzle the oil along with lemon juice over the chicken. Cook in the oven for 30 to 40 minutes until cooked through. 5. Baste the breasts with fluid from the bottom of the pan. Turn on the broil setting and broil it for 5-10 minutes, watching closely, until the skin has crisped up to your liking. 6. Remove from the oven, break apart the onion, and enjoy the chicken with the onions and caramelized garlic cloves alongside your favorite vegetable.
Per Serving: Calories 392; Fat 32g; Sodium 766mg; Carbs 6g; Fiber 1g; Sugar 1g; Protein 20g

Smoked Paprika Drumsticks

Prep time: 5 minutes| Cook time: 45 minutes| Serves: 6

Oil or cooking spray, for greasing	½ teaspoon freshly ground black pepper
1 tablespoon smoked paprika	
1 tablespoon garlic powder	¼ teaspoon cayenne pepper
1 tablespoon onion powder	2 tablespoons nutritional yeast
1 teaspoon baking powder	6 chicken drumsticks, patted dry
1 teaspoon sea salt	2 tablespoons butter, melted

1. Preheat the oven to 300°F/149°C. Prepare a baking sheet by lining aluminum foil. 2. Place the rack on the sheet and grease it with oil. 3. In a resealable plastic bag, add the paprika powder, garlic powder, onion powder, baking powder, salt, pepper, cayenne, and nutritional yeast and shake well until well combined. 4. Add the chicken drumsticks to the spiced mix bag and shake well until coated. 5. Place the drumsticks on rack and cook for 20-25 minutes. 6. After 25 minutes, raise the oven to 400°F/204°C temperature setting. 7. Grease the drumsticks with the melted butter and bake for an additional 20 minutes or until crispy.
Per Serving: Calories 200; Fat 12g; Sodium 985mg; Carbs 3g; Fiber 1g; Sugar 1g; Protein 20g

Roasted Chicken Thighs And Zucchini In Wine

Prep time: 10 minutes| Cook time: 30 minutes| Serves: 4

2 tablespoons coconut oil	cut into 1-inch pieces
8 bone-in, skin-on chicken thighs	1 teaspoon minced fresh thyme
Sea salt	½ cup dry red wine
Freshly ground black pepper	3 tablespoons cold butter, cut into pieces
2 zucchinis, halved lengthwise,	

1. Preheat the oven to 400°F/204°C. 2. Melt the coconut oil in the ovenproof pan over medium heat. 3. Pat dry the chicken thighs with paper towels. Season generously with salt and pepper. 4. Place the chicken skin-side down in the ovenproof pan, and cook for 5 to 7 minutes, until a crispy skin develops. Flip the chicken, and add the zucchini and thyme to the pan. 5. Transfer the pan to the oven and bake for 20 minutes, or until the chicken is cooked through. 6. Transfer the chicken and zucchini to individual serving plates. Using pot holders, return the pan to the stove top. 7. Pour the red wine into the pan and simmer over medium heat until reduced by half, about 5 minutes. 8. Remove the pan from the heat. Whisk butter in 1 tablespoon at a time. The sauce will become thick and glossy. Drizzle the sauce around the chicken and zucchini.
Per Serving: Calories 490; Fat 34g; Sodium 698mg; Carbs 5g; Fiber 1g; Sugar 1g; Protein 36g

"Roasted" Duck

Prep time: 15 minutes| Cook time: 7 to 8 hours| Serves: 8

3 tablespoons extra-virgin olive oil, divided
1 (2½-pound) whole duck, giblets removed
Salt, for seasoning
Freshly ground black pepper, for seasoning

4 garlic cloves, crushed
6 thyme sprigs, chopped
1 cinnamon stick, broken into several pieces
1 sweet onion, coarsely chopped
¼ cup chicken broth

1. Lightly grease the slow cooker with 1 tablespoon of olive oil. 2. Rub the remaining 2 tablespoons of olive oil all over the duck and season with salt and pepper—stuff the garlic, thyme, and cinnamon into the duck's cavity. 3. Spread the onion quarters on the bottom of the slow cooker and place the duck on top so it does not touch the base of the insert, and pour in the broth. 4. Cover it and cook on low temp setting for 7 to 8 hours, or until the internal temperature reaches 180°F/82°C on an instant-read thermometer. 5. Serve warm.
Per Serving: Calories 364; Fat 28g; Sodium 752mg; Carbs 2g; Fiber 1g; Sugar 0g; Protein 29g

Hot Chicken Wings

Prep time: 15 minutes| Cook time: 6 hours| Serves: 8

1 (12-ounce) bottle hot pepper sauce
¾ cup melted grass-fed butter
1 tablespoon dried oregano

2 teaspoons garlic powder
1 teaspoon onion powder
3 pounds chicken wing sections

1. In a bowl mix hot sauce, butter, oregano, garlic powder, and onion powder until blended. 2. Add the pat dry chicken wings and toss to coat well in sauce. Pour the mixture into a slow cooker. 3. Cover it and cook on low temperature setting for 6 hours. Serve.
Per Serving: Calories 375; Fat 23g; Sodium 1283mg; Carbs 1.6g; Fiber 0g; Sugar 0g; Protein 38g

Chicken Thighs with Tangy Lemon Sauce

Prep time: 15 minutes| Cook time: 20 minutes| Serves: 4

1 tablespoon butter
1 tablespoon minced shallots
1 cup sour cream
2 tablespoons freshly squeezed lemon juice

½ teaspoon salt, divided
¼ teaspoon freshly ground black pepper, divided
1 pound bone-in chicken thighs

1. Preheat the oven to 425°F/218°C. Melt the butter in a cooking pan. 2. Add the shallots—cook for 3-4 minutes, or until tender. 3. Lower the heat and add the sour cream, lemon juice, ¼ teaspoon of salt, and ⅛ teaspoon of pepper. Mix well to combine. 4. Refrigerate until ready to serve—Season the chicken with the remaining ¼ teaspoon of salt and ⅛ teaspoon of pepper. Place the chicken into a 9-inch-square baking dish. 5. Bake for about 18 minutes or it reaches 165°F/74°C. Plate the chicken, spooning an equal amount of lemon cream sauce on each thigh.
Per Serving: Calories 393; Fat 32g; Sodium 698mg; Carbs 3g; Fiber 0g; Sugar 1g; Protein 22g

Herb-Infused Chicken Thighs

Prep time: 15 minutes| Cook time: 35 minutes| Serves: 4

3 tablespoons extra-virgin olive oil, divided
4 (7-ounce) bone-in chicken thighs
½ cup green olives
Juice of 2 lemons

1 teaspoon lemon zest
1 teaspoon minced garlic
1 teaspoon chopped fresh tarragon
1 teaspoon chopped fresh thyme
1 teaspoon chopped fresh rosemary

1. Preheat the oven to 450°F/232°C. 2. In a large ovenproof pan add olive oil and sear the chicken thighs for 4 minutes per side. 3. With help of fork prick the chicken thighs. 4. In a small bowl, stir the olive oil with the green olives, garlic, lemon juice, lemon zest, tarragon, thyme, and rosemary. 5. Add the herbed olive oil mixture to the chicken, cover the pan, and place it in the oven. 6. Braise the herbed chicken until they are cooked through and tender for about 25 minutes, and serve hot.
Per Serving: Calories 435; Fat 36g; Sodium 985mg; Carbs 2g; Fiber 1g; Sugar 1g; Protein 26g

Mustardy Chicken Drumsticks

Prep time: 15 minutes| Cook time: 20 minutes| Serves: 4

1½ pounds chicken drumsticks
¼ teaspoon salt
¼ teaspoon freshly ground black pepper
2 tablespoons butter
3 tablespoons finely chopped shallots
2 fresh thyme sprigs
1 tablespoon balsamic vinegar

¼ cup dry white wine
1 teaspoon Worcestershire sauce
½ cup chicken broth
2 teaspoons tomato paste
½ cup heavy (whipping) cream
1 tablespoon Dijon mustard
2 tablespoons finely chopped fresh parsley

1. Season the drumsticks with salt and pepper. Set aside. In a large pan melt the butter, and cook the drumsticks for 6-7 minutes, until browned. 2. Transfer the cooked drumsticks to a serving dish. Keep warm. Add the shallots with thyme to the same pan and cook for 1 minutes until tender. 3. Add the vinegar, and Worcestershire sauce and white wine. Bring the wine mixture to a boil. Stir the chicken broth in the wine mix. Return the mixture to a boil. 4. Add the tomato paste. Stir to combine well with the wine mix and cook for 5-6 minutes, until the mixture reduces. 5. Add the heavy cream in the sauce and boil it. 6. Whisk the mustard in the wine sauce. Pour the delicious sauce over the drumsticks. Serve topped with the chopped parsley and enjoy.
Per Serving: Calories 420; Fat 21g; Sodium 654mg; Carbs 3g; Fiber 0g; Sugar 0g; Protein 48g

Traditional Jamaican Jerk Chicken

Prep time: 10 minutes plus 4 hours to marinate| Cook time: 60 minutes| Serves: 4

1 onion, finely chopped
½ cup finely chopped scallions
3 tablespoons soy sauce
1 tablespoon apple cider vinegar
1 tablespoon olive oil
2 teaspoons chopped fresh thyme
2 teaspoons Splenda, or another sugar substitute
1 teaspoon liquid smoke

1 teaspoon salt
1 teaspoon allspice
1 teaspoon cayenne pepper
1 teaspoon freshly ground black pepper
½ teaspoon nutmeg
½ teaspoon cinnamon
1 whole chicken, quartered

1. In a bowl, mix the onion, scallion, soy sauce, cider vinegar, olive oil, thyme, Splenda, liquid smoke, salt, allspice, cayenne pepper, black pepper, nutmeg, and cinnamon. 2. Place the chicken pieces in a baking dish, skin-side down. Pour the marinade over it. Place the marinate covered, in the refrigerator, for at least 4 hours. 3. Preheat the oven to 425°F/218°C. Cook for 30 minutes. Remove the baking dish from the oven. 4. Turn the chicken skin-side up. Return the pan to the oven—cook for 20 to 30 minutes more, or until the internal temperature reaches 165°F/74°C.
Per Serving: Calories 557; Fat 36g; Sodium 965mg; Carbs 4g; Fiber 1g; Sugar 1g; Protein 43g

Southern Crispy Baked Chicken

Prep time: 20 minutes plus 4 hours to chill| Cook time: 50 minutes| Serves: 8

½ cup sour cream
¼ cup unsweetened almond milk
2 teaspoons hot sauce
8 bone-in, skin-on chicken thighs
Avocado oil
1 cup almond flour
1 cup crushed pork rinds
⅓ cup grated Parmesan cheese

1 teaspoon paprika
1 teaspoon kosher salt
½ teaspoon garlic powder
½ teaspoon freshly ground black pepper
¼ teaspoon cayenne pepper
2 eggs, lightly beaten

1. In a gallon-size zip-top bag, combine the sour cream, almond milk, and hot sauce. Add the chicken thighs, seal the bag, and shake until the chicken is thoroughly coated. 2. Cool for 4 hours and up to 24 hours—preheat the oven to 400°F/204°C. Prepare a baking sheet with parchment paper, brush with avocado oil, and set aside. 3. Stir the almond flour, pork rinds, Parmesan cheese, paprika, salt, garlic powder, black pepper, and cayenne in a shallow dish. 4. Place the eggs in another shallow bowl. 5. Dip the chicken into the egg and dredge it in the almond flour mixture, coating all sides. Place the coated chicken, skin-side down, on the baking sheet—bake for 35 minutes. 6. Flip the chicken and bake for 15 minutes more, or until the chicken reaches 165°F/74°C on an instant-read thermometer. Serve warm
Per Serving: Calories 395; Fat 31g; Sodium 786mg; Carbs 3g; Fiber 1g; Sugar 2g; Protein 26g

Roasted Whole Chicken with Jicama

Prep time: 15 minutes| Cook time: 60 minutes| Serves: 4

1 shallot, minced
2 fresh thyme sprigs, chopped
2 fresh rosemary sprigs, chopped
2 garlic cloves, minced
2 fresh sage sprigs, chopped
2 tablespoons chopped fresh parsley

1 (5-pound) chicken
¼ cup olive oil
1 cup roughly chopped jicama
½ teaspoon salt
¼ teaspoon freshly ground black pepper

1. Preheat the oven to 425°F/218°C. Add the shallot, thyme, rosemary, and garlic to a food processor or blender—pulse to chop. 2. Add the sage and parsley. Pulse lightly until mixed. On a flat surface, place the chicken breast side up. Carefully separate the skin, creating a pocket of the meat. 3. Stuff the herb mixture in equal amount under the skin of the chicken. Place the herb stuffed chicken in a baking dish. 4. Grease the herbed chicken with olive oil. 5. Place the dish in the preheated oven—bake for 15 minutes. 6. Spread the jicama all around the chicken, and spiced with salt and pepper. Return back the pan to the oven. Lower the heat to 375°F. Cook the chicken again for 1 hour. Remove the chicken from the oven. 7. Rest for 15 minutes before serving.
Per Serving: Calories 604; Fat 49g; Sodium 632mg; Carbs 3g; Fiber 2g; Sugar 1g; Protein 39g

Crispy Fried Chicken

Prep time: 15 minutes| Cook time: 45 minutes| Serves: 8

3 cups lard, coconut oil, or avocado oil, for frying
8 chicken thighs, bone-in, skin-on (about 3 pounds)
2 teaspoons salt, divided
1½ cups whey protein isolate, unflavored
1 teaspoon garlic powder

1 teaspoon freshly ground black pepper
1 teaspoon baking powder
1 teaspoon baking soda
½ cup buttermilk
½ cup almond milk
3 large eggs

1. Preheat your oven to 325°F/163°C, and put a cooling rack on a baking sheet. Place a large pan on the stove, and fill it with the lard or oil. 2. Spice the chicken thighs with 1 teaspoon of salt. Put two shallow bowls on the counter beside the stove. 3. Combine the whey protein, garlic powder, remaining teaspoon of salt, and pepper in one bowl, and mix well. In the other bowl, combine the baking powder and baking soda, and mix. 4. Add the buttermilk, almond milk, and eggs. Whisk well with a fork. 5. Heat the oil to 350°F/177°C. Dredge one of the thighs in the whey protein mixture, then dredge the chicken thigh in the egg mixture, coat well, and then back to the whey protein mixture until fully coated. 6. Pick up the thigh and carefully lay in the hot oil. When the edges around the thigh are golden brown, use tongs to turn the thigh over and cook for 2 or 3 minutes, until golden brown. 7. Transfer the thigh onto the cooling rack on the baking sheet. One at a time, repeat coating and frying with each thigh, and then place the baking sheet in the oven for 15 to 20 minutes. Remove from the oven and serve.
Per Serving: Calories 418; Fat 24g; Sodium 874mg; Carbs 2g; Fiber 0g; Sugar 0g; Protein 49g

Chicken White Chili

Prep time: 15 minutes| Cook time: 6 to 8 hours| Serves: 12

½ cup butter
2 cups chopped onion
2 cups peeled, cubed turnips
1½ cups diced red bell pepper
½ cup diced orange or yellow bell pepper
1 (3-ounce) can diced green chiles
4 garlic cloves, minced
2 pounds ground chicken
5 cups chicken broth

2 teaspoons chili powder (or to taste)
2 teaspoons cumin
2 teaspoons oregano
1 teaspoon cayenne pepper
1 teaspoon salt
1 teaspoon freshly ground black pepper
16 ounces sour cream
2 cups shredded cheddar cheese

1. In a pot over high heat, melt butter and cook the onion for 8-10 minutes. 2. Add the red bell pepper, orange bell pepper, turnips, green chiles, and garlic. Sauté for 5-6 minutes. 2. Add the ground chicken. Stir to break up the meat, searing for 6-8 minutes. 3. Pour in the chicken broth and stir well. 4. Add the chili powder, oregano, cumin, and cayenne pepper and boil it on low. 5. Cook the chili for 6-8 hours until thickened and reduced. Season with salt and black pepper. Serve with sour cream and cheddar cheese.
Per Serving: Calories 413; Fat 28g; Sodium 666mg; Carbs 8g; Fiber 2g; Sugar 3g; Protein 31g

Regular Chicken Adobo

Prep time: 5 minutes| Cook time: 35 minutes| Serves: 4

2 tablespoons canola oil
4 bone-in, skin-on chicken leg and thighs
Sea salt
Freshly ground black pepper
6 garlic cloves, smashed

½ cup rice vinegar
⅓ cup low-sodium soy sauce
½ cup chicken broth
2 bay leaves
1 scallion, thinly sliced

1. Preheat the oven to 400°F/204°C. Heat a large ovenproof pan. Heat the oil until it shimmers. Pat dry the chicken and season generously with salt and pepper. Place the chicken into the pan and sear for 7 to 10 minutes until it gets a nice, brown crust. Flip the chicken. 2. Cook the garlic to the pan for 1 minute. Stir in the rice vinegar, soy sauce, chicken broth, and bay leaves, and bring to a simmer. 3. Transfer the cooking pan to the oven and cook for another 25 minutes until the chicken is well cooked. Garnish with scallions just before serving.
Per Serving: Calories 392; Fat 25g; Sodium 578mg; Carbs 3g; Fiber 0g; Sugar 0g; Protein 36g

Traditional Keto Chicken Quesadillas

Prep time: 10 minutes| Cook time: 10 minutes| Serves: 4

2 tablespoons butter
2 tablespoons cream cheese
2 low-carb tortillas
6 ounces grilled chicken, chopped (or canned or rotisserie)
½ cup grated cheddar cheese

½ cup grated mozzarella cheese
2 teaspoons taco seasoning
½ cup sour cream
½ avocado, peeled, pitted, and chopped

1. Melt a butter in a pan. 2. Evenly spread the cream cheese on one side of the tortillas. Place one tortilla in the pan, cream cheese–side up. Add the chicken, cheddar, and mozzarella evenly over the tortilla, and season with the taco seasoning. 3. Place the other tortilla on the chicken, cream cheese–side down, and cook for 3 to 4 minutes, or until the bottom is golden brown. 4. Carefully flip the tortilla and cook another 3 to 4 minutes until golden brown. 5. Slice the quesadilla into 8 wedges, and serve with sour cream and avocado.
Per Serving: Calories 384; Fat 27g; Sodium 774mg; Carbs 15g; Fiber 7g; Sugar 2g; Protein 21g

Potluck Chicken Squash Casserole

Prep time: 30 minutes| Cook time: 50 minutes| Serves: 8

Olive oil
1 spaghetti squash, halved lengthwise and seeded
Kosher salt
5 tablespoons butter
1 cup diced celery
½ cup diced onion
1 cup diced green bell pepper
½ cup diced poblano pepper
4 garlic cloves, minced
1 can diced tomatoes, drained

⅓ cup chicken stock
1 cup heavy (whipping) cream
5 ounces cream cheese, at room temperature
1 teaspoon ground cumin
½ teaspoon garlic powder
¼ teaspoon freshly ground black pepper
1½ cups shredded Colby cheese
4 cups shredded cooked chicken

1. Preheat the oven to 400°F/204°C. Prepare a baking sheet with parchment paper. 2. Grease a 9-by-13-inch pan with olive oil. Set aside. Poke the squash several times with a knife or fork. Microwave the whole squash for 5 to 7 minutes to soften it slightly. Drizzle the squash with oil and season lightly with salt. Place the squash, cut-side down, on the baking sheet—roast for 30 minutes. 3. While the squash roasts melt the butter in a large pan over medium-high heat. Add the celery, onion, green bell pepper, and poblano. Cook for 7 minutes until softened. 4. Add in the garlic and cook it for 1 to 2 minutes more. Stir in the tomatoes along with green chilies and chicken stock. Cook until reduced by half. 5. Add the heavy cream to the veggies and simmer for 3 to 4 minutes until reduced and thickened. 6. End the cooking and transfer the veggie mixture to a bowl. Stir in the cream cheese, cumin, garlic powder, pepper, and season with salt. Stir well combined with the cream cheese. 7. Once squash cooked, carefully flip it over. It should be tender on top but not thoroughly done all the way through. Using a fork, scrape across the spaghetti squash to create strands—lower the oven temperature to 350°F/177°C. 8. Gently mix the squash with veggie mixture. Stir in ½ cup of Colby cheese and the chicken. Transfer the mixture to the baking pan. 9. Top with the remaining 1 cup of Colby cheese. Bake for 20 minutes, or until warmed through and the cheese is melted and bubbly.
Per Serving: Calories 530; Fat 38g; Sodium 658mg; Carbs 17g; Fiber 3g; Sugar 2g; Protein 30g

Avocado Burger with Chicken

Prep time: 5 minutes| Cook time: 15 minutes| Serves: 4

1 pound ground chicken
½ cup almond flour
2 garlic cloves, minced
1 teaspoon onion powder
¼ teaspoon salt

⅛ teaspoon freshly ground black pepper
1 avocado, diced
2 tablespoons olive oil
4 low-carb buns or lettuce wraps

1. Mix the ground chicken, almond flour, garlic, onion powder, salt, and pepper in a large bowl. Add the avocado, gently incorporating it into the meat while forming four patties. Set aside. 2. Heat the oil in a pan for about 1 minute. Add the patties to the pan—cook for about 8 minutes per side, or until golden brown and cooked through. 3. Serve on a low-carb bun, in a lettuce wrap (if using), or on its own.
Per Serving: Calories 413; Fat 26g; Sodium 547mg; Carbs 8g; Fiber 5g; Sugar 2g; Protein 34g

Lettuce-Wrapped Burger

Prep time: 5 minutes| Cook time: 10 minutes| Serves: 1

1 tablespoon avocado oil
6 ounces ground chicken
1 avocado, pitted, peeled, and sliced

4 Bibb lettuce leaves
salt, to taste
black pepper, freshly ground

1. In a pan, heat the oil. Form the ground chicken into a patty and season with salt and freshly ground black pepper. 2. Add the chicken patty to the pan and cook until it is nicely browned and no longer pink in the center about 3 to 5 minutes on each side. Top the patty with the sliced avocado, and wrap it in the lettuce leaves.
Per Serving: Calories 682; Fat 54g; Sodium 698mg; Carbs 16g; Fiber 12g; Sugar 5g; Protein 33g

Spicy Kung Pao

Prep time: 20 minutes plus 10 minutes to marinate| Cook time: 10 minutes| Serves: 6

1½ pounds chicken breast, boneless, cut into bite-size pieces
6 tablespoons soy sauce
4 tablespoons sesame oil
3 teaspoons sriracha sauce
2 teaspoons granulated erythritol blend
1 teaspoon fish sauce
1 teaspoon apple cider vinegar
½ teaspoon minced fresh ginger

1 medium red pepper, chopped
1 medium zucchini, cut into ½-inch half moons
2 tablespoons olive oil
½ teaspoon xanthan gum
2 ounces (20 to 25) cashews, halved
1 tablespoon sesame seeds, for garnish
2 scallions, chopped, for garnish

1. Place the chicken in a medium bowl. Whisk the soy sauce, sesame oil, sriracha, sweetener, fish sauce, vinegar, and ginger in a small bowl. 2. Pour 2 tablespoons of the soy sauce mixture over the chicken, stir, cover, and marinate for at least 10 minutes or overnight. 3. In a pan, heat the olive oil. Cook the chicken, occasionally stirring, for 3 to 5 minutes, until cooked through. Add the red pepper and zucchini, and stir for another 2 or 3 minutes. Stir in the remainder of the sauce. Add the xanthan gum, mix well with the sauce; then add the cashews. 4. Stir for 2 to 3 minutes as the sauce thickens, and then remove from heat. Sprinkle with the sesame seeds and scallions, and serve.
Per Serving: Calories 287; Fat 15g; Sodium 753mg; Carbs 9g; Fiber 1g; Sugar 0.6g; Protein 29g

Delicious Chicken Potstickers

Prep time: 15 minutes| Cook time: 50 minutes| Serves: 6

For the pot stickers
1 large head cabbage
1 pound ground chicken
2 garlic cloves, minced
1 tablespoon soy sauce
1 teaspoon sesame oil
1 teaspoon sriracha sauce

2 tablespoons olive oil
For the sauce
¼ cup soy sauce
2 tablespoons peanut butter
1 teaspoon rice wine vinegar
1 teaspoon sesame oil
1 teaspoon sriracha sauce

1. In a pot add water to fill the pot halfway over medium heat. When the water begins boiling, place the head of cabbage in the water, core-side down, cover, and cook for 15 minutes. 2. Remove the cabbage, and when cool enough to handle, scoop or cut out the core. Carefully peel off the leaves. 3. Choose 12 of the best leaves and place on paper towels. Cut ½ inch off the cupped part (part of the leaf close to the core), and use the knife to shave across the rib/vein (without cutting

the leaf in half) so it's easier to roll. 4. Stir the chicken, garlic, soy sauce, 1 teaspoon of sesame oil, and sriracha in a medium bowl. Scoop the mixture into the cupped part of one of the leaves. Roll over once, fold in the edges, and continue rolling up. 5. Repeat with the remaining mixture and leaves. Add 2 inches of water to the large pot. Lightly grease a steamer, and set it in the pot of water. 6. When the water is hot, place the rolls in the steamer, cover, and steam over medium-low heat for 25 minutes. Place a plate lined with paper towels by the stove. 7. In a nonstick pan over medium-high heat, heat the olive oil and add 2 or 3 rolls and panfry for 2 to 3 minutes, rolling them back and forth occasionally to get a good char on each side, and then transfer to the paper towel–lined plate. 8. Repeat with the remaining rolls. Mix the soy sauce, peanut butter, vinegar, 1 teaspoon of sesame oil, and sriracha in a small bowl. Serve the sauce with the rolls.
Per Serving: Calories 229; Fat 10g; Sodium 548mg; Carbs 15g; Fiber 5g; Sugar 4g; Protein 22g

Jamaican Curry Chicken

Prep time: 10 minutes. | Cooking time: 20 minutes. | Serves: 4

1½ pounds chicken drumsticks
1 teaspoon salt
1 tablespoon Jamaican curry powder

½ medium onion, diced
½ teaspoon dried thyme
1 cup chicken broth

1. Sprinkle salt and curry powder over drumsticks. 2. Place rest of ingredients into Instant Pot.
Hit the manual button and adjust time for almost 20 minutes. 3. Turn the pot's lid to close. 4. When the pot beeps, quick-release the pressure. Serve warm.
Per Serving: Calories 412; Total Fat 23.6g; Sodium 1495mg; Total Carbs 4.8g; Fiber 1.3g; Sugars 1.7g; Protein 37.9g

Chicken Quesadillas with Cheese

Prep time: 5 minutes| Cook time: 15 minutes| Serves: 4

1 tablespoon olive oil
2 cups cooked chicken, diced or shredded
4 (8-inch) low-carb tortillas

1 cup shredded Mexican blend cheese
2 jalapeños, seeded and sliced
4 teaspoons hot sauce

1. Heat the oil on medium flame. Spoon ½ cup of chicken onto one side of a tortilla. Top with ¼ cup of cheese. Add some jalapeños and hot sauce if using. 2. Add to the pan and cook for 2 minutes, pressing down lightly. Flip and cook for 2 minutes, or until the cheese has melted warmed through. Place the cooked quesadilla on a plate and cover with aluminum foil to keep warm. Repeat with the remaining tortillas.
Per Serving: Calories 383; Fat 23g; Sodium 876mg; Carbs 19g; Fiber 15g; Sugar 4g; Protein 25g

Chicken Cutlets with Garlic Cream Sauce

Prep time: 10 minutes. | Cooking time: 25 minutes. | Serves: 4

¾ cup canned coconut milk
Juice and zest of 1 lime
1 tablespoon swerve
2 teaspoons minced garlic
1 teaspoon soy sauce
½ cup almond flour
2 large eggs, beaten

¾ cup unsweetened shredded coconut
¼ cup almond meal
4 (3-ounce) boneless, skinless chicken breasts, pounded to about ⅓-inch thick
3 tablespoons olive oil

1. Mix the coconut milk, lime juice, lime zest, swerve, garlic, and soy sauce in a suitable saucepan over medium heat. 2. Cook the sauce to a boil, then reduce its heat to low and simmer until thickened, for almost 5 minutes. 3. Remove the sauce from the heat, pour into a container, and refrigerate until chilled, for almost 2 hours. 4. At 350°F/177°C, preheat your oven. 5. Layer a suitable baking sheet with parchment paper. 6. Put the almond flour in a suitable bowl. 7. Put the beaten eggs in another suitable bowl. 8. In a third bowl, mix the coconut and almond meal.
Line up the bowls with the almond flour, eggs, then the coconut. 9. Pat the chicken pieces dry with paper towels and dredge each piece in the almond flour, then the egg mixture, and finally the coconut mixture to coat. 10. Place the coated chicken on the baking sheet. 11. Brush the cutlets carefully with the olive oil. 12. Bake the chicken until golden brown and cooked through, turning once. for almost 20 minutes in total. 13. Serve with chilled dipping sauce.
Per Serving: Calories 319; Total Fat 15.6g; Sodium 99mg; Total Carbs 4.8g; Fiber 0.7g; Sugars 2.9g; Protein 38.5g

Greek Chicken Salad

Prep time: 10 minutes. | Cooking time: 15 minutes. | Serves: 4

Marinade
2 (6-ounces) boneless, skinless chicken breasts
2 garlic cloves, minced
2 tablespoons avocado oil
Juice of 1 lemon
½ teaspoon dried oregano
½ teaspoon dried thyme
¼ teaspoon salt
¼ teaspoon pepper
1 cup chicken broth
Salad

¼ cup halved Kalamata olives
¼ cup sliced pepperoncini
½ cup cherry tomatoes, halved
1 cup chopped cucumber
½ cup crumbled feta cheese
Dressing
½ cup mayo
¼ cup white or red wine vinegar
¼ teaspoon dried oregano
¼ teaspoon garlic powder
½ teaspoon Dijon mustard

1. Mix all marinade ingredients and chicken in resealable bag or covered container. 2. Place in fridge to marinate for almost 2 hours. 3. Hit the sauté button on the Instant Pot and add chicken to Instant Pot. 4. Sear chicken for almost 3–5 minutes or until each side is browned. 5. Add broth to pot and hit the cancel button. 6. Place lid on Instant Pot and click to close. 7. Hit the manual button and set timer for almost 10 minutes. 8. When the pot beeps, allow a natural release for almost 10 minutes and quick-release the remaining pressure. 9. To prepare salad, cut chicken into 1-inch bite-sized cubes. 10. Add chicken and all salad ingredients except feta to a suitable bowl and keep it aside. 11. In suitable bowl, beat dressing ingredients and pour on top of salad, tossing to cover. Sprinkle feta on top.
Per Serving: Calories 654; Total Fat 46.8g; Sodium 845mg; Total Carbs 9.9g; Fiber 3.5g; Sugars 3.5g; Protein 56.9g

Lazy Ranch Chicken

Prep time: 10 minutes. | Cooking time: 20 minutes. | Serves: 6

1 teaspoon salt
¼ teaspoon pepper
¼ teaspoon dried oregano
½ teaspoon garlic powder
3 (6-ounces) skinless chicken

breasts
1 cup chicken broth
1 dry ranch packet
8 ounces cream cheese
1 stick butter

1. Mix seasoning in a suitable bowl and sprinkle over both sides of chicken. 2. Place chicken breasts in bottom of Instant Pot. 3. Place cream cheese brick and stick of butter on top of chicken breast. 4. Turn the pot's lid to close. Hit the manual button and adjust time for almost 20 minutes.
When the pot beeps, allow a 10-minute natural release. 5. Quick-release the remaining pressure.
Remove chicken and shred with fork. Return to Instant Pot. 6. Use rubber spatula to stir. Serve warm.
Per Serving: Calories 375; Total Fat 19.8g; Sodium 2105mg; Total Carbs 9g; Fiber 0.7g; Sugars 24.8g; Protein 24.3g

Herbed Roasted Chicken

Prep time: 15 minutes| Cook time: 1 hour 30 minutes| Serves: 6

½ cup (1 stick) butter, room temperature
2 tablespoons olive oil or avocado oil
3 garlic cloves, minced
1 tablespoon rosemary
1 tablespoon thyme
1 teaspoon garlic salt

1 teaspoon freshly ground black pepper
Juice of ½ lemon
5- to 6-pound whole chicken, room temperature, patted dry, and giblets and neck removed
Chopped parsley, for garnish

1. Preheat the oven to 425°F/218°C. 2. Prepare a roasting pan with aluminum foil. Mix the butter, oil, garlic, rosemary, thyme, garlic salt, pepper, and lemon juice in a small bowl. 3. Gently lose the chicken skin, and rub the mixture under each area as far as you can reach and all over the outer skin and bottom. 4. Tie the chicken legs together with string. Place a rack on a roasting pan and the chicken, breast-side up. Roast for 90 minutes, basting every 30 minutes using the juices in the bottom of the pan. If it starts to brown too much toward the end, lay a piece of foil loosely over the top. 5. The chicken should be 165°F/74°C in the internal. Garnish with chopped parsley, and serve.
Per Serving: Calories 549; Fat 37g; Sodium 689mg; Carbs 0g; Fiber 0g; Sugar 0g; Protein 54g

Garlic Parmesan Wings

Prep time: 10 minutes. | Cooking time: 12 minutes. | Serves: 4

2 pounds chicken wings
1 teaspoon seasoned salt

½ teaspoon pepper
½ teaspoon garlic powder
1 cup water

3 tablespoons butter
1 teaspoon lemon pepper
¼ cup grated parmesan cheese

1. Pat wings dry and sprinkle with seasoning. 2. Pour water into Instant Pot and place steam rack on bottom. 3. Place wings on steam rack and Turn the pot's lid to close. 4. Hit the manual button and adjust time for almost 10 minutes. 5. When the pot beeps, quick-release the pressure.
For crispy wings: 1. place on foil-lined baking sheet and broil for almost 3–5 minutes. 2. Pour water out of Instant Pot. Add butter to pot and hit the sauté button. 3. Add lemon pepper to melted butter. Hit the cancel button. 4. Return wings to pot and toss with tongs to completely cover with lemon pepper butter mixture. Sprinkle with parmesan. Serve warm.
Per Serving: Calories 413; Total Fat 24.5g; Sodium 962mg; Total Carbs 6.9g; Fiber 1.1g; Sugars 2.9g; Protein 39.1g

Sweet and Sour Meatballs

Prep time: 10 minutes. | Cooking time: 10 minutes. | Serves: 4

1 pound ground chicken
1 egg
1 teaspoon salt
1 teaspoon pepper
1 teaspoon garlic powder
½ medium onion, diced

1 cup water
2 teaspoons erythritol
1 teaspoon rice vinegar
2 teaspoons reduced-sugar ketchup
½ teaspoon sriracha

1. Mix chicken, egg, salt, pepper, garlic powder, and onion. Form into small balls. 2. Pour water into Instant Pot and place steam rack on bottom. 3. Place meatballs on steam rack. 4. Turn the pot's lid to close. Hit the manual button and adjust time for almost 10 minutes. 5. In suitable bowl, mix erythritol, vinegar, ketchup, and sriracha. 6. When the pot beeps, quick-release the pressure. Toss meatballs in sauce. Serve warm.
Per Serving: Calories 596; Total Fat 24.6g; Sodium 316mg; Total Carbs 6.8g; Fiber 15.6g; Sugars 9.5g; Protein 58.8g

Lemon Herb Whole Chicken

Prep time: 10 minutes. | Cooking time: 25 minutes. | Serves: 4

3 teaspoons salt
3 teaspoons garlic powder
2 teaspoons dried rosemary
2 teaspoons dried parsley
1 teaspoon pepper

1 (4–5-pound) whole chicken
2 tablespoons coconut oil
1 cup chicken broth
1 lemon, zested and quartered

1. In a suitable bowl, mix salt, garlic, rosemary, parsley, and pepper. 2. Rub herb mix over chicken. Hit the sauté button on the Instant Pot and add coconut oil to preheat. 3. Place chicken in pot to brown for almost 5–7 minutes. 4. Hit the cancel button and carefully remove chicken with tongs. 5. Add broth and scrape bottom of pot with rubber spatula or wooden spoon until no seasoning is stuck to pot. Place steam rack in pot. 6. Grate lemon zest over chicken. Place lemon quarters inside chicken. 7. Place chicken back into Instant Pot. Turn the pot's lid to close.
Hit the meat button and adjust time to 25 minutes. 8. When the pot beeps, allow a 10-minute natural release and quick-release the remaining steam. Slice or shred chicken (and skin if desired). Serve warm.
Per Serving: Calories 388; Total Fat 21.8g; Sodium 787mg; Total Carbs 5.4g; Fiber 1.5g; Sugars 1.4g; Protein 49.3g

Barbecue Wings

Prep time: 10 minutes. | Cooking time: 12 minutes. | Serves: 4

1 pound chicken wings
1 teaspoon salt
½ teaspoon pepper

¼ teaspoon garlic powder
1 cup sugar-free barbecue sauce
1 cup water

1. In bowl, toss wings in salt, pepper, garlic powder, and half of barbecue sauce. Pour water into Instant Pot. Place steam rack on bottom of pot. 2. Place wings on steam rack and turn the pot's lid to close. Hit the manual button and adjust time for almost 12 minutes. When the pot beeps, quick-release the steam. Toss in remaining sauce. 3. For crispier wings, place on foil-lined baking sheet and broil for almost 5–7 minutes.
Per Serving: Calories 618; Total Fat 13.5g; Sodium 96mg; Total Carbs 8.7g; Fiber 5.3g; Sugars 0.5g; Protein 24.4g

Easy Chicken for Meal Prep

Prep time: 10 minutes. | Cooking time: 10 minutes. | Serves: 4

1 tablespoon coconut oil	½ teaspoon dried oregano
½ teaspoon garlic powder	2 (6-ounces) boneless, skinless
½ teaspoon salt	chicken breasts
½ teaspoon dried basil	1 cup water
½ teaspoon pepper	

1. Hit the sauté button on the Instant Pot and add coconut oil to preheat. Mix seasoning in suitable bowl and sprinkle evenly over chicken. Once oil is sizzling, carefully add chicken to the Instant Pot. 2. Sear chicken for almost 4 minutes until golden per side. Remove chicken and add water to Instant Pot. Remove any seasoning stuck to the bottom of the pot using a rubber spatula. 3. Place steam rack inside Instant Pot and add chicken on top of steam rack. 4. Lock lid and hit the manual button. Set timer for almost 10 minutes. 5. When the pot beeps, allow a natural release for almost 5 minutes then quick-release the remaining pressure. 6. Shred, cube, or slice chicken for salads, soups, or easy meal prep.
Per Serving: Calories 402; Total Fat 19.9g; Sodium 1387mg; Total Carbs 4g; Fiber 8g; Sugars 12.7g; Protein 32.1g

BLT Chicken Salad

Prep time: 10 minutes. | Cooking time: 15 minutes. | Serves: 4

4 slices bacon	1 cup water
2 (6-ounce) chicken breasts	⅓ cup mayo
1 teaspoon salt	1 ounce chopped pecans
½ teaspoon garlic powder	½ avocado, diced
¼ teaspoon pepper	½ cup diced roma tomatoes
¼ teaspoon dried thyme	1 tablespoon lemon juice
¼ teaspoon dried parsley	2 cups chopped romaine lettuce

1. Hit the sauté button on the Instant Pot and hit the adjust button to set heat to less. 2. Add bacon to Instant Pot and allow the fat to render for almost 3–5 minutes. 3. Hit the cancel button. 4. Hit the sauté button on the Instant Pot and hit the adjust button to set heat to normal. 5. Finish crisping bacon; remove and keep it aside. Hit the cancel button. 6. Sprinkle seasoning over chicken. 7. Pour water into Instant Pot; use a wooden spoon to ensure nothing is stuck to the bottom. 8. Place steam rack in pot and place chicken on top. Turn the pot's lid to close. 9. Hit the manual button and adjust time for almost 10 minutes. 10. While chicken is cooking, prepare sauce. 11. In a suitable bowl, mix mayo, pecans, avocado, roma tomatoes, and lemon juice. When the pot beeps, quick-release the pressure. 12. Remove chicken and let cool for almost 10 minutes. Then cut into cubes and add to bowl. 13. Mix until chicken is fully coated. Mix in lettuce right before eating.
Per Serving: Calories 408; Total Fat 23.1g; Sodium 412mg; Total Carbs 7.7g; Fiber 7.2g; Sugars 19.2g; Protein 24.4g

Pesto Chicken

Prep time: 10 minutes. | Cooking time: 20 minutes. | Serves: 2

2 (6-ounces) boneless, skinless	1 cup water
chicken breasts, butterflied	¼ cup whole-milk ricotta
½ teaspoon salt	¼ cup pesto
¼ teaspoon pepper	¼ cup shredded whole-milk
¼ teaspoon garlic powder	mozzarella cheese
¼ teaspoon dried parsley	Chopped parsley for garnish
2 tablespoons coconut oil	

1. Sprinkle seasonings on chicken breasts. 2. Hit the sauté button on the Instant Pot and add coconut oil to preheat. 3. Sauté chicken for almost 3–5 minutes or until golden brown. 4. Remove chicken and place into 7-cup glass bowl. 5. Pour water into pot and use wooden spoon or rubber spatula to make sure no seasoning is stuck to bottom of pot. 6. Place spoonful of ricotta onto chicken pieces. Pour pesto over chicken. 7. Sprinkle mozzarella over chicken. Cover with foil. 8. Place steam rack into Instant Pot and carefully put bowl on top. 9. Turn the pot's lid to close. Hit the manual button and adjust time for almost 20 minutes. 10. When the pot beeps, allow a natural release. Serve with chopped parsley if desired.
Per Serving: Calories 343; Total Fat 20.1g; Sodium 903mg; Total Carbs 0.2g; Fiber 0.1g; Sugars 0.2g; Protein 37.1g

White Chicken Casserole

Prep time: 10 minutes. | Cooking time: 15 minutes. | Serves: 4

1 cup broccoli florets	1½ cups alfredo sauce
½ cup fresh spinach	½ teaspoon salt
¼ cup whole-milk ricotta	¼ teaspoon pepper

1 pound thin-sliced deli chicken	mozzarella cheese
1 cup shredded whole-milk	1 cup water

1. Place broccoli in a suitable bowl. 2. Add spinach, ricotta, alfredo sauce, salt, and pepper to bowl and mix. 3. Use a spoon to separate into three sections. 4. Layer chicken in bottom of 7-cup glass bowl. 5. Place one section of the veggie mix on top in an even layer and top with a layer of mozzarella. Repeat until all veggie mix has been used and finish casserole with a layer of mozzarella. 6. Cover dish with foil sheet. 7. Pour water into Instant Pot and place steam rack in bottom of pot. 8. Place foil-covered dish on steam rack. Turn the pot's lid to close. 9. Hit the manual button and adjust time for almost 15 minutes. 10. When the pot beeps, quick-release the pressure. If desired, broil in oven for almost 3–5 minutes until golden.
Per Serving: Calories 585; Total Fat 39.5g; Sodium 1687mg; Total Carbs 0.4g; Fiber 2.7g; Sugars 3.1g; Protein 43.2g

Spicy Chicken Enchilada Casserole

Prep time: 30 minutes| Cook time: 45 minutes| Serves: 8

3 cups chicken broth	1 tablespoon minced garlic
1½ pounds chicken thighs,	½ teaspoon salt
boneless	½ teaspoon freshly ground black
2 cups roasted green chiles,	pepper
chopped	¼ teaspoon cayenne pepper
1 cup sour cream	1 tablespoon olive oil
2 cups Monterey Jack cheese,	1 bunch fresh cilantro, chopped
shredded	2 low-carb tortillas, cut into
½ cup diced onion	½-inch-wide strips

1. Preheat the oven to 400°F/204°C. 2. To a pot, bring the chicken broth to a boil. Reduce the heat to a simmer. Add the chicken thighs—cook for 12 minutes. 3. Remove the chicken and set it to cool. 4. Shred the chicken into bite-size pieces. 5. Transfer to a large bowl. Add the green chiles, Monterey Jack cheese, sour cream, garlic, onion, salt, black pepper, and cayenne pepper to the shredded chicken. 6. Mix thoroughly to combine. In a pan, heat the olive oil. 7. Add the tortilla and crisp for 2-3 minutes. 8. Transfer the chicken mix to a large baking dish. Apply the cilantro to the top of the chicken mixture, then add the tortilla strips. Place the dish in the oven. 9. Cook it for 15-20 minutes, or until golden brown. Remove from the oven. Cool the casserole for 5 minutes before serving.
Per Serving: Calories 383; Fat 23g; Sodium 855mg; Carbs 19g; Fiber 15g; Sugar 4g; Protein 25g

Loaded Buffalo Wings

Prep time: 10 minutes. | Cooking time: 12 minutes. | Serves: 4

2 pounds chicken wings	¼ cup buffalo sauce
1 teaspoon seasoned salt	⅓ cup blue cheese crumbles
½ teaspoon garlic powder	2 stalks green onion, sliced
¼ teaspoon pepper	¼ cup cooked bacon crumbles
¾ cup chicken broth	

1. Pat wings dry and sprinkle with salt, garlic, and pepper. 2. Pour broth and buffalo sauce into Instant Pot and place wings in bottom. 3. Turn the pot's lid to close. Hit the manual button and adjust time for almost 12 minutes. 4. When the pot beeps, quick-release the pressure. Gently stir to coat wings with sauce. 5. For crispier wings: place on foil-lined baking sheet and broil for almost 3–5 minutes until skin is crispy. Brush with leftover sauce and top with blue cheese, green onions, and bacon.
Per Serving: Calories 326; Total Fat 12g; Sodium 779mg; Total Carbs 8.3g; Fiber 2.9g; Sugars 1.3g; Protein 46.9g

Italian Chicken Thighs

Prep time: 10 minutes. | Cooking time: 15 minutes. | Serves: 4

4 bone-in chicken thighs	¼ teaspoon dried basil
2 cloves garlic, minced	¼ teaspoon dried parsley
1 teaspoon salt	½ teaspoon dried oregano
¼ teaspoon pepper	1 cup water

1. Place chicken thighs in suitable bowl. Sprinkle with remaining ingredients except water and toss to evenly coat. 2. Pour water into Instant Pot and place steam rack in bottom. Place chicken thighs on steam rack and turn the pot's lid to close. 3. Hit the manual button and adjust time for almost 15 minutes. When the pot beeps, quick-release the pressure. For crispy skin: broil chicken in oven for almost 3–5 minutes or until golden.
Per Serving: Calories 232; Total Fat 8.4g; Sodium 300mg; Total Carbs 8.6g; Fiber 0.9g; Sugars 0.1g; Protein 30.1g

Balsamic Caprese-Stuffed Chicken Breasts

Prep time: 10 minutes. | Cooking time: 40 minutes. | Serves: 4

½ cup olive oil, extra-virgin
2 boneless, skinless chicken breasts (about 6 ounces each)
4 ounces frozen spinach, thawed and drained well
1 cup shredded fresh mozzarella cheese
¼ cup chopped fresh basil
2 tablespoons chopped sun-dried tomatoes (preferably marinated in oil)
1 teaspoon salt
1 teaspoon black pepper, freshly ground
½ teaspoon garlic powder
1 tablespoon balsamic vinegar

1. At 375°F/191°C, preheat your oven. 2. Drizzle 1 tablespoon olive oil in a suitable deep baking dish and swirl to coat the bottom. 3. Make a deep incision about 3 to 4 inches long along the length of each chicken breast to create a pocket. 4. Using your knife or fingers, carefully increase the size of the pocket without cutting through the chicken breast. 5. In a suitable bowl, mix the spinach, mozzarella, basil, sun-dried tomatoes, 2 tablespoons olive oil, ½ teaspoon salt, ½ teaspoon pepper, and the garlic powder and mix well with a fork. 6. Stuff half of the filling mixture into the pocket of each chicken breast. 7. Hit the opening and secure with toothpicks. 8. In a suitable skillet, heat 2 tablespoons of olive oil over medium-high heat. 9. Carefully sear the chicken breasts until browned, 3 to 4 minutes per side. 10. Transfer to the prepared baking dish, incision-side up. 11. Scrape up any filling that fell out in the skillet and add it to the baking dish. 12. Cover this pan with foil and bake until the chicken is cooked through, 30 to 40 minutes, depending on the thickness of the breasts. 13. Remove from your oven and rest, covered, for almost 10 minutes. 14. Meanwhile, in a suitable bowl, whisk the remaining 3 tablespoons olive oil, balsamic vinegar, ½ teaspoon salt, and ½ teaspoon pepper. 15. To serve, remove the toothpicks cut each chicken breast in half, widthwise, and serve a half chicken breast drizzled with oil and vinegar.
Per serving: Calories: 238; Total fat 10.6g; Sodium 149mg; Total carbs 0.6g; Fiber 0.4g; Sugars 0.2g; Protein 33g

Bacon Chicken Alfredo

Prep time: 10 minutes. | Cooking time: 20 minutes. | Serves: 4

2 (6-ounce) boneless, skinless chicken breasts, butterflied
¼ teaspoon salt
⅛ teaspoon pepper
½ teaspoon garlic powder
¼ teaspoon dried thyme
¼ teaspoon dried parsley
2 tablespoons coconut oil
1 cup water
1 stick butter
¼ cup heavy cream
2 cloves garlic, finely minced
½ cup grated parmesan cheese
¼ cup cooked crumbled bacon

1. Sprinkle seasoning on chicken breasts. 2. Hit the sauté button on the Instant Pot and add coconut oil to preheat. 3. Sear chicken 3–5 minutes until golden brown on both sides. Hit the cancel button. 4. Remove chicken carefully using tongs, and keep it aside. 5. Pour water into Instant Pot and place steam rack in bottom. 6. Place chicken on steam rack and turn the pot's lid to close. 7. Hit the manual button and adjust time for almost 20 minutes. 8. When the pot beeps, quick-release the pressure. Remove chicken and keep it aside on clean dish. 9. Pour water out of Instant Pot, reserving ½ cup; keep it aside. 10. Hit the sauté button on the Instant Pot and add butter to pot. 11. When butter is melted add heavy cream, garlic, parmesan, and reserved water. 12. Reduce for almost 4 minutes until it begins to thicken, stirring frequently. 13. Hit the cancel button and add in cooked bacon. Pour over chicken to serve.
Per Serving: Calories 347; Total Fat 15.7g; Sodium 999mg; Total Carbs 1.8g; Fiber 1.1g; Sugars 7g; Protein 39.6g

Chicken Enchilada Bowl

Prep time: 10 minutes. | Cooking time: 25 minutes. | Serves: 4

2 (6-ounce) boneless, skinless chicken breasts
½ teaspoon salt
½ teaspoon garlic powder
¼ teaspoon pepper
2 teaspoons chili powder
2 tablespoons coconut oil
¾ cup red enchilada sauce
¼ cup store-bought chicken broth
¼ cup diced onion
1 (4-ounce) can green chilies
2 cups cooked cauliflower rice
1 avocado, diced
½ cup sour cream
1 cup shredded cheddar cheese

1. Sprinkle chicken with salt, garlic powder, pepper, and chili powder. 2. Hit the sauté button on the Instant Pot and add coconut oil to preheat. 3. Sear each side of chicken breast. Hit the cancel button. 4. Pour enchilada sauce and broth over chicken. 5. Add onion and chilies to pot. Turn the pot's lid to close. Hit the manual button and adjust time for almost 25 minutes. 6. When the pot beeps, quick-release the

pressure and shred chicken. 7. Serve chicken with cauliflower rice, diced avocado, sour cream, and cheddar.
Per Serving: Calories 372; Total Fat 16.3g; Sodium 742mg; Total Carbs 6.8g; Fiber 0.8g; Sugars 1.8g; Protein 42.3g

Basic Taco Shredded Chicken with Fried Cheese Shells

Prep time: 10 minutes. | Cooking time: 20 minutes. | Serves: 6

Chicken
1 cup chicken broth
4 (6-ounce) boneless, skinless chicken breasts
1 teaspoon salt
¼ teaspoon pepper
1 tablespoon chili powder
2 teaspoons cumin
2 teaspoons garlic powder
Fried cheese shells
1½ cups shredded whole-milk mozzarella cheese

1. Place all chicken ingredients into Instant Pot. Turn the pot's lid to close. 2. Hit the manual button and adjust time for almost 20 minutes. 3. When the pot beeps, quick-release the pressure. Shred chicken and serve in bowls or in cheese shells. 4. To make cheese shells, preheat nonstick skillet over medium on stovetop. 5. Sprinkle ¼ cup of cheese in pan and let fry until golden. Flip and turn off heat. 6. Allow cheese to get brown. Fill with chicken and fold. It will harden as it cools. 7. Repeat with remaining cheese and filling. Serve warm.
Per Serving: Calories 236; Total Fat 10.4g; Sodium 713mg; Total Carbs 9.8g; Fiber 0.5g; Sugars 0.1g; Protein 25.7g

Chicken Vegetable Hash

Prep time: 10 minutes. | Cooking time: 40 minutes. | Serves: 4

¼ cup coconut oil
14 ounces boneless, skinless chicken thighs, diced
1 onion, chopped
1 red bell pepper, diced
2 teaspoons minced garlic
1 cup diced raw or frozen
pumpkin
½ cup shredded cabbage
1 teaspoon chopped fresh thyme
Sea salt
Black pepper
1 cup pumpkin seeds
½ cup shredded kale

1. Heat the oil in a suitable skillet over medium-high heat. 2. Sauté the chicken until it is cooked through, for almost 15 minutes. 3. Transfer the prepared chicken to a plate using a slotted spoon. 4. Add the bell pepper, onion, and garlic and sauté until softened, for almost 5 minutes. 5. Stir in the pumpkin, cabbage, and thyme and sauté until the vegetables are tender. for almost 15 minutes. 6. Return the chicken back in the skillet and season with black pepper and salt. 7. Add the pumpkin seeds and kale and sauté until the greens are wilted, for almost 5 minutes.
Per Serving: Calories 344; Total Fat 10g; Sodium 251mg; Total Carbs 4.7g; Fiber 0.5g; Sugars 2.2g; Protein 55.7g

Loaded Chicken And Cauliflower Nachos

Prep time: 10 minutes. | Cooking time: 25 to 30 minutes. | Serves: 4

¼ cup olive oil
1 tablespoon onion powder
1 teaspoon paprika
1 teaspoon ground cumin
1 large head cauliflower (about 1 pound)
Salt
Black pepper
1 cup cooked chicken, diced or shredded
¾ cup shredded Mexican blend cheese
¼ cup low-carb salsa

1. At 375°F/191°C, preheat your oven. 2. Layer a suitable baking sheet with aluminum sheet. 3. In a suitable bowl, mix the oil, onion powder, paprika, and cumin. Keep it aside. 4. Cut the cauliflower into quarters and remove any leaves and thick stem. 5. Cut the quarters crosswise into even ½-inch-thick slices. 6. Add the cauliflower to the bowl with the spice mixture and turn to coat. 7. Transfer the cauliflower to the prepared baking sheet and spread in a single layer. 8. Season with black pepper and salt. Roast for almost 20 minutes, then remove from your oven. 9. Top with the chicken and cheese and return to your oven for almost 5 to 10 minutes, until the cheese has melted. Remove from your oven, top with the salsa, and serve.
Per Serving: Calories 349; Total Fat 15.1g; Sodium 157mg; Total Carbs 5.6g; Fiber 2.6g; Sugars 22.5g; Protein 29.7g

Chicken Bacon Ranch Casserole

Prep time: 10 minutes. | Cooking time: 20 minutes. | Serves: 4

4 slices bacon
4 (6-ounces) boneless, skinless chicken breasts
½ teaspoon salt
¼ teaspoon pepper

1 tablespoon coconut oil
½ cup ranch dressing
½ cup chicken broth
2 ounces cream cheese
½ cup shredded cheddar cheese

1. Hit the sauté button on the Instant Pot and cook bacon until crispy; remove, and place on paper towel. 2. While bacon is cooking, cut chicken into 1-inch bite-sized cubes, sprinkle with black pepper and salt, and keep it aside. 3. When bacon is finished cooking, add coconut oil and chicken breasts to Instant Pot. 4. Sauté chicken in coconut oil and bacon grease until golden brown. Hit the cancel button. 5. Add ranch and broth. Turn the pot's lid to close; hit the manual button and set time for almost 20 minutes. 6. When the pot beeps, quick-release the pressure and stir in cream cheese and cheddar. 7. Crumble cooked bacon and sprinkle on top. Serve warm.
Per Serving: Calories 427; Total Fat 18.1g; Sodium 676mg; Total Carbs 3.7g; Fiber 7.5g; Sugars 1.7g; Protein 51.2g

Chicken Tenders

Prep time: 10 minutes. | Cooking time: 30 minutes. | Serves: 4

2 cups crushed pork rinds
¼ cup grated parmesan cheese
1 teaspoon garlic powder
1 teaspoon black pepper
1 large egg

½ cup heavy (whipping) cream
1 pound boneless chicken tenderloins (10 to 12 tenderloins), patted dry

1. At 425°F/218°C, preheat your oven. 2. Layer a suitable baking sheet with parchment paper and keep it aside. 3. In a shallow bowl, mix the pork rinds, parmesan cheese, garlic powder, and pepper. 4. In another shallow bowl, whisk the egg and heavy cream. 5. Dip a tenderloin entirely in the egg mixture, then lay the tenderloin in the pork rind mixture, turning to coat both sides. 6. Lay the coated tenderloin on the prepared baking sheet and repeat with the remaining tenderloins. 7. Bake for almost 25 to 30 minutes.
Per Serving: Calories 309; Total Fat 17.4g; Sodium 348mg; Total Carbs 4.8g; Fiber 1.9g; Sugars 0.6g; Protein 33.4g

Barbecue Shredded Chicken

Prep time: 10 minutes. | Cooking time: 25 minutes. | Serves: 4

1 (5-pound) whole chicken
3 teaspoons salt
1 teaspoon pepper
1 teaspoon garlic powder
1 teaspoon dried parsley

½ medium onion, cut into 4 large pieces
1 cup water
½ cup low-carb barbecue sauce

1. Sprinkle chicken with salt, pepper, garlic, and parsley. 2. Place onion pieces inside chicken cavity. 3. Pour water into Instant Pot and place steam rack in bottom. 4. Carefully place seasoned chicken on steam rack. 5. Brush with half of barbecue sauce. Turn the pot's lid to close. 6. Hit the manual button and adjust time for almost 25 minutes. 7. When the pot beeps, using a clean brush, add remaining sauce to chicken. 8. For crispy skin or thicker sauce: broil in oven for almost 5 minutes or until slightly brown.
Per Serving: Calories 314; Total Fat 8.7g; Sodium 337mg; Total Carbs 1.2g; Fiber 4.1g; Sugars 16g; Protein 37.9g

Shredded Chicken

Prep time: 10 minutes. | Cooking time: 8 minutes. | Serves: 6

1 cup chicken broth
¼ cup tomato sauce
1 teaspoon salt

4 large boneless, skinless chicken breasts (about 6 ounces each)

1. Pour the broth, tomato sauce, and salt into an electric pressure cooker and stir to mix. 2. Add the chicken breasts and cover in the sauce. 3. Lock the pressure cooker lid in place with the steam vent set to sealing. 4. Select high pressure and set the timer for almost 8 minutes. 5. After cooking, allow a 10-minute natural pressure release. 6. Open the pressure release valve and let out any remaining steam. 7. Carefully open the pressure cooker and use two forks to shred the chicken into the broth. 8. Let sit for almost 5 minutes, then use a slotted spoon to remove the chicken.
Per Serving: Calories 271; Total Fat 19.2g; Sodium 124mg; Total Carbs 7.2g; Fiber 2.9g; Sugars 0.5g; Protein 18.6g

Roast Chicken with Cilantro Mayonnaise

Prep time: 10 minutes. | Cooking time: 1 hour 30 minutes. | Serves: 6

1 (3-pound) whole roasting chicken
Sea salt, for seasoning
1 onion, cut into 8 wedges
¼ cup olive oil

Black pepper
½ mayonnaise
1 tablespoon chopped fresh cilantro

1. At 350°F/177°C, preheat your oven. 2. Wash the chicken in cold water, inside and out, and pat it completely dry with paper towels. Set the chicken in a baking dish and lightly salt the cavity. 3. Place the onion in the cavity. Brush the chicken skin all over with olive oil and season the skin with the black pepper and salt. Roast the chicken until it is golden brown and cooked through (to an internal temperature of 185°F/85°C.), for almost 90 minutes. Remove the chicken from your oven and let it sit for almost 15 minutes. 4. In a suitable bowl, mix the mayonnaise and cilantro. Carve the chicken and serve with the mayonnaise.
Per Serving: Calories 309; Total Fat 5.1g; Sodium 245mg; Total Carbs 3g; Fiber 9.6g; Sugars 14.2g; Protein 25.8g

Chicken Paprikash

Prep time: 10 minutes. | Cooking time: 30 minutes. | Serves: 4

¼ cup olive oil
¾ pound boneless chicken breasts, cut into ½-inch strips
1 medium onion, sliced
1 red bell pepper, diced
1 tablespoon minced garlic
½ cup low-sodium chicken stock
½ cup canned coconut milk

¼ cup no-salt-added tomato paste
3 tablespoons smoked paprika
½ cup sour cream
Sea salt
Black pepper, freshly ground
2 tablespoons chopped fresh parsley

1. Preheat 2 tablespoons of olive oil in a suitable skillet over medium-high heat. 2. Brown the chicken until cooked through. for almost 10 minutes, and transfer to a plate using a slotted spoon. 3. Add the remaining olive oil and sauté the onion, bell pepper, and garlic until softened, for almost 4 minutes. 4. Stir in the reserved cooked chicken, chicken stock, coconut milk, tomato paste, and paprika. 5. Cover the skillet and simmer, stirring occasionally, until the chicken and vegetables are very tender. for almost 15 minutes. 6. Stir in the sour cream and simmer an additional 1 minute. 7. Season with black pepper and salt and serve topped with parsley.
Per Serving: Calories 481; Total Fat 14.6g; Sodium 285mg; Total Carbs 7.5g; Fiber 7.3g; Sugars 1g; Protein 31.1g

Chicken Milanese

Prep time: 10 minutes. | Cooking time: 40 minutes. | Serves: 4

2 tablespoons butter
½ scallion, chopped, green part only
¼ cup dry white wine
½ cup chicken stock
½ cup heavy (whipping) cream
1 teaspoon thyme
1 teaspoon freshly squeezed lemon juice

2 (8-ounce) boneless chicken breasts, halved lengthwise
¾ cup almond flour
¼ cup parmesan cheese
1 large egg
1 tablespoon water
¼ cup olive oil
¼ cup chopped fresh parsley

1. In a suitable saucepan over medium-high heat, melt the butter. 2. Sauté the scallion until it is bright green, for almost 2 minutes. 3. Add the wine, chicken stock, and cream. 4. Cook the sauce to a boil, then reduce its heat to low, and simmer until the sauce reduces to about 1 cup, for almost 20 minutes. 5. Remove the sauce from the heat, and stir in the thyme and lemon juice. 6. Use a mallet to pound the chicken pieces out thin without ripping through. 7. Pat the pieces dry with paper towels. In a suitable bowl, mix the almond flour and parmesan cheese. 8. In another suitable bowl, mix the egg and water. 9. Dip the prepared chicken pieces in the egg mixture, and then dredge them in the almond-cheese mixture to coat. 10. In a suitable skillet over medium heat, heat the olive oil. 11. In a suitable skillet, cook the breaded chicken pieces until the bottom is golden brown. for almost 3 minutes. 12. Flip the cutlets, and cook until the chicken is cooked through and the second side is golden brown. for almost 4 minutes. 13. Top the cutlets with the parsley, and serve with the sauce.
Per serving: Calories: 389; Total fat 12.7g; Sodium 685mg; Total Carbs 0.9g; Fiber 3.5g; Sugars 6.5g; Protein 47.2g

Paprika Chicken with Broccoli

Prep time: 10 minutes. | Cooking time: 40 minutes. | Serves: 6

6 boneless, skinless chicken breasts (6 ounces each)	2 teaspoons onion powder
6 tablespoons mayonnaise	Salt
2 tablespoons paprika	Black pepper
	1 pound broccoli florets

1. At 375°F/191°C, preheat your oven. 2. Layer a suitable baking sheet with foil sheet. 3. Meanwhile, in a suitable resealable bag or a bowl, mix the chicken, mayonnaise, paprika, and onion powder and massage the spices into the meat. 4. Let marinate in the refrigerator for almost 30 minutes. 5. Transfer the chicken to the prepared baking sheet and season with black pepper and salt. 6. Discard the remaining marinade. Cook for almost 40 minutes. 7. While the chicken cooks, bring a suitable saucepan of water to a boil. Add the broccoli. 8. Cook for almost 6 to 8 minutes, until tender. 9. Drain, season with black pepper and salt to taste, and serve with the chicken.
Per Serving: Calories 322; Total Fat 15.9g; Sodium 104mg; Total Carbs 5.1g; Fiber 0.9g; Sugars 2.9g; Protein 38.4g

Chicken Parmesan

Prep time: 10 minutes. | Cooking time: 35 minutes. | Serves: 6

3 large boneless chicken breasts, halved	⅛ teaspoon black pepper
¾ cup grated parmesan cheese	1 large egg
½ cup almond flour	¼ cup olive oil
1 teaspoon Italian seasoning	6 tablespoons sugar-free pasta sauce
½ teaspoon garlic powder	1 cup shredded mozzarella cheese
¼ teaspoon salt	

1. At 350°F/177°C, preheat your oven. 2. Keep the chicken between two pieces of plastic wrap.
Pound the chicken and flatten until all pieces are about ½ inch thick. 3. In a suitable bowl, mix the almond flour, ½ cup of parmesan cheese, Italian seasoning, garlic powder, salt, and pepper.
In another bowl, beat the egg. 4. Dip each piece of chicken into the egg wash, then thoroughly coat in the "breading." Keep it aside. In a suitable skillet over medium-high heat, heat the olive oil for almost 2 minutes. 5. Add the "breaded" chicken. Cook for almost 5 to 7 minutes per side.
Remove from the skillet and place on a parchment-lined baking sheet. 6. Top with 1 tablespoon of pasta sauce. 7. And divide a cup of mozzarella cheese among the chicken. 8. Sprinkle each with the rest of the parmesan cheese. 9. Place the baking sheet in your oven. 10. Bake for almost 20 minutes, until the cheese is thoroughly melted.
Per Serving: Calories 384; Total Fat 23.6g; Sodium 80mg; Total Carbs 0.7g; Fiber 8.3g; Sugars 3.5g; Protein 24.6g

Coconut Chicken

Prep time: 10 minutes. | Cooking time: 25 minutes. | Serves: 4

2 tablespoons olive oil	1 tablespoon curry powder
4 (4-ounce) boneless chicken breasts, cut into 2-inch chunks	1 teaspoon ground cumin
½ cup chopped sweet onion	1 teaspoon ground coriander
1 cup coconut milk	¼ cup chopped fresh cilantro

1. Place a suitable saucepan over medium-high heat and add the olive oil. 2. Sauté the chicken until almost cooked through. for almost 10 minutes. 3. Add the onion and sauté for an additional 3 minutes. 4. In a suitable bowl, whisk the coconut milk, curry powder, cumin, and coriander. 5. Pour the sauce into the saucepan with the chicken and bring the liquid to a boil. 6. Reduce its heat and simmer until the chicken is tender and the sauce has thickened, for almost 10 minutes. 7. Serve the chicken with the sauce, topped with cilantro.
Per Serving: Calories 314; Total Fat 8.7g; Sodium 337mg; Total Carbs 1.2g; Fiber 4.1g; Sugars 16g; Protein 37.9g

Breaded Chicken Strip Lettuce Wraps

Prep time: 10 minutes. | Cooking time: 5 minutes. | Serves: 1

1 large egg	2 boneless chicken thighs, cut into thin strips
1 teaspoon Italian seasoning	2 bibb lettuce leaves
1 tablespoon avocado oil	

1. In a suitable bowl, whisk the egg and Italian seasoning. 2. Season with a little salt and black pepper. In a suitable skillet, heat the oil over medium heat. 3. Coat the chicken strips in the egg mixture. 4. Add the chicken strips to the skillet and cook for almost 5 minutes, turning

occasionally, until fully cooked. Wrap the chicken in the lettuce leaves.
Per Serving: Calories 422; Total Fat 7.3g; Sodium 1093mg; Total Carbs 6.9g; Fiber 5.9g; Sugars 2.4g; Protein 58.5g

Chopped Chicken-Avocado Lettuce Wraps

Prep time: 10 minutes. | Cooking time: 0 minutes. | Serves: 4

½ avocado, peeled and pitted	breast, chopped
⅓ cup mayonnaise	Sea salt
1 teaspoon freshly squeezed lemon juice	Black pepper
2 teaspoons chopped fresh thyme	8 large lettuce leaves
1 (6-ounces) cooked chicken	¼ cup chopped walnuts

1. In a suitable bowl, mash the avocado with the mayonnaise, lemon juice, and thyme until well combined. 2. Stir in the chopped chicken and season the filling with black pepper and salt. 3. Spoon the chicken salad into the lettuce leaves and top with the walnuts. 4. Serve 2 lettuce wraps per person.
Per Serving: Calories 393; Total Fat 11.7g; Sodium 591mg; Total Carbs 6.4g; Fiber 4.3g; Sugars 6.6g; Protein 56.4g

BBQ Chicken Wraps

Prep time: 10 minutes. | Cooking time: 0 minutes. | Serves: 4

2 cups cooked chicken, diced or shredded	8 (8-inch) low-carb tortillas
½ cup low-carb barbecue sauce	1 cup chopped or shredded iceberg lettuce

1. In a suitable bowl, mix the chicken and barbecue sauce. 2. Divide the prepared mixture among the tortillas, then add the lettuce. 3. Roll up the tortillas and place them on a serving plate, seam-side down.
Per Serving: Calories 428; Total Fat 29g; Sodium 546mg; Total Carbs 0.8g; Fiber 3.1g; Sugars 0.2g; Protein 30.6g

Bacon-Wrapped Jalapeño Chicken

Prep time: 10 minutes. | Cooking time: 20 minutes. | Serves: 4

4 (4-ounce) boneless chicken breasts	2 garlic cloves, minced
¾ cup cream cheese, at room temperature	8 bacon slices
4 jalapeño peppers, halved	¼ teaspoon salt
1 teaspoon onion powder	⅛ teaspoon black pepper
	2 tablespoons olive oil

1. At 400°F/204°C, preheat your oven. 2. On a flat surface, cut each chicken breast in half horizontally. 3. Do not cut all the way through the other side. Open the breasts flat. 4. Spread an equal amount of cream cheese over each of the butterflied breasts. 5. Top each with two jalapeño halves. Sprinkle with onion powder and garlic. 6. Fold the breasts closed. Wrap each breast with two bacon slices. Secure with toothpicks. 7. Season the outside of the breasts with the black pepper and salt. 8. Place the bacon-wrapped chicken in a baking pan. Drizzle with the olive oil. 9. Bake the chicken for almost 20 minutes, or until the internal temperature is 165°F/74°C. Remove this pan from your oven. Allow the chicken to rest for almost 2 to 3 minutes. 10. Remove the toothpicks from the meat and serve.
Per Serving: Calories 539; Total Fat 35.2g; Sodium 3880mg; Total Carbs 4g; Fiber 5.4g; Sugars 5.9g; Protein 48g

Crispy Chicken Paillard

Prep time: 10 minutes. | Cooking time: 10 minutes. | Serves: 4

½ cup grated parmesan cheese	ground
¼ cup almond flour	4 (6-ounces) boneless chicken breasts
1 teaspoon garlic powder	2 tablespoons canola oil
½ teaspoon sea salt	
½ teaspoon black pepper, freshly	

1. Mix the parmesan cheese, almond flour, garlic powder, salt, and pepper in a shallow dish. 2. Place the chicken breasts one at a time between two sheets of parchment paper. 3. Pound with the flat side of a meat mallet until the chicken is about ½-inch thick. 4. Heat the canola oil in a suitable skillet over medium-high heat. 5. Lightly coat the chicken pieces in the parmesan and flour mixture, and sear for almost 5 minutes per side.
Per Serving: Calories 342; Total Fat 13.7g; Sodium 678mg; Total Carbs 2.3g; Fiber 4.5g; Sugars 22.1g; Protein 26.7g

Chicken Breast Tenders with Riesling Cream Sauce

Prep time: 10 minutes. | Cooking time: 30 minutes. | Serves: 4

4 (about 6-ounces) boneless, skinless chicken breasts
½ cup almond flour
2 tablespoons coconut flour
1 teaspoon garlic powder
Sea salt
Black pepper, freshly ground

2 tablespoons canola oil
½ cup Riesling or sauvignon Blanc
½ cup chicken bone broth
½ cup heavy (whipping) cream
4 cups mixed greens

1. At 250°F/121°C, preheat your oven. Slice the chicken into 4-by-2-inch pieces. 2. In a shallow dish, mix the almond flour, coconut flour, garlic powder, salt, and pepper. 3. Dredge the chicken pieces in the flour mixture. 4. Heat the canola oil in a suitable skillet over medium-high heat. 5. Sear the chicken pieces for almost 2 to 3 minutes per side until well browned. 6. Transfer to a baking dish and place in your oven to keep warm. 7. Add the Riesling to the skillet and cook until reduced to about ¼ cup, for almost 3 minutes. 8. Add the broth and heavy cream, and cook over medium-low heat to thicken the sauce for almost 5 minutes. 9. Place the chicken onto serving plates and garnish with the mixed greens. 10. Serve the Riesling cream sauce on the side.
Per Serving: Calories 385; Total Fat 13.2g; Sodium 929mg; Total Carbs 1.6g; Fiber 4.2g; Sugars 2.6g; Protein 36.4g

Almond Chicken Fingers

Prep time: 10 minutes. | Cooking time: 20 minutes. | Serves: 4

Nonstick cooking spray
1 cup almond meal
1 teaspoon garlic powder
½ teaspoon ground cumin
½ teaspoon paprika
¼ teaspoon cayenne pepper
2 large eggs

1½ tablespoon olive oil, to brush on the fingers before basting
1 pound boneless, skinless chicken tenders
Fresh spinach leaves, for serving
Sugar-free ketchup, barbecue sauce

1. At 425°F/218°C, preheat your oven. 2. Line a suitable baking sheet with foil sheet and coat with nonstick spray. 3. In a shallow bowl, mix the almond meal, garlic powder, cumin, paprika, and cayenne. 4. Beat the eggs into another shallow bowl. 5. Working one at a time, dip the chicken tenders into the egg mixture, letting the excess drip off. 6. Dredge in the almond meal mixture to fully coat, then place on the prepared baking sheet. 7. Bake the chicken tenders for almost 20 minutes, checking them periodically and flipping about halfway through. Serve on a bed of spinach.
Per Serving: Calories 307; Total Fat 15.5g; Sodium 720mg; Total Carbs 6.6g; Fiber 1g; Sugars 2.8g; Protein 36.6g

Chicken Kebabs with Spicy Almond Sauce

Prep time: 10 minutes. | Cooking time: 12 minutes. | Serves: 4

½ cup almond butter
1 tablespoon soy sauce
1 tablespoon finely chopped fresh cilantro
1 teaspoon swerve
1 teaspoon minced garlic
Juice of 1 lime

Pinch red pepper flakes
Juice of 1 lime
¼ cup olive oil
2 tablespoons soy sauce
1 tablespoon minced garlic
¾ pound boneless, skinless chicken breast, cut into strips

1. Whisk the almond butter, soy sauce, cilantro, swerve, garlic, lime juice, and red pepper flakes in a suitable bowl until well combined. 2. Keep it aside, covered, in the refrigerator. In a suitable bowl, mix the lime juice, olive oil, soy sauce, garlic, and chicken until well mixed. 3. Marinate at least 1 hour and up to 24 hours, covered, in the refrigerator. 4. Preheat your oven to broil. Remove the chicken strips from the marinade and thread them onto wooden skewers that have been soaked in water. 5. Arrange the kebabs on a suitable baking sheet and broil, turning once, until the meat is cooked through but still juicy, 10 to 12 minutes total. Serve with almond butter sauce.
Per Serving: Calories 353; Total Fat 18.5g; Sodium 682mg; Total Carbs 2.3g; Fiber 0.8g; Sugars 1g; Protein 45.8g

Chicken Pot Pie

Prep time: 10 minutes. | Cooking time: 1 hour 5 minutes. | Serves: 6

3 tablespoons olive oil
1½ pounds boneless, skinless

chicken thighs, cut into 1-inch pieces

¼ cup diced white onion
⅓ cup diced zucchini
⅓ cup diced celery
1 garlic clove, minced
1 teaspoon sea salt
½ teaspoon dried thyme
½ teaspoon dried parsley

1 cup low-sodium chicken broth
¼ cup heavy (whipping) cream
¼ teaspoon cream of tartar
Cooking spray
Formed into 2 balls, chilled
1 large egg, beaten

1. In a suitable skillet over medium heat, warm the olive oil until shimmering. 2. Add the chicken and cook until browned. for almost 3 minutes per side. 3. Drop the heat to medium and add the onion, zucchini, and celery. 4. Cook, stirring frequently, until the onions and celery are soft and the zucchini is beginning to brown. for almost 7 minutes. 5. Stir in the garlic, salt, thyme, and parsley. Cook for almost 1 more minute. 6. Pour in the broth and scrape the bottom of this pan to release any brown bits. 7. Cook to a boil and then reduce its heat to low and simmer for almost 20 minutes or until the liquid reduces and the prepared mixture thickens. 8. Slowly pour in the cream and sprinkle in the cream of tartar, whisking constantly. 9. Simmer for another 5 to 10 minutes, until thickened. 10. At 350°F/177°C, preheat your oven. 11. Spray a 9-inch pie pan with cooking spray. 12. Remove the prepared dough from the refrigerator. 13. Place 1 dough ball at a time between 2 pieces of parchment paper and roll out to ⅛-inch-thick circles. 14. Lay 1 dough circle in the bottom of the pie dish. 15. Pour the pie filling into the dish and then top with the remaining dough circle. 16. Crimp the edges of the prepared dough and use a fork to poke holes all over the top of the prepared dough. 17. Brush the prepared dough with the egg (if using), for a darker pie crust. 18. Bake until the prepared dough is just golden on top, 20 to 25 minutes. 19. Let cool for almost 5 minutes. Serve immediately.
Per Serving: Calories 223; Total Fat 10.6g; Sodium 646mg; Total Carbs 4.1g; Fiber 2.4g; Sugars 1.6g; Protein 29.5g

Chicken and Dumplings

Prep time: 10 minutes. | Cooking time: 15 minutes. | Serves: 4

1 tablespoon avocado oil
⅓ cup diced white onion
¼ cup chopped carrots
½ cup chopped celery
2 garlic cloves, minced

1½ cups shredded cooked chicken breast
1 teaspoon dried thyme
4 cups low-sodium chicken broth

1. Heat the oil in a suitable saucepan over medium heat. 2. Add the onion, carrots, and celery. 3. Cook, stirring frequently, until the onion is translucent, for 5 to 6 minutes. 3. Stir in the minced garlic and cook for 2 minutes. Stir in the chicken and thyme. 4. Pour in the broth and cook to a boil. Reduce its heat to low and simmer while you make the dumplings. 5. Roll the prepared dough into a square ¼ inch thick. 6. Slice the prepared dough into long pieces and then tear into 1-inch chunks. 7. Drop the dumpling pieces into the simmering soup and stir to incorporate. 8. Cook, stirring frequently so the dumplings don't bind, for another 3 to 5 minutes or until the dumplings are cooked through. Serve immediately.
Per Serving: Calories 282; Total Fat 15.4g; Sodium 646mg; Total Carbs 6.4g; Fiber 7g; Sugars 6.5g; Protein 22.5g

Chicken Enchiladas

Prep time: 10 minutes. | Cooking time: 20 minutes. | Serves: 4

4 cups cooked chicken, diced or shredded
½ cup low-carb salsa
1 cup tomato sauce
1 teaspoon paprika

1 teaspoon onion powder
1 teaspoon dried oregano
4 (8-inch) low-carb tortillas
½ cup shredded Mexican blend cheese

1. At 350°F/177°C, preheat your oven. 2. In a resealable bag, mix the chicken and salsa. 3. Massage the bag to blend, seal, and refrigerate for almost 30 minutes to marinate. 4. In a bowl, mix the tomato sauce, paprika, onion powder, and oregano. 5. Spread half the prepared mixture on the bottom of a 9-by-13-inch baking dish. 6. Place the tortillas on a suitable cutting board. Divide the chicken mixture evenly among them. Roll each tortilla up and place them in the dish, seam-side down. 7. Cover the enchiladas with the remaining tomato sauce mixture, then sprinkle the cheese on top. Cook uncovered for almost 15 to 20 minutes, until the meat is fully warmed through and the cheese has melted.
Per Serving: Calories 476; Total Fat 37.7g; Sodium 742mg; Total Carbs 5.3g; Fiber 6g; Sugars 5g; Protein 24.8g

Chicken Fajitas

Prep time: 10 minutes. | Cooking time: 20 minutes. | Serves: 4

1 pound boneless, skinless chicken breasts and/or thighs, sliced into thin strips
1 teaspoon salt
1 teaspoon dried oregano
1 teaspoon garlic powder
½ teaspoon black pepper, freshly ground
1 teaspoon ground cumin
½ teaspoon red pepper flakes
½ teaspoon paprika
¼ teaspoon ground cinnamon
2 tablespoons avocado oil or

butter
½ white onion, sliced
½ red bell pepper, sliced into strips
½ green bell pepper, sliced into strips
2 tablespoons chicken broth
2 to 4 coconut or almond flour wraps, or grain-free chips
1 cup shredded romaine lettuce
Sugar-free salsa, guacamole, sour cream, and shredded cheese, for serving

1. In a suitable bowl, mix the chicken with the salt, oregano, garlic powder, pepper, cumin, red pepper flakes, paprika, cinnamon, and 1 tablespoon of oil. 2. Heat the remaining tablespoon of oil in a suitable skillet over medium-high heat. 3. Sauté the onion for almost 3 to 5 minutes, until translucent. 4. Add the bell peppers and sauté for almost 5 minutes, until tender. 5. Add the chicken mixture and sauté for almost 2 to 3 minutes, then reduce its heat to medium, cover, and cook for almost 5 minutes, or until the chicken is cooked through. 6. Let the chicken mixture cool a bit. 7. Divide the wraps or chips among plates, sprinkle the shredded romaine on top, and spoon the chicken fajita mixture on top of the lettuce. 8. Serve the fajitas with salsa, guacamole, sour cream, and cheese, if desired.
Per Serving: Calories 260, Fat 20.2g, Sodium 408mg, Carbs 4.9g, Fiber 1.6g, Sugars 1.3g, Protein 15.3g

Caprese Balsamic Chicken

Prep time: 10 minutes. | Cooking time: 25 minutes. | Serves: 4

3 tablespoons balsamic vinegar
1 tablespoon butter
2 (6-ounces) boneless, skinless chicken breasts, halved lengthwise
Sea salt

Black pepper
1 tablespoon olive oil
¼ cup herb pesto
1 tomato, cut into 4 slices
1 cup shredded mozzarella cheese

1. At 400°F/204°C, preheat your oven. 2. In a suitable saucepan over medium heat, bring the balsamic vinegar and butter to a boil; then reduce its heat to low and simmer until thickened. For almost 5 minutes. Keep it aside. 3. Season the chicken breasts with black pepper and salt.
In a suitable skillet over medium heat, heat the olive oil. 4. Cook the chicken, turning once, until just cooked through, for almost 10 minutes total. 5. Place the cooked chicken in a 9-by-13-baking dish. 6. Spread 1 tablespoon of pesto over each piece of chicken, top each with tomato slices, and evenly divide the cheese between the pieces. 7. Bake in your oven until the cheese is melted and golden. For almost 5 minutes. 8. Serve with a drizzle of the reduced balsamic vinegar.
Per serving: Calories: 441; Total fat 33.9g; Sodium 759mg; Total Carbs 4.9g; Fiber 2.2g; Sugars 3.6g; Protein 21.4g

Bacon Ranch Cheesy Chicken Breasts

Prep time: 10 minutes. | Cooking time: 55 minutes. | Serves: 4

Cooking spray for the baking dish
3 tablespoons olive oil
4 boneless chicken breasts
½ teaspoon salt
¼ teaspoon black pepper, freshly ground
1 tablespoon garlic powder
8 bacon slices sliced into ½-inch pieces

¼ cup butter
¼ cup ranch dressing, or purchased bottled dressing
½ cup shredded cheddar cheese
½ cup shredded mozzarella cheese
½ cup grated parmesan cheese
½ teaspoon dried parsley

1. At 350°F/177°C, preheat your oven and prepare a baking dish with cooking spray. 2. In a suitable skillet over medium-high heat, heat the olive oil for almost 1 minute. 3. Season the chicken breasts with the salt, pepper, and garlic powder. Add them to the skillet. Sear each breast for almost 5 minutes per side. 4. Place the chicken into the prepared dish. 5. Spread 1 tablespoon of butter and 1 tablespoon of ranch dressing over each breast. 6. Top the chicken with the bacon, covering each breast completely. 7. Place the dish in the preheated

oven. Bake for almost 30 minutes. 8. Remove from your oven. Sprinkle equal amounts of the cheddar, mozzarella, and parmesan cheeses over the bacon-topped breasts. 9. Season with the dried parsley. Return the dish to your oven. 10. Bake for another 10 to 12 minutes, or until the cheese melts.
Per serving: Calories: 314; Total fat 13.3g; Sodium 194mg; Total Carbs 4.9g; Fiber 6.8g; Sugars 16g; Protein 26g

Chicken Piccata

Prep time: 10 minutes. | Cooking time: 20 minutes. | Serves: 4

4 (6-ounces) boneless, skinless chicken breasts
½ teaspoon salt
¼ teaspoon pepper
½ teaspoon garlic powder
2 tablespoons coconut oil

1 cup water
4 tablespoons butter
Juice of 1 lemon
2 tablespoons capers
2 cloves garlic, minced
¼ teaspoon xanthan gum

1. Sprinkle salt, black pepper, and garlic powder on chicken breast. 2. Hit the sauté button on the Instant Pot and add coconut oil to preheat. 3. Sear chicken until golden per side. for almost 5–7 minutes. Hit the cancel button. 4. Remove chicken and keep it aside. Pour water into Instant Pot; scrape bottom of pan with wooden spoon if necessary to remove any stuck-on seasoning or meat. 5. Place steam rack in pot and add chicken. 6. Turn the pot's lid to close. Hit the manual button and adjust time for almost 10 minutes. 7. When the pot beeps, allow a 10-minute natural release, then quick-release the remaining pressure. 8. Remove chicken and keep it aside. Strain broth from Instant Pot into suitable bowl and return to pot. 9. Hit the sauté button on the Instant Pot and add butter, lemon juice, capers, garlic, and xanthan gum. 10. Stir frequently, and reduce sauce until desired thickness for at least 5 minutes. Serve over chicken.
Per Serving: Calories 416; Total Fat 23.6g; Sodium 934mg; Total Carbs 6g; Fiber 2g; Sugars 0.6g; Protein 37.9g

Creamy Chicken and Spinach Bake

Prep time: 10 minutes. | Cooking time: 30 minutes. | Serves: 4

Nonstick cooking spray
1 pound boneless, skinless chicken breasts, cubed
10 ounces baby spinach
8 ounces cream cheese, at room temperature
¾ cup shredded mozzarella

cheese
¼ cup sour cream
2 teaspoons minced garlic
Salt
Black pepper

1. At 400°F/204°C, preheat your oven. 2. Grease a 9-by-13-inch baking dish with cooking spray. Spread out the chicken in the dish. 3. Layer the spinach over the top, keeping it as flat as possible. 4. In a suitable bowl, mix the cream cheese, ¼ cup of mozzarella, the sour cream, and garlic. Season with black pepper and salt. Spoon the prepared mixture on top of the spinach. 5. Cover with foil sheet and bake for almost 20 minutes. 6. Remove from your oven, uncover, and top with the remaining ½ cup of mozzarella. 7. Bake for another 10 to 15 minutes, until the chicken has reached an internal temperature of 165°F/74°C.
Per Serving: Calories 476, Fat 27.6g, Sodium 992mg, Carbs 4.5g, Fiber 4g, Sugars 4.3g; Protein 16.8g

Spinach and Feta Stuffed Chicken

Prep time: 10 minutes. | Cooking time: 20 minutes. | Serves: 4

4 (6-ounce) boneless, skinless chicken breasts, butterflied
½ cup frozen spinach
⅓ cup crumbled feta cheese
1¼ teaspoons salt
¼ teaspoon pepper

¼ teaspoon garlic powder
¼ teaspoon dried oregano
¼ teaspoon dried parsley
2 tablespoons coconut oil
1 cup water

1. Pound the chicken breasts to ¼-inch thickness. 2. In a suitable bowl, mix frozen spinach, feta, and add ¼ teaspoon salt. 3. Divide mixture and spoon onto chicken breasts. 4. Seal the chicken breasts and secure with toothpicks or butcher's string. 5. Sprinkle remaining seasonings onto chicken. 6. Hit the sauté button on the Instant Pot and add coconut oil to preheat. 7. Sear each chicken breast until golden brown. Hit the cancel button. 8. Remove chicken and keep it aside briefly. 9. Pour water into Instant Pot and scrape bottom to remove any chicken or seasoning that is stuck on. Place steam rack into pot. 10. Place chicken on steam rack and turn the pot's lid to close. 11. Adjust time for almost 15 minutes. Serve warm.
Per Serving: Calories 227; Total Fat 8.8g; Sodium 302mg; Total Carbs 8.9g; Fiber 2.1g; Sugars 3.3g; Protein 28.5g

Buffalo Chicken Wings

Prep time: 10 minutes. | Cooking time: 50 minutes. | Serves: 4

1 tablespoon olive oil
1 teaspoon salt
½ teaspoon black pepper
2 pounds chicken wings

¼ cup hot sauce
1 tablespoon butter, melted
¼ teaspoon cayenne pepper
1 cup blue cheese sauce

1. At 400°F/204°C, preheat your oven. 2. In a suitable bowl, mix the olive oil, ½ teaspoon of salt, and ¼ teaspoon of black pepper. 3. Add the wings and stir to coat. Evenly divide the wings between two baking sheets. 4. Place the sheets in your oven. Bake for almost 45 to 50 minutes, or until the outer skin is crispy. 5. In another suitable bowl, mix the hot sauce, butter, cayenne pepper, the remaining ½ teaspoon of salt, and remaining ¼ teaspoon of black pepper. 6. Add the cooked wings. Toss them in the sauce for almost 1 minute to coat. 7. Serve with blue cheese sauce or ranch dressing.

Per Serving: Calories 217; Total Fat 5.1g; Sodium 624mg; Total Carbs 6.8g; Fiber 0.8g; Sugars 1.8g; Protein 31.1g

Curried Chicken Salad

Prep time: 10 minutes. | Cooking time: 0 minutes. | Serves: 4

½ cup mayonnaise
1 tablespoon lemon juice
1 teaspoon curry powder
Sea salt
Black pepper, freshly ground

16 ounces shredded cooked chicken, light and dark meat
¼ cup chopped toasted cashews
1 celery stalk, minced
¼ cup diced red onion

1. In a suitable bowl, whisk the mayonnaise, lemon juice, and curry powder. 2. Season with black pepper and salt. Fold in the chicken, cashews, celery, and red onion. Serve.

Per Serving: Calories 342; Total Fat 13.7g; Sodium 678mg; Total Carbs 2.3g; Fiber 4.5g; Sugars 22.1g; Protein 26.7g

Regular Salmon Patties

Prep time: 5 minutes| Cook time: 8 minutes| Serves: 4

12 ounces pouched pink salmon
3 tablespoons mayonnaise
⅓ cup blanched finely ground almond flour
½ teaspoon Cajun seasoning
1 medium avocado, peeled, pitted, and sliced

1. Mix salmon, mayonnaise, flour, and Cajun seasoning in a medium bowl. Form mixture into four patties. 2. Place patties into an ungreased air fryer basket. Set the temperature setting to 400°F/204°C and the timer for 8 minutes, turning patties halfway through cooking. Cakes will be made when firm and golden brown. 3. Transfer patties to four medium plates and serve warm with avocado slices.
Per Serving: Calories 263; Fat 18g; Sodium 589mg; Carbs 5g; Fiber 3g; Sugar 0g; Protein 20g

Crispy Fish Sticks

Prep time: 15 minutes| Cook time: 12 minutes| Serves: 4

1 large egg
½ teaspoon old bay seasoning
1½ ounces plain pork rinds, finely
crushed
4 (4-ounce) cod fillets, cut into 1" × 2" sticks

1. In a medium bowl, whisk egg. In a separate medium bowl, combine old bay seasoning and pork rinds. 2. Dip each fish stick into the egg, then gently press it into the pork rind mixture to coat all sides. Place fish sticks into an ungreased air fryer basket. 3. Set the temperature setting to 400°F/204°C and the timer for 12 minutes, turning fish sticks halfway through cooking. 4. When done, fish sticks will be golden brown and have an internal temperature of at least 145°F/63°C when done. Serve warm.
Per Serving: Calories 156; Fat 5g; Sodium 605mg; Carbs 0g; Fiber 0g; Sugar 0g; Protein 25g

Ahi Tuna Steaks with Bagel Seasoning

Prep time: 5 minutes| Cook time: 14 minutes| Serves: 2

2 (6-ounce) ahi tuna steaks
2 tablespoons olive oil
3 tablespoons of everything bagel seasoning

1. Drizzle each steak with olive oil. Place seasoning on a medium plate and press each side of tuna steaks into seasoning to form a thick layer. 2. Place steaks into an ungreased air fryer basket. 3. Set the temperature setting to 400°F/204°C and the timer for 14 minutes, turning steaks halfway through cooking. Steaks will be done when the internal temperature is at least 145°F/63°C for well-done. Serve warm.
Per Serving: Calories 385; Fat 14g; Sodium 1513mg; Carbs 0g; Fiber 0g; Sugar 0g; Protein 40g

Instant Shrimp

Prep time: 2 minutes| Cook time: 5 minutes| Serves: 4

1-pound medium shrimp, peeled and deveined
2 tablespoons salted butter,
melted
¼ teaspoon salt
¼ teaspoon ground black pepper

1. Toss shrimp in butter in a large bowl, then sprinkle with salt and pepper. 2. Place shrimp into an ungreased air fryer basket. 3. Set the temperature setting to 400°F/204°C and the timer for 5 minutes, shaking the basket halfway through cooking. 4. Shrimp will be pink when done. Serve warm.
Per Serving: Calories 119; Fat 6g; Sodium 736mg; Carbs 1g; Fiber 0g; Sugar 0g; Protein 13g

Hot and Tangy Shrimp

Prep time: 5 minutes| Cook time: 5 minutes| Serves: 4

1-pound medium shrimp, peeled and deveined
1 tablespoon salted butter, melted
2 teaspoons chili powder
¼ teaspoon garlic powder
¼ teaspoon salt
¼ teaspoon ground black pepper
½ small lime, zested and juiced, divided

1. In a medium bowl, toss shrimp with butter, then sprinkle with chili

powder, garlic powder, salt, pepper, and lime zest. 2. Place shrimp into an ungreased air fryer basket. 3. Set the temperature setting to 400°F/204°C and the timer for 5 minutes. Shrimp will be firm and form a "C" shape when done. 4. Transfer shrimp to serving dish and drizzle with lime juice. Serve warm.
Per Serving: Calories 98; Fat 4g; Sodium 752mg; Carbs 2g; Fiber 1g; Sugar 0g; Protein 13g

Crispy Coconut Shrimp

Prep time: 5 minutes| Cook time: 8 minutes| Serves: 2

8 ounces jumbo shrimp, peeled and deveined
2 tablespoons salted butter, melted
½ teaspoon old bay seasoning
¼ cup unsweetened shredded coconut
¼ cup coconut flour

1. In a large bowl, toss shrimp in butter and old bay seasoning. 2. In a medium bowl, combine shredded coconut with coconut flour. Coat each piece of shrimp in coconut mixture. 3. Place shrimp into an ungreased air fryer basket. Set the temperature setting to 400°F/204°C and the timer for 8 minutes, gently turning the shrimp halfway through cooking. The shrimp will be pink and C-shaped when done. Serve warm.
Per Serving: Calories 296; Fat 19g; Sodium 786mg; Carbs 13g; Fiber 7g; Sugar 4g; Protein 17g

Wrapped Scallops

Prep time: 5 minutes| Cook time: 10 minutes| Serves: 4

8 (1-ounce) sea scallops, cleaned and patted dry
8 slices of sugar-free bacon
¼ teaspoon salt
¼ teaspoon ground black pepper

1. Wrap scallop in 1 slice of bacon and secure with a toothpick. Sprinkle with salt and pepper. 2. Place scallops into an ungreased air fryer basket. 3. Set the temp setting to 360°F/182°C and the timer for 10 minutes. When done, scallops will be opaque and firm and have an internal temperature of 130°F/54°C. Serve warm.
Per Serving: Calories 125; Fat 6g; Sodium 691mg; Carbs 2g; Fiber 0g; Sugar 0g; Protein 14g

Garlic Scallops

Prep time: 5 minutes| Cook time: 10 minutes| Serves: 4

4 tablespoons salted butter, melted
4 teaspoons peeled and finely minced garlic
½ small lemon, zested and juiced
8 (1-ounce) sea scallops, cleaned and patted dry
¼ teaspoon salt
¼ teaspoon ground black pepper

1. Mix butter, garlic, lemon zest, and lemon juice in a small bowl. Place scallops in an ungreased 6" round nonstick baking dish. Pour butter mixture over scallops, then sprinkle with salt and pepper. 2. Place dish into air fryer basket. Set the temperature setting to 360°F/182°C and the timer for 10 minutes. When done, scallops will be opaque and firm and have an internal temperature of 130°F/54°C. Serve warm.
Per Serving: Calories 145; Fat 11g; Sodium 458mg; Carbs 3g; Fiber 0g; Sugar 0g; Protein 7g

Crab-Stuffed Boats

Prep time: 5 minutes| Cook time: 7 minutes| Serves: 4

2 medium avocados, halved and pitted
8 ounces cooked crab meat
¼ teaspoon old bay seasoning
2 tablespoons peeled and diced yellow onion
2 tablespoons mayonnaise

1. Scoop out avocado flesh in each avocado half, leaving ½" around the edges to form a shell. Chop scooped-out avocado. 2. Combine crab meat, old bay seasoning, onion, mayonnaise, and chopped avocado in a medium bowl. Place ¼ mixture into each avocado shell. 3. Place avocado boats into an ungreased air fryer basket. Set the temperature to 350°F/177°C and the timer for 7 minutes. The avocado will be browned on the top, and the mixture will be bubbling when done. Serve warm.
Per Serving: Calories 209; Fat 15g; Sodium 307mg; Carbs 1g; Fiber 5g; Sugar 0g; Protein 12g

Traditional Lobster Tails

Prep time: 5 minutes| Cook time: 9 minutes| Serves: 4

4 (6-ounce) lobster tails	minced garlic
2 tablespoons salted butter, melted	¼ teaspoon salt
	¼ teaspoon ground black pepper
1 tablespoon peeled and finely	2 tablespoons lemon juice

1. Carefully cut open lobster tails with scissors and pull back the shell to expose the meat. Pour butter over each tail, then sprinkle with garlic, salt, and pepper. 2. Place tails into an ungreased air fryer basket. Set the temperature setting to 400°F/204°C and the timer for 9 minutes. The lobster, will be firm and opaque when done. 3. Transfer tails to four medium plates and pour lemon juice over lobster meat. Serve warm.
Per Serving: Calories 186; Fat 7g; Sodium 910mg; Carbs 1g; Fiber 0g; Sugar 0g; Protein 28g

Delicious Tuna Cakes

Prep time: 10 minutes| Cook time: 10 minutes| Serves: 4

4 (3-ounce) pouches tuna, drained	white onion
1 large egg, whisked	½ teaspoon old bay seasoning
2 tablespoons peeled and chopped	

1. In a large bowl, mix all patties ingredients and form into four beautiful patties. 2. Place patties into an ungreased air fryer basket. 3. Set the temperature setting to 400°F/204°C and the timer for 10 minutes. Cakes will be browned and crispy when done. Let cool for 5 minutes before serving.
Per Serving: Calories 100; Fat 2g; Sodium 432mg; Carbs 1g; Fiber 0g; Sugar 0g; Protein 21g

Yummy Italian Baked Cod

Prep time: 5 minutes| Cook time: 12 minutes| Serves: 4

4 (6-ounce) cod fillets	1 teaspoon Italian seasoning
2 tablespoons salted butter, melted	¼ teaspoon salt
	½ cup low-carb marinara sauce

1. Place cod into an ungreased 6" round nonstick baking dish. Pour butter over cod and sprinkle with Italian seasoning and salt. Top with marinara. 2. Place dish into air fryer basket. Set the temperature to 350°F/177°C and the timer for 12 minutes. Fillets will be lightly browned, easily flake, and have an internal temperature of at least 145°F/63°C when done. Serve warm.
Per Serving: Calories 193; Fat 8g; Sodium 811mg; Carbs 2g; Fiber 0g; Sugar 0g; Protein 27g

Mediterranean-Style Cod Steak

Prep time: 5 minutes| Cook time: 12 minutes| Serves: 4

4 (6-ounce) cod fillets	6 cherry tomatoes, halved
3 tablespoons fresh lemon juice	¼ cup pitted and sliced Kalamata olives
1 tablespoon olive oil	
¼ teaspoon salt	

1. Place cod into an ungreased 6" round nonstick baking dish. Pour lemon juice into the dish and drizzle cod with olive oil. Sprinkle with salt—place tomatoes and olives around the baking dish in between fillets. 2. Place dish into air fryer basket. Set the temperature to 350°F/177°C and the timer for 12 minutes, carefully turning the cod halfway through cooking. Fillets will be lightly browned, easily flake, and have an internal temperature of at least 145°F/63°C when done. Serve warm.
Per Serving: Calories 189; Fat 8g; Sodium 891mg; Carbs 2g; Fiber 0g; Sugar 1g; Protein 26g

Delicious Rainbow Salmon Kebabs

Prep time: 10 minutes| Cook time: 8 minutes| Serves: 2

6 ounces boneless, skinless salmon, cut into 1" cubes	½ medium zucchini, trimmed and cut into ½" slices
¼ medium red onion, peeled and cut into 1" pieces	1 tablespoon olive oil
½ yellow bell pepper, seeded and cut into 1" pieces	½ teaspoon salt
	¼ teaspoon ground black pepper

1. Using one 6" skewer, skewer 1 piece salmon, then 1 piece onion, 1 piece bell pepper, and finally 1 piece zucchini. Repeat this pattern with additional skewers to make four kebabs total. Grease with olive oil and sprinkle with salt and black pepper. 2. Place kebabs into an ungreased air fryer basket. Set the temperature setting to 400°F/204°C and the timer for 8 minutes, turning kebabs halfway through cooking. Salmon will easily flake and have an internal temperature of at least 145°F/63°C when done; vegetables will be tender. Serve warm.
Per Serving: Calories 183; Fat 9g; Sodium 642mg; Carbs 6g; Fiber 1g; Sugar 2g; Protein 17g

Spicy Fish Bowl

Prep time: 10 minutes| Cook time: 12 minutes| Serves: 4

½ teaspoon salt	cabbage
¼ teaspoon garlic powder	⅓ cup mayonnaise
¼ teaspoon ground cumin	¼ teaspoon ground black pepper
4 (4-ounce) cod fillets	¼ cup chopped pickled jalapeños
4 cups finely shredded green	

1. Sprinkle salt, garlic powder, and cumin over cod and place them into an ungreased air fryer basket. Set the temperature to 350°F/177°C and the timer for 12 minutes, turning fillets halfway through cooking. Cod will flake easily and have an internal temperature of at least 145°F/63°C when done. 2. In a large bowl, toss cabbage with mayonnaise, pepper, and jalapeños until fully coated. Serve cod warm over cabbage slaw on four medium plates.
Per Serving: Calories 221; Fat 14g; Sodium 850mg; Carbs 4g; Fiber 2g; Sugar 2g; Protein 18g

Delicious Cajun Salmon

Prep time: 5 minutes| Cook time: 7 minutes| Serves: 2

2 (4-ounce) boneless, skinless salmon fillets	⅛ teaspoon cayenne pepper
	½ teaspoon garlic powder
2 tablespoons salted butter, softened	1 teaspoon paprika
	¼ teaspoon ground black pepper

1. Brush each fillet with butter. Mix all other ingredients except butter and rub them into the fish on both sides. 2. Place fillets into an ungreased air fryer basket. Set the temperature setting to 390°F/199°C and the timer for 7 minutes. The internal temperature will be 145°F/63°C when done. Serve warm.
Per Serving: Calories 248; Fat 14g; Sodium 174mg; Carbs 1g; Fiber 1g; Sugar 0g; Protein 23g

Southern-Style Catfish Steak

Prep time: 10 minutes| Cook time: 12 minutes| Serves: 4

4 (7-ounce) catfish fillets	almond flour
⅓ cup heavy whipping cream	2 teaspoons old bay seasoning
1 tablespoon lemon juice	½ teaspoon salt
1 cup blanched finely ground	¼ teaspoon ground black pepper

1. Place catfish fillets into a large bowl with cream and pour lemon juice. Stir to coat. 2. In a separate bowl, mix flour along with old bay seasoning. Remove each fillet and gently shake off excess cream. Sprinkle with salt and pepper. Press each fillet gently into the flour mixture on both sides to coat. 3. Place fillets into an ungreased air fryer basket. Set the temperature setting to 400°F/204°C and the timer for 12 minutes, turning fillets halfway through cooking. Catfish will be golden brown and have an internal temperature of at least 145°F/63°C when done. Serve warm.
Per Serving: Calories 284; Fat 14g; Sodium 625mg; Carbs 1g; Fiber 1g; Sugar 1g; Protein 32g

Sweet Buttery Salmon

Prep time: 5 minutes| Cook time: 12 minutes| Serves: 4

2 tablespoons salted butter, melted	4 (4-ounce) boneless, skinless salmon fillets
1 teaspoon low-carb maple syrup	½ teaspoon salt
1 teaspoon yellow mustard	

1. In a small bowl, whisk together butter, syrup, and mustard—brush ½ mixture over each fillet on both sides. Sprinkle fillets with salt on both sides. 2. Place salmon into an ungreased air fryer basket. Set the temperature setting to 400°F/204°C and the timer for 12 minutes. Halfway through cooking, brush fillets on both sides with the remaining syrup mixture. Salmon will easily flake and have an internal temperature of at least 145°F/63°C when done. Serve warm.
Per Serving: Calories 193; Fat 9g; Sodium 435mg; Carbs 1g; Fiber 0g; Sugar 0g; Protein 23g

Cheesy Lobster Tails

Prep time: 5 minutes| Cook time: 7 minutes| Serves: 4

4 (4-ounce) lobster tails
2 tablespoons salted butter, melted
1½ teaspoons Cajun seasoning, divided

¼ teaspoon salt
¼ teaspoon ground black pepper
¼ cup grated Parmesan cheese
½ ounce plain pork rinds, finely crushed

1. Cut lobster tails open carefully with scissors and gently pull the meat away from the shells, resting meat on top of the shells. 2. Grease lobster meat with butter and spice with 1 teaspoon of Cajun seasoning, ¼ teaspoon per tail. Mix remaining Cajun seasoning, salt, pepper, Parmesan, and pork rinds in a small bowl. Gently press ¼ mixture onto the meat on each lobster's tail. 3. Carefully place tails into an air fryer basket. Set the temperature setting to 400°F/204°C and the timer for 7 minutes. 4. Lobster tails will be crispy and golden on top and have an internal temperature of at least 145°F/63°C when done. Serve warm.
Per Serving: Calories 184; Fat 0g; Sodium 931mg; Carbs 1g; Fiber 0g; Sugar 0g; Protein 23g

Lemon Butter Cod Steak

Prep time: 5 minutes| Cook time: 12 minutes| Serves: 4

4 (4-ounce) cod fillets
2 tablespoons salted butter, melted

1 teaspoon old bay seasoning
½ medium lemon, cut into 4 slices

1. Place cod fillets into an ungreased 6" round nonstick baking dish. Brush tops of fillets with butter and sprinkle with old bay seasoning. Lay 1 lemon slice on each fillet. 2. Cover the spiced fillet with aluminum foil and place into air fryer basket. Set the temperature to 350°F/177°C and the timer for 12 minutes, turning fillets halfway through cooking. When done, fish will be opaque and have an internal temperature of at least 145°F/63°C when done. Serve warm.
Per Serving: Calories 128; Fat 6g; Sodium 529mg; Carbs 0g; Fiber 0g; Sugar 0g; Protein 17g

Tuna Tomatoes

Prep time: 5 minutes| Cook time: 5 minutes| Serves: 2

2 medium beefsteak tomatoes, tops removed, seeded, membranes removed
2 (2.6-ounce) pouches tuna packed in water, drained
1 medium stalk celery, trimmed and chopped

2 tablespoons mayonnaise
¼ teaspoon salt
¼ teaspoon ground black pepper
2 teaspoons coconut oil
¼ cup shredded mild cheddar cheese

1. Scoop pulp out of each tomato, leaving ½" shell. 2. Mix tuna, celery, mayonnaise, salt, and pepper in a medium bowl. Drizzle with coconut oil. Spoon ½ mixture into each tomato and top each with 2 tablespoons of cheddar. 3. Place tomatoes into an ungreased air fryer basket. Set the temperature setting to 320°F/160°C and the timer for 5 minutes. The cheese will be melted when done. Serve warm.
Per Serving: Calories 219; Fat 15g; Sodium 697mg; Carbs 4g; Fiber 1g; Sugar 2g; Protein 18g

Nut-Crusted Mahi Mahi

Prep time: 5 minutes| Cook time: 15 minutes| Serves: 4

Coconut oil, for greasing
4 (4-ounce) Mahi Mahi fillets, rinsed and patted dry
1 teaspoon sea salt, plus a pinch
½ teaspoon black pepper, plus a pinch
½ cup macadamia nuts, salted,

roasted, coarsely chopped
2 tablespoons almond flour (or crushed pork rinds)
½ teaspoon garlic powder
½ teaspoon onion powder
4 tablespoons mayonnaise

1. Preheat the oven to 400°F/204°C. 2. With coconut oil, grease an 8-inch square baking dish. 3. Place the mahi-mahi in the prepared baking dish. 4. Spice fillet with salt and pepper on both sides. In small bowl, mix the macadamia nuts, almond flour, garlic powder, onion powder, and a pinch salt and pepper. 4. Spread 1 tablespoon of mayonnaise on each fillet. Divide the nut mixture among the top of the 4 fillets, gently patting it down to adhere to the mayonnaise. 5. Bake for about 15 minutes until golden brown and cooked through.
Per Serving: Calories 364; Fat 28g; Sodium 689mg; Carbs 4g; Fiber 2g; Sugar 1g; Protein 24g

Salmon-Stuffed Mushrooms

Prep time: 5 minutes| Cook time: 25 minutes| Serves: 4

4 portabella mushroom caps
2 (6-ounce) cans wild-caught salmon (or freshly cooked wild-caught salmon)
4 ounces cream cheese, at room temperature
¼ cup mayonnaise
2 scallions, chopped

½ teaspoon paprika
½ teaspoon garlic powder
½ teaspoon sea salt
¼ teaspoon freshly ground black pepper
1 cup freshly grated Parmesan cheese

1. Preheat the oven to 350°F/177°C. 2. Prepare a baking sheet with parchment paper. Clean the mushrooms, remove the stems, and carefully scrape the gills away with a spoon. Place them top down on the baking sheet. 3. Combine the salmon, cream cheese, mayonnaise, scallions, paprika, garlic powder, salt, and pepper in a large bowl. Mix well to combine. 4. Spoon the salmon mixture into the mushroom caps, dividing equally. 5. Sprinkle with the Parmesan and bake for 20 to 25 minutes until the mushrooms are tender and the cheese is bubbly.
Per Serving: Calories 385; Fat 29g; Sodium 468mg; Carbs 5g; Fiber 1g; Sugar 2g; Protein 26g

Halibut in a Blanket

Prep time: 10 minutes| Cook time: 20 minutes| Serves: 4

Coconut oil, for greasing
4 (4-ounce) halibut fillets, about 1-inch thick
½ cup (1 stick) butter, cut into squares
2 tablespoons finely chopped

scallion
1 tablespoon minced garlic
½ lemon
Sea salt
Freshly ground black pepper

1. Preheat the oven to 400°F/204°C. 2. Cut out four 12-inch squares of aluminum foil, and grease them with coconut oil. Place one halibut fillet on each foil square. Place two pats of butter on each fillet. Sprinkle the scallion and garlic over the fillets, dividing equally, and then squeeze the lemon half over the fillets, finally topping with a healthy sprinkle of salt and pepper. 3. Pull the sides of each foil square up to create a pouch around the halibut, and then roll the top like a paper lunch bag. The fish should be thoroughly enclosed, but there should be room in the foil pouches to allow steam to circulate and cook the fish. Place the foil pouches on a large baking sheet. 4. Bake it for 20 minutes until it opaque throughout. Remove the fish from the foil pouches before serving but save the "juice" to serve over any veggies you choose to serve with the dish.
Per Serving: Calories 313; Fat 25g; Sodium 632mg; Carbs 1g; Fiber 0g; Sugar 0g; Protein 21g

Crispy Fish with Tartar Sauce

Prep time: 10 minutes| Cook time: 15 minutes| Serves: 4

For the fish sticks
Avocado or coconut oil, for greasing
1 egg, lightly beaten
1 scoop unflavored MCT powder (or collagen powder)
Pinch sea salt
Pinch freshly ground black pepper
1 cup freshly grated Parmesan cheese
½ cup crushed pork rinds
1 teaspoon garlic powder
1 teaspoon onion powder
1 teaspoon paprika

1-pound cod fillets, rinsed, patted dry, and cut into 1-by-4-inch pieces
For the sauce
4 tablespoons mayonnaise
1 pickle spear, finely chopped
1 teaspoon freshly squeezed lemon juice
½ teaspoon onion powder
½ teaspoon garlic powder
Pinch sea salt
Pinch freshly ground black pepper
1 teaspoon chopped fresh dill
Dash low-carb sweetener

To make the fish sticks: 1. Preheat the oven to 400°F/204°C. Prepare a rimmed baking tray with aluminum foil. Place a wire rack over the baking sheet and lightly grease the rack with oil. 2. Put the lightly beaten egg in a shallow bowl. Combine the MCT powder, salt, and pepper in another shallow bowl. 3. Combine the Parmesan, pork rinds, garlic powder, onion powder, and paprika in a third bowl. 4. Dip the fish in the MCT mixture to coat both sides, shaking off the excess. Next, dip in the egg and then into the Parmesan mixture, patting to help the coating adhere. Place the fish on the wire rack. 5. Bake the fish for 12 - 15 minutes until golden brown.
To make the sauce: 1. Mix together the mayonnaise, chopped pickle, lemon juice, onion powder, and garlic powder in a small bowl. Add the salt, pepper, dill, and sweetener. Serve immediately
Per Serving: Calories 314; Fat 20g; Sodium 698mg; Carbs 2g; Fiber 0g; Sugar 0g; Protein 31g

Shrimp Alfredo and Zoodles

Prep time: 10 minutes| Cook time: 25 minutes| Serves: 5

For zoodles
3 medium zucchinis
1 teaspoon salt
For shrimp and sauce
2 tablespoons ghee
3 garlic cloves, minced
1-pound shrimp, peeled and
deveined
4 ounces cream cheese, at room

temperature
½ cup heavy (whipping) cream
½ teaspoon sea salt
¼ teaspoon freshly ground black
pepper
1 cup freshly grated Parmesan
cheese
¼ teaspoon cayenne pepper

To make the zoodles: 1. Trim off the ends of the zucchinis. Swirl the zucchini into noodle shapes (zoodles) using a vegetable spiral slicer. 2. Lay the zoodles on a kitchen towel and sprinkle with the salt. 3. While the sauce is simmering, fold the zoodles up in the towel and squeeze out as much water as possible.

To make the shrimp and sauce: 1. In a cooking pan melt the ghee and cook the garlic for 3 minutes until fragrant. 2. Add the shrimp in it and cook for 4-6 minutes, until the shrimp turn pink. 3. Remove the cooked shrimp to a plate. 4. In the same cooking pan, add the cream cheese and whisk until melted. 5. Pour in the cream, whisking constantly. 6. Spice with the salt and pepper. 7. Let the creamy sauce simmer for 5-10 minutes, often whisking, until thickened. 8. Remove the cooking pan from the heat and stir in the Parmesan and cayenne. Adjust the seasoning as per taste. 8. Add the zoodles, cover, and cook for 5 minutes. 9. The zoodles will release a bit of water, thin out the thick sauce a bit. 10. Add the cooked shrimp and toss before serving.
Per Serving: Calories 329; Fat 25g; Sodium 489mg; Carbs 6g; Fiber 1g; Sugar 2g; Protein 20g

Regular Crab Cakes

Prep time: 10 minutes| Cook time: 10 minutes| Serves: 4

8 ounces fresh lump crabmeat
2 tablespoons mayonnaise
1 teaspoon old bay seasoning
½ ounce plain pork rinds, finely

crushed
¼ cup seeded and chopped red
bell pepper

1. In a large bowl, mix all ingredients. Separate into four equal sections and form into patties. 2. Cut a piece of parchment to fit the air fryer basket. Place patties onto ungreased parchment and into an air fryer basket. Set the temperature setting to 380°F/193°C and the timer for 10 minutes, turning the patties halfway through cooking. Crab cakes will be golden when done. Serve warm.
Per Serving: Calories 116; Fat 7g; Sodium 561mg; Carbs 0g; Fiber 0g; Sugar 0g; Protein 12g

Spiced Snow Crab Legs

Prep time: 5 minutes| Cook time: 15 minutes| Serves: 4

8 pounds fresh shell-on snow crab
legs
2 tablespoons coconut oil
2 teaspoons old bay seasoning

4 tablespoons salted butter,
melted
2 teaspoons lemon juice

1. Place crab legs into an ungreased air fryer basket, working in batches if needed. Drizzle legs with coconut oil and sprinkle with old bay seasoning. 2. Set the temperature setting to 400°F/204°C and the timer for 15 minutes, shaking the basket three times during cooking. Legs will turn a bright red-orange when done. Serve warm. 3. In a separate small bowl, whisk butter and lemon juice for dipping. Serve on the side.
Per Serving: Calories 284; Fat 13g; Sodium 1186mg; Carbs 0g; Fiber 0g; Sugar 0g; Protein 38g

Cajun Crab Legs And Veggies

Prep time: 15 minutes| Cook time: 30 minutes| Serves: 6

Coconut oil, for greasing
2 zucchinis, halved lengthwise
and sliced
3 cups roughly chopped
cauliflower
10 tablespoons butter or ghee,
melted, divided
2 tablespoons Cajun seasoning

1 tablespoon mince or chopped
garlic
6 ounces sausages or bratwurst,
cut into rounds ½-inch thick2
pounds of frozen snow crab legs
(about two clusters)
½ lemon
Chopped fresh parsley for garnish

1. Preheat the oven to 450°F/232°C temperature setting. Prepare a large baking sheet by lining it with aluminum foil and then grease the foil with oil. 2. Arrange the zucchini halves cut-side up on the baking sheet. Spread the cauliflower in an even layer. In a bowl, stir 5 tablespoons of melted butter with Cajun seasoning, and garlic. 3. Pour half of the spiced butter mixture over the veggies. 4. Bake the veggies for 15-20 minutes until tender. 5. Place the sausage slices on the vegetables. 6. Break the crab legs and put them in a pan. Drizzle with the remaining spiced butter mixture—bake them all for another 10 minutes. 7. Squeeze the lemon juice and sprinkle parsley, and serve immediately with the remaining butter for dipping.
Per Serving: Calories 415; Fat 29g; Sodium 845mg; Carbs 5g; Fiber 2g; Sugar 0g; Protein 33g

BBQ Chicken Skewers

Prep time: 10 minutes. | Cooking time: 20 minutes. | Serves: 4

4 boneless, skinless chicken
breasts (6 ounces each)
1 cup low-carb barbecue sauce
1 red bell pepper cut into 2-inch
chunks
2 medium zucchini cut into

½-inch rounds
1 (8-ounce) package white
mushrooms, stems removed
Salt
Black pepper

1. Cut the chicken into even 2-inch pieces. 2. Set ¼ cup of barbecue sauce aside for basting. 3. Mix the remaining ¾ cup of barbecue sauce and the chicken in a resealable bag. 4. Seal and place in the refrigerator for at least 30 minutes. Preheat the grill to medium-high. 5. Remove the chicken from the marinade. Thread each skewer, alternating the ingredients. 6. Each skewer should have 3 pieces of chicken, 1 slice of zucchini, 1 or 2 mushrooms, and 1 or 2 pieces of bell pepper. Season with salt and black pepper. 7. Cook the skewers on the grill, turning occasionally, for almost 20 minutes. 8. Brush the cooked skewers with the reserved ¼ cup of barbecue sauce before serving.
Per Serving: Calories 275; Total Fat 2.2g; Sodium 486mg; Total Carbs 7.3g; Fiber 0.4g; Sugars 17.5g; Protein 36.3g

Delicious Shrimp Scampi

Prep time: 5 minutes| Cook time: 10 minutes| Serves: 4

4 tablespoons butter or ghee
4 garlic cloves, minced
½ cup bone broth
½ teaspoon sea salt
¼ teaspoon freshly ground black
pepper

2 pounds shrimp, peeled and
deveined
¼ cup freshly squeezed lemon
juice
Chopped fresh parsley, for garnish

1. Cook garlic in the butter for 3 minutes until fragrant over medium heat. 2. Add the bone broth, salt, and pepper, and bring to a simmer for about 2 minutes. 3. Add the shrimp and cook for 4- 6 minutes, until the shrimp turn pink. Add the lemon juice. Sprinkle parsley over the shrimp to serve.
Per Serving: Calories 253; Fat 13g; Sodium 698mg; Carbs 3g; Fiber 0g; Sugar 0g; Protein 31g

Crispy Keto Baked Fish

Prep time: 10 minutes| Cook time: 20 minutes| Serves: 4

½ cup extra-virgin olive oil,
divided
1-pound flaky white fish (such as
cod, haddock, or halibut), skin
removed
½ cup shelled finely chopped
pistachios
½ cup ground flaxseed

Zest and juice of 1 lemon, divided
1 teaspoon ground cumin
1 teaspoon ground allspice
½ teaspoon salt (use 1 teaspoon if
pistachios are unsalted)
¼ teaspoon freshly ground black
pepper

1. Preheat the oven to 400°F/204°C. 2. Manage a baking sheet with parchment lining and drizzle 2 tablespoons olive oil over the sheet, spreading to coat the bottom evenly. 3. Cut the fish into 4 dense pieces. Place on the prepared baking sheet. Combine the pistachios, flaxseed, lemon zest, cumin, allspice, salt, and pepper in a small bowl. 4. Drizzle in ¼ cup olive oil and stir well. Divide the nut mixture evenly atop the fish pieces. Drizzle the lemon juice and remaining 2 tablespoons oil over the fish and bake until cooked for about 15 -20 minutes.
Per Serving: Calories 509; Fat 41g; Sodium 745mg; Carbs 9g; Fiber 2g; Sugar 2g; Protein 26g

Nut-Crusted Catfish

Prep time: 20 minutes| Cook time: 25 minutes| Serves: 4

4 catfish fillets, about 4 ounces each, rinsed and dry
2 cups chopped pecans
1½ teaspoons gluten-free Worcestershire sauce
1¼ teaspoons garlic powder
1¼ teaspoons paprika
1 teaspoon salt, plus more for seasoning
½ teaspoon black pepper, plus more for seasoning
¼ teaspoon onion powder
¼ teaspoon cayenne pepper
2 eggs, lightly beaten
1 teaspoon hot sauce
Chopped fresh parsley, for serving
Lemon wedges, for serving

1. Preheat the oven to 375°F/191°C. Prepare a baking sheet with parchment paper. Set aside. Combine the pecans, Worcestershire sauce, garlic powder, paprika, salt, black pepper, onion powder, and cayenne in a food processor. 2. Pulse until the pecans are finely chopped. Pour the mixture into a shallow pie plate and set aside. In a separate shallow dish, whisk the eggs and hot sauce. 3. Dip each catfish fillet into the egg, coating it on both sides, and dredge in the pecan mixture, pressing the pecan coating onto the fish to make sure the top of the fillet is well coated. Place the fillets onto the baking sheet. 4. Bake for 20-25 minutes until done and the pecan crust is golden brown and fragrant. The thickest part of the fish should flake easily and will be opaque all the way through. 5. Garnish with parsley and lemon wedges for squeezing.
Per Serving: Calories 647; Fat 55g; Sodium 1104mg; Carbs 11g; Fiber 7g; Sugar 5g; Protein 27g

Traditional Fish Tacos

Prep time: 15 minutes| Cook time: 20 minutes| Serves: 4

1 large egg, beaten
½ cup coconut flour, divided
1 teaspoon salt
1 teaspoon ground cumin
¼ teaspoon paprika
⅛ teaspoon chili powder
1-pound skinless, boneless cod,
cut into 1-inch pieces, patted dry
8 large butter lettuce leaves
½ cup coleslaw, divided
1 sliced avocado
¼ cup Pico de Gallo, divided
1 lime, quartered

1. Preheat the oven to 400°F/204°C. Prepare a baking sheet with parchment paper. Pour the egg into a small bowl. Pour ¼ cup of coconut flour into a medium bowl. 2. In a second medium bowl, thoroughly combine the remaining ¼ cup of coconut flour, salt, cumin, paprika, and chili powder. 3. Dip the cod pieces into the plain coconut flour, the egg, and finally the seasoned flour. Place the cod on the baking sheet in a single layer. Bake for 10 minutes, flip, and then bake for another 10 minutes. Let cool for 2 minutes. 4. To assemble the tacos, lay out the lettuce leaves and top with equal amounts of cod, coleslaw, avocado, and Pico de Gallo. Squeeze lime juice on top. Serve immediately.
Per Serving: Calories 344; Fat 22g; Sodium 478mg; Carbs 19g; Fiber 9g; Sugar 4g; Protein 25g

Crispy Fried Cod Sticks

Prep time: 15 minutes| Cook time: 15 minutes| Serves: 4

1 cup crushed pork rinds
¼ cup grated Parmesan cheese
½ cup heavy (whipping) cream
1 large egg
4 (4-ounce) cod fillets, patted dry
Extra-virgin olive oil, for frying
1 (10-ounce) can original Ro-Tel (drained)
2 tablespoons lemon juice

1. Combine the pork rinds and grated Parmesan. In another bowl, whisk the heavy cream and egg. 2. Dip each cod fillet thoroughly in the egg mixture, then dip on both sides into the pork rind mixture, making sure the entire fillet is covered. 3. Put the fillet in fridge to refrigerate while the oil heats. Heat the oil to 365°F/185°C. Working in batches if necessary, fry each fillet for about 2 minutes on each side or until the outside is golden brown. 4. Drain on a paper towel if needed, then plate and serve, topping each fillet with one-quarter of the can of Ro-Tel.
Per Serving: Calories 375; Fat 28g; Sodium 455mg; Carbs 6g; Fiber 0g; Sugar 0g; Protein 36g

Mustard-Crusted Cod with Roasted Veggies

Prep time: 5 minutes| Cook time: 25 minutes| Serves: 4

1-pound broccoli, cut into florets
2 tablespoons olive oil
Salt
½ cup Dijon mustard
4 skinless cod fillets (4 ounces each)

¾ cup pork rind crumbs
Parsley leaves, for garnish

1. Preheat the oven to 400°F/204°C. 2. Combine the broccoli, oil, and ½ teaspoon salt in a medium bowl and toss to combine. 3. Spread the broccoli in one side of the baking sheet—roast for 15 minutes. Meanwhile, spread the mustard onto one side of each fillet. 4. Press the pork rind crumbs onto the mustard. Place the cod on the empty side of the baking sheet. Roast for 8 to 10 minutes until the fish is opaque and flakes easily with a fork. 5. Season the broccoli with salt to taste. Serve the broccoli with the cod, garnished with the parsley.
Per Serving: Calories 337; Fat 17g; Sodium 369mg; Carbs 5g; Fiber 4g; Sugar 2g; Protein 37g

Cod with Green Pistou

Prep time: 15 minutes| Cook time: 10 minutes| Serves: 4

1 cup roughly chopped fresh Italian parsley
1 to 2 garlic cloves, minced
Zest and juice of 1 lemon
1 teaspoon salt
½ teaspoon freshly ground black
pepper
1 cup extra-virgin olive oil, divided
1-pound cod fillets, cut into 4 equal-sized pieces

1. Pulse the parsley, garlic, lemon zest and juice, salt, and pepper in a food processor. While the food processor is blending, slowly stream in ¾ cup of olive oil until well combined. 2. In a large pan, heat the remaining ¼ cup of olive oil over medium-high heat. Add the cod fillets, cover, and cook for 4 to 5 minutes on each side, or until cooked through. 3. Remove from the heat and keep warm. Add the pistou to the pan and heat over medium-low heat. Return the cooked fish to the pan, flipping to coat in the sauce. Serve warm, covered with pistou.
Per Serving: Calories 581; Fat 55g; Sodium 714mg; Carbs 3g; Fiber 1g; Sugar 1g; Protein 21g

Oven-Fried Catfish

Prep time: 10 minutes plus 3 hours to soak| Cook time: 30 minutes| Serves: 4

4 catfish fillets
2 teaspoons baking soda
Avocado oil
½ cup almond flour
¼ cup crushed pork rinds
¼ teaspoon paprika
¼ teaspoon garlic powder
¼ teaspoon kosher salt
⅛ teaspoon cayenne pepper
2 eggs, lightly beaten

1. Place the catfish in a large bowl of cold water, add the baking soda, and stir to combine. Let it marinate for overnight. 2. Preheat the oven to 350°F/177°C. Manage a baking sheet with parchment lining and brush it liberally with avocado oil. Drain the catfish, rinse it, and pat it dry with a paper towel. 3. Stir the almond flour, pork rinds, paprika, garlic powder, salt, and cayenne in a shallow pie plate. Whisk the beaten eggs and 1 tablespoon water to combine in another shallow dish. 4. Coat each catfish fillet in the egg mixture and dredge it in the almond flour mixture, coating both sides well. Place the fillets, not touching, on the baking sheet. 5. Bake the fish for 25-30 minutes until the fish is cooked through and flaky, turning the fish halfway through the baking time. Serve with tartar sauce.
Per Serving: Calories 308; Fat 20g; Sodium 689mg; Carbs 2g; Fiber 1g; Sugar 1g; Protein 30g

Nutty Halibut Curry

Prep time: 5 minutes| Cook time: 35 minutes| Serves: 4

1 tablespoon avocado oil
½ cup finely chopped celery
½ cup frozen butternut squash cubes
1 cup full-fat canned coconut milk
½ cup seafood stock
1½ tablespoons curry powder
1 tablespoon dried cilantro
½ tablespoon garlic powder
½ tablespoon ground turmeric
1 teaspoon ground ginger
1-pound skinless halibut fillet, cut into chunks
Cooked cauliflower rice, for serving

1. Heat the avocado oil in a saucepan with a lid. Add the celery and cook for about 3 minutes. Add the squash and cook for 5 minutes. Add the coconut milk and seafood stock and cook, stirring, for 3 minutes. 2. Stir in the curry powder, cilantro, garlic, turmeric, and ginger. Add the halibut to the pot, reduce the heat to medium, cover, and cook for 15 -20 minutes until the fish is thoroughly white and flakes easily with a fork. Serve the halibut curry over cauliflower rice if you'd like, or just eat it by itself!
Per Serving: Calories 362; Fat 22g; Sodium 986mg; Carbs 8g; Fiber 3g; Sugar 1g; Protein 33g

Roasted Cod with Garlic Butter

Prep time: 5 minutes| Cook time: 20 minutes| Serves: 2

2 (8-ounce) cod fillets	lengthwise
¼ cup (½ stick) butter, thinly sliced	¼ teaspoon salt
1 tablespoon minced garlic	¼ teaspoon freshly ground black pepper
½ pound baby bok choy, halved	

1. Preheat the oven to 400°F/204°C temperature setting. 2. Make a pouch with aluminum foil. Place the cod inside the pouch. 3. Top the cod with slices of butter and the garlic, evenly divided. Tuck the bok choy around the fillets. Season with salt and pepper. 4. Close the aluminum pouch with the two ends of the foil so the butter remains in it. Place the sealed pouches in a baking dish. Bake the fish pouches for 15 to 20 minutes, depending on the thickness of the fillets. Serve immediately.
Per Serving: Calories 317; Fat 24g; Sodium 478mg; Carbs 4g; Fiber 1g; Sugar 2g; Protein 23g

Poached Cod with Veggie Noodles

Prep time: 15 minutes| Cook time: 15 minutes| Serves: 2

1 teaspoon olive oil	1 enormous turnip, spiralized
1 garlic clove, smashed	1 large zucchini, spiralized
1 small shallot, thinly sliced	3 or 4 radishes, spiralized
1½ cups chicken broth	1 to 2 tablespoons chopped fresh parsley, for garnish
2 (6-ounce) fillets cod	Lemon wedges, for serving
Salt	
Freshly ground black pepper	

1. Heat the olive oil in saucepan (big enough to hold the fish) over medium heat. Sauté the garlic and shallot for 2 to 3 minutes until fragrant. 2. Pour in the broth and simmer. Spice the fish with salt and pepper and gently add to the broth. 3. Cover the pan and cook for about 10 minutes, or until the flesh is opaque and flakes easily with a fork. 4. Assemble the bowls by evenly dividing the turnip, zucchini, and radish noodles. Top each with cooked fish and ladle the broth over each bowl. 5. Serve with parsley and a lemon wedge on the side for squeezing.
Per Serving: Calories 203; Fat 4g; Sodium 541mg; Carbs 14g; Fiber 4g; Sugar 1g; Protein 29g

Crispy Cod Cakes

Prep time: 5 minutes| Cook time: 20 minutes| Serves: 2

3 tablespoons extra-virgin olive oil	2 tablespoons ground flaxseed
¼ medium onion, chopped	1 tablespoon freshly squeezed lemon juice
1 garlic clove, minced	1 teaspoon dried dill
1 cup cauliflower rice	½ teaspoon ground cumin
1-pound cod fillets	½ teaspoon pink Himalayan sea salt
½ cup almond flour	
1 large egg	¼ teaspoon freshly ground black pepper
2 tablespoons chopped fresh parsley	Tartar sauce

1. Heat oil and cook the onion and garlic for about 7 minutes, until tender over medium heat. Add in the cauliflower rice stir for 5 to 7 minutes, until warmed through and tender. Transfer to a large bowl. Heat 1 teaspoon of olive oil in the same pan over medium-high heat. Cook the cod for 4 to 5 minutes on each side, until cooked through. 2. Let the cod cool for a couple of minutes. Add the almond flour, egg, parsley, flaxseed, lemon juice, dill, cumin, salt, and pepper to the bowl with the cauliflower rice. Mix until the ingredients are well combined. 3. Add the fish to the bowl and mix well. Heat the remaining 1 tablespoon of olive oil in the pan over medium heat. 4. Using a ½ cup measuring cup, form 4 fish cakes by packing the mixture into the cup, then slipping the cake out of the cup onto a plate. Place the fish cakes in the hot oil and cook for about 5 minutes per side, flipping once, until golden brown on both sides. Place the cod cakes on serving plates, and do help with tartar sauce.
Per Serving: Calories 531; Fat 34g; Sodium 359mg; Carbs 12g; Fiber 6g; Sugar 2g; Protein 45g

Baked Halibut Steak with Herb Sauce

Prep time: 15 minutes| Cook time: 18 minutes| Serves: 4

4 (5-ounce) halibut fillets	Freshly ground black pepper
1 tablespoon extra-virgin olive oil	½ cup plain Greek yogurt
Sea salt	¼ cup mayonnaise

2 tablespoons sour cream	1 teaspoon chopped fresh basil
Juice and zest of 1 lemon	1 teaspoon chopped fresh chives
1 tablespoon chopped fresh dill	

1. Preheat the oven to 400°F/204°C. Prepare a baking sheet with parchment paper. 2. Pat dry fish with paper towels and lightly oil with olive oil. Season both sides of the fish with salt and pepper. 3. Place the spiced fillets on the baking sheet, and bake until cooked through about 15 to 18 minutes. While the fish is cooking, stir the yogurt, mayonnaise, sour cream, lemon juice, lemon zest, dill, basil, and chives in a small bowl. 4. Serve the fish with a generous dollop of sauce.
Per Serving: Calories 374; Fat 25g; Sodium 236mg; Carbs 2g; Fiber 0g; Sugar 0g; Protein 33g

Pesto Flounder with Greens

Prep time: 10 minutes| Cook time: 10 minutes| Serves: 6

2 pounds bok choy (about 1 large head)	Parmesan cheese
	Freshly ground black pepper
6 skinless flounder fillets (4 ounces each)	2 tablespoons olive oil
	1 garlic clove, minced
6 tablespoons pesto	Salt
6 tablespoons finely grated	

1. Preheat the broiler to high. Prepare a baking sheet with aluminum foil. Trim off the thick root end of the bok choy. 2. Slice stalks into quarters, then cut into rough chunks. 3. Pat dry the fish with paper towels and place it on the baking sheet. 4. Spread a tablespoon pesto over each fillet. Sprinkle 1 tablespoon of Parmesan on each fillet. 5. Spice it with pepper. Cook it under the broiler for 5 to 7 minutes until is opaque. Heat the olive oil and cook bok choy with garlic, frequently stirring, for about 5 minutes. 6. When done, remove it from the broiler and transfer to serving plates. Add cooked garlicky bok choy and season with salt.
Per Serving: Calories 264; Fat 17g; Sodium 354mg; Carbs 10g; Fiber 4g; Sugar 3g; Protein 19g

Baked Haddock

Prep time: 10 minutes| Cook time: 27 minutes| Serves: 4

2 tablespoons olive oil	½ teaspoon ground cumin
1 onion, thinly sliced	Sea salt
1 tablespoon minced garlic	Freshly ground black pepper
4 (3-ounce) haddock fillets	2 tablespoons chopped fresh cilantro
2 cups canned coconut milk	
1 teaspoon ground coriander	

1. Preheat the oven to 350°F/177°C. Heat the olive oil in ovenproof pan over medium-high heat. Sauté the onion and garlic until lightly caramelized, about 7 minutes. 2. Pan sear the fish, turning once, about 8 minutes. Add the coconut milk, coriander, and cumin, stirring carefully. 3. Cover and bake until the fish flake with a fork, for about 12 minutes. Season with salt and pepper, and serve topped with cilantro.
Per Serving: Calories 381; Fat 29g; Sodium 632mg; Carbs 6g; Fiber 1g; Sugar 1g; Protein 23g

Cheesy Fried Haddock

Prep time: 15 minutes| Cook time: 12 minutes| Serves: 4

1-pound boneless haddock fillets, cut into 4 equal pieces	¼ cup flaxseed meal
	¼ teaspoon freshly ground black pepper
¼ cup almond flour, divided	
1 large egg	Pinch ground cayenne pepper
1 tablespoon water	½ cup extra-virgin olive oil
½ cup Parmesan cheese	Lemon wedges, for garnish

1. Put 2 tablespoons of almond flour in a small bowl, and set it next to the fish. 2. Stir the eggs and water in another small bowl, and set the mixture next to the almond flour. 3. Stir the remaining 2 tablespoons of almond flour with the Parmesan cheese, flaxseed meal, black pepper, and cayenne pepper in a medium bowl. 4. Set the bowl next to the egg mixture. Dredge the fish pieces in the almond flour, the egg mixture, and the flour mixture, in that order, until all 4 pieces are coated. 5. Heat the olive oil. When the oil is hot, fry the fish, turning once, until both sides are golden and crispy for about 6 minutes per side, depending on the thickness of the fish. Transfer the fish to a paper towel-lined plate, and use paper towels to blot off the excess oil. Serve with lemon wedges.
Per Serving: Calories 349; Fat 25g; Sodium 741mg; Carbs 4g; Fiber 3g; Sugar 1g; Protein 27g

Crispy Haddock

Prep time: 20 minutes| Cook time: 12 minutes| Serves: 4

16 ounces boneless, skinless haddock fillet, cut into 4 pieces
1 cup almond flour
½ teaspoon paprika
⅛ teaspoon ground cardamom
⅛ teaspoon sea salt
Pinch freshly ground black pepper
½ cup heavy (whipping) cream
¼ cup coconut oil

1. Rinse the fillets and pat them thoroughly dry with paper towels. In a medium bowl, stir the almond flour, paprika, cardamom, salt, and pepper until well blended. 2. Pour the cream into another medium bowl and set it beside the almond flour mixture. Dredge one fish fillet in the flour mixture, shaking off the excess. 3. Then dip the fillet into the cream, shaking off the excess liquid. Finally, dredge the fish in the flour again to coat thoroughly and set aside. 4. Repeat with the remaining fillets. Fry the fillets until the fish is golden and crispy, turning once about 12 minutes total.
Per Serving: Calories 475; Fat 39g; Sodium 845mg; Carbs 7g; Fiber 3g; Sugar 2g; Protein 28g

Teriyaki Halibut

Prep time: 5 minutes| Cook time: 15 minutes| Serves: 1

1 tablespoon balsamic vinegar
1 tablespoon coconut aminos
1 teaspoon grated ginger root
1 tablespoon avocado oil
1 (6-ounce) halibut fillet
Pink Himalayan salt
Freshly ground black pepper

1. In a saucepan heat the balsamic vinegar, coconut aminos, and grated ginger until bubbling. Reduce the heat to low and simmer for 5 minutes. 2. Transfer to a bowl and set aside. Heat the oil in a sauté pan or pan. 3. Season the halibut with salt and pepper and add the fish to the pan. Sear the halibut for about 3 minutes and then flip and sear the other side for 3 more minutes. 4. Flip once more and brush 1 tablespoon of teriyaki sauce over the top and sides of the fish. Lower the heat to medium flame and cook for another 2 minutes on each side, or until the center is opaque. 5. Remove the halibut from the pan and top with the remaining sauce before serving.
Per Serving: Calories 393; Fat 19g; Sodium 698mg; Carbs 5g; Fiber 0g; Sugar 0g; Protein 45g

Baked Keto Halibut

Prep time: 20 minutes| Cook time: 15 minutes| Serves: 4

½ cup heavy (whipping) cream
½ cup finely chopped pecans
¼ cup finely chopped almonds
4 (4-ounce) boneless halibut fillets
Sea salt
Freshly ground black pepper
2 tablespoons extra-virgin olive oil

1. Preheat the oven to 400°F/204°C. Prepare a baking sheet with parchment. Pour the heavy cream into a bowl and set it on your work surface. 2. Stir the pecans and almonds in another bowl and set beside the cream. Pat dry the halibut fillets with paper towels and lightly season with salt and pepper. 3. Dip the fillets in the cream, shaking off the excess; then dredge the fish in the nut mixture so that both sides of each piece are thickly coated. 4. Place the fish on the prepared baking sheet and brush both sides of the pieces generously with olive oil. Bake the fish until the topping is golden, and the fish flakes easily with a fork, for 12 to 15 minutes. Serve.
Per Serving: Calories 392; Fat 31g; Sodium 698mg; Carbs 3g; Fiber 2g; Sugar 1g; Protein 26g

Halibut with Tangy Basil Sauce

Prep time: 10 minutes| Cook time: 20 minutes| Serves: 4

½ cup extra-virgin olive oil, divided
2 large garlic cloves, minced
1-pint grape tomatoes halved
¼ cup dry white wine
Juice of 1 lemon
½ cup roughly chopped fresh basil
Sea salt
Freshly ground black pepper
1¼ pounds halibut, cut into 4 (5-ounce) fillets

1. Heat olive oil in a saucepan. Cook the garlic until fragrant. 2. Cook the tomatoes for 10 minutes until they partially break down. Stir in the wine and simmer for 1 to 2 minutes to cook off the alcohol. 3. Stir in basil along with lemon juice and season generously with salt and pepper. While the sauce is cooking, heat the remaining 2 tablespoons of olive oil in a large pan over medium-high heat. 4. Season the

halibut fillets liberally with salt and pepper. Sear on each side for 3 to 4 minutes, or until the fish flakes easily with a fork.
Per Serving: Calories 467; Fat 31g; Sodium 412mg; Carbs 5g; Fiber 0g; Sugar 0g; Protein 38g

Pan-Fried Salmon and Bok Choy In Miso Vinaigrette

Prep time: 10 minutes. | Cooking time: 25 minutes. | Serves: 4

¼ cup miso paste
2 tablespoons rice wine vinegar or dry white wine
6 tablespoons toasted sesame oil
2 tablespoons ground ginger
1 teaspoon red pepper flakes
2 garlic cloves, minced
1 pound wild-caught salmon fillet, skin removed
½ cup avocado oil or olive oil, extra-virgin
8 heads baby bok choy, quartered
2 tablespoons tamari or water
2 tablespoons sesame seeds

1. In a suitable bowl, mix the miso, vinegar, 2 tablespoons of sesame oil, ginger, red pepper flakes, and garlic and whisk until smooth. 2. In a glass baking dish or resealable storage bag, place the salmon and pour the marinade over it. 3. Refrigerate for 30 minutes or up to overnight. To cook the fish, in a suitable skillet heat 4 tablespoons of avocado oil over medium-high heat. Remove the salmon from the marinade, reserving the liquid, and fry for almost 3 to 5 minutes per side, until the fish is crispy and golden brown. The time depends on your desired doneness and the thickness of the fish. 4. Transfer the fish to a suitable platter and keep warm. 5. In the same skillet, add the remaining 4 tablespoons of avocado oil over medium-high heat. Add the bok choy and fry for almost 7 minutes, until it is crispy and just tender. Transfer it to the platter with the salmon. 6. Reduce its heat to low. Add the reserved miso marinade and tamari to the oil in the skillet and whisk to mix well. Simmer, uncovered, for almost 4 to 5 minutes, until slightly thickened. Whisk in the remaining 4 tablespoons of sesame oil until smooth. 7. Serve the salmon and bok choy drizzled with the warm miso vinaigrette and sprinkled with the sesame seeds.
Per serving: Calories: 305; Total fat 5.7g; Sodium 307mg; Total Carbs 4g; Fiber 1.8g; Sugars 4.4g; Protein 20.8g

Thai-Inspired Seafood Chowder

Prep time: 10 minutes. | Cooking time: 15 minutes. | Serves: 4

2 tablespoons coconut oil
1 red bell pepper, coarsely chopped
1 (2-inch) piece fresh ginger, peeled and minced
6 garlic cloves, sliced
1 jalapeño, finely chopped (seeded for less heat, if preferred)
2 teaspoons Thai green curry paste
2 (13.5-ounce) cans full-fat coconut milk
¼ cup tamari (or 2 tablespoons miso paste and 2 tablespoons water)
1 to 2 teaspoons monk fruit extract
8 ounces wild-caught shrimp, peeled and deveined
8 ounces cod fillet, skinned and cut into bite-size chunks
Grated zest and juice of 1 lime
½ to 1 cup sliced fresh basil
Sliced jalapeño, for garnish

1. In a suitable stockpot, heat the coconut oil over medium heat. Add the bell pepper, ginger, garlic, and jalapeño and sauté for almost 4 to 5 minutes, until the vegetables are tender. 2. Add the curry paste and sauté for almost 1 minute, then add the coconut milk and tamari and whisk to mix well. Stir in the monk fruit extract (if using). 3. Bring the prepared mixture to a boil, reduce its heat to low, add the shrimp and cod, cover and simmer for almost 3 to 4 minutes, until the seafood is cooked through but not overly done. 4. Remove the shrimp from the heat and stir in the lime zest and juice and basil. Serve warm, garnished with the jalapeño (if using).
Per serving: Calories: 232; Total fat 9.7g; Sodium 389mg; Total carbs 1.1g; Fiber 0.5g; Sugars 0.2g; Protein 33.1g

Grandma Bev's Ahi Poke

Prep time: 10 minutes. | Cooking time: 0 minutes. | Serves: 6

3 scallions, both white and green parts diced
½ cup soy sauce
2 teaspoons sesame oil
1 tablespoon sesame seeds
¼ teaspoon ground ginger
1 teaspoon garlic powder
1 teaspoon salt
2 pounds fresh ahi tuna, cut into ½-inch cubes

1. In a suitable bowl, mix the scallions, soy sauce, sesame oil, sesame seeds, ginger, garlic powder, and salt. 2. Mix the soy sauce mixture with the tuna, and toss well. Serve immediately.
Per serving: Calories: 339; Total fat: 23g; saturated fat: 3g; cholesterol: 80mg; carbohydrates: 1g; Fiber: 1g; Protein: 30g

Sautéed Shrimp with Arugula Pesto

Prep time: 10 minutes. | Cooking time: 5 minutes. | Serves: 4

2 cups packed arugula
1 cup packed whole fresh basil leaves
½ cup chopped walnuts
½ cup freshly shredded parmesan cheese
2 garlic cloves, peeled
1 teaspoon salt
½ teaspoon black pepper, freshly ground
¾ cup olive oil, extra-virgin
1 pound wild-caught shrimp, peeled and deveined

1. In a food processor, mix the arugula, basil, walnuts, parmesan, and garlic and blend until very finely chopped. Add ½ teaspoon of salt and the pepper. 2. With the processor running, stream in ½ cup of olive oil until well blended. If the prepared mixture seems too thick, add warm water, 1 tablespoon at a time, until the texture is smooth and creamy. Keep it aside. 3. In a suitable skillet, heat the remaining ¼ cup of olive oil over medium-high heat. Add the shrimp, sprinkle with the remaining ½ teaspoon of salt, and sauté for almost 3 to 4 minutes, until the shrimp are just pink. 4. Remove the shrimp from the heat and stir in the pesto to mix well. Serve warm.
Per serving: Calories: 256; Total fat 11.6g; Sodium 695mg; Total carbs 1.4g; Fiber 0.3g; Sugars 0.5g; Protein 34.4g

Mediterranean Poached Cod

Prep time: 10 minutes. | Cooking time: 25 minutes. | Serves: 4

1 pound cod fillet, cut into 4 equal pieces
1 teaspoon salt
½ teaspoon black pepper, freshly ground
½ cup olive oil, extra-virgin
1 red bell pepper, sliced
1 (14-ounce) can artichoke hearts, quartered
1 (6 ounces) can large pitted green or black olives, drained and halved
4 large garlic cloves, peeled and crushed
2 tablespoons chopped fresh rosemary
¼ cup white wine vinegar or rice vinegar

1. Sprinkle the cod with black pepper and salt. 2. In a suitable skillet, heat 2 tablespoons of olive oil over medium-high heat. 3. Sear the cod for almost 1 to 2 minutes per side. 4. Transfer this fish to a serving dish and keep warm. 5. In the same skillet, add the remaining 6 tablespoons of olive oil over medium heat. 6. Add the bell pepper, artichokes, olives, garlic, and rosemary and sauté for almost 2 to 3 minutes, or until very fragrant. 7. Reduce its heat to low, stir in the vinegar, return the cod to the skillet, cover and poach for almost 10 to 12 minutes, until the fish is cooked through and the vegetables are tender. 8. Serve the cod and vegetables warm, drizzled with the cooking oil.
Per serving: Calories: 259; Total fat 9.6g; Sodium 111mg; Total carbs 7.3g; Fiber 2.1g; Sugars 3.4g; Protein 34.8g

Snapper Piccata

Prep time: 10 minutes. | Cooking time: 20 minutes. | Serves: 4

¼ cup almond flour
1 teaspoon salt
½ teaspoon black pepper, freshly ground
1 pound red snapper fillet, skinned and cut into 4 equal pieces
2 tablespoons olive oil, extra-virgin
½ cup (1 stick) unsalted butter
2 tablespoons minced shallot or red onion
2 tablespoons dry white wine
3 tablespoons coarsely chopped capers
Juice of 1 lemon (about 2 tablespoons)
¼ cup chopped parsley

1. In a shallow dish, mix the almond flour, salt, and pepper. Dredge the fish in the flour, shaking off any excess. 2. In a suitable skillet, heat the olive oil and 2 tablespoons of butter over medium-high heat. Sear the fish for almost 2 to 3 minutes per side, until browned and cooked through. Transfer to a serving dish and keep warm. 3. In the same skillet, melt 2 tablespoons of butter. Add the shallot and sauté for almost 1 to 2 minutes, until just tender. Whisk in the wine, bring to a simmer, then reduce its heat to low. Add the capers and lemon juice and simmer for almost 1 to 2 minutes. 4. Remove this skillet from the heat and whisk in the remaining 4 tablespoons of butter until melted. Stir in the parsley. 5. To serve, spoon the sauce over each piece of fish.
Per serving: Calories: 265; Total fat 12.7g; Sodium 826mg; Total carbs 9.9g; Fiber 1.5g; Sugars 5.6g; Protein 32.6g

Seared Cod with Coconut-Mushroom Sauce

Prep time: 10 minutes. | Cooking time: 20 minutes. | Serves: 4

1 pound cod fillet
½ teaspoon salt
¼ teaspoon black pepper, freshly ground
½ cup coconut oil
Grated zest and juice of 1 lime
4 ounces shiitake mushrooms, sliced
2 garlic cloves, minced
1 (13.5-ounce) can full-fat coconut milk
1 teaspoon ground ginger
1 teaspoon red pepper flakes
2 tablespoons tamari (or 1 tablespoon miso paste and 1 tablespoon water)
2 tablespoons toasted sesame oil

1. Cut the cod into four equal pieces and season with black pepper and salt. 2. In a suitable skillet, heat 4 tablespoons of coconut oil over high heat until just before smoking. 3. Add the cod, skin-side up, cover to prevent splattering and sear for almost 4 to 5 minutes, until it's golden brown. Remove the fish from the skillet, drizzle with the juice of ½ lime, and let rest. 4. In the same skillet, add the remaining 4 tablespoons of coconut oil and heat over medium. Add the mushrooms and sauté for almost 5 to 6 minutes, until they are just tender. Add the garlic and sauté for almost 1 minute, until fragrant. 5. Whisk in the coconut milk, ginger, red pepper flakes, tamari, and remaining lime zest and juice and reduce its heat to low. Return the cod to the skillet, skin-side down, cover and simmer for almost 3 to 4 minutes, until the fish is cooked through. 6. To serve, place the cod on rimmed plates or in shallow bowls and spoon the sauce over the fish. Drizzle with the sesame oil.
Per serving: Calories: 456; Total fat 26.2g; Sodium 119mg; Total Carbs 3.5g; Fiber 1.5g; Sugars 2.3g; Protein 28.8g

Seared Citrus Scallops with Mint and Basil

Prep time: 10 minutes. | Cooking time: 10 minutes. | Serves: 4

1 pound sea scallops, patted dry
1 teaspoon salt
½ teaspoon black pepper, freshly ground
¼ cup olive oil, extra-virgin
4 tablespoons unsalted butter
Grated zest and juice of 1 orange
Grated zest and juice of 1 lemon
2 tablespoons chopped fresh mint
2 tablespoons chopped fresh basil

1. Sprinkle the scallops with ½ teaspoon of salt and the pepper. 2. In a suitable skillet, heat the olive oil over medium-high heat. Place the scallops, one by one, into the hot oil and sear for almost 2 to 3 minutes per side, or until the scallops are lightly golden. Using a slotted spoon, remove from the skillet and keep warm. 3. Add the butter to the skillet and reduce its heat to medium low. Once the butter has melted, whisk in the citrus zests and juices, mint, basil, and the remaining ½ teaspoon of salt. Cook for almost 1 minute. 4. Remove it from the heat and return the seared scallops to the skillet, tossing to coat them in the butter sauce. 5. Serve the scallops warm, drizzled with sauce.
Per serving: Calories: 423; Total fat 23.2g; Sodium 340mg; Total carbs 2.7g; Fiber 0.5g; Sugars 0.5g; Protein 57.7g

Pan-Fried Shrimp Balls over Garlicky Greens

Prep time: 10 minutes. | Cooking time: 25 minutes. | Serves: 4

1 pound wild-caught shrimp, peeled, deveined, and finely chopped
¼ cup coconut or almond flour
1 large egg, lightly beaten
1 (2-inch) piece fresh ginger, peeled and minced
¼ cup minced scallion, green part only
1 teaspoon garlic powder
Grated zest of 1 lime
½ teaspoon salt
¼ to ½ teaspoon red pepper flakes
10 tablespoons olive oil, plus more for frying as needed
8 cups kale or spinach, torn into bite-size pieces
6 garlic cloves, minced
¼ cup soy sauce
2 tablespoons rice vinegar
2 tablespoons sesame oil

1. In a suitable bowl, mix the shrimp, coconut flour, egg, ginger, 2 tablespoons of scallion, garlic powder, lime zest, salt, and red pepper flakes, mixing well with a fork. Using your hands, form the shrimp mixture into about a dozen (1-inch) balls and place them on a cutting board or baking sheet lined with parchment paper. Allow to rest for almost 10 minutes. 2. In a suitable skillet or saucepan, heat 4 tablespoons of olive oil over medium-high heat. Working in batches of three to four balls, panfry them for almost 5 to 7 minutes total, carefully turning to brown all sides. Repeat until all the shrimp balls have been fried, adding additional oil with each batch as needed. Keep the shrimp balls warm. 3. In a suitable skillet, heat 2 tablespoons of olive oil over medium-high heat. Add the greens and sauté for almost 5 minutes. Add the garlic and sauté for almost 2 to 4 minutes, or until the greens are wilted. 4. In a suitable bowl, beat the soy sauce, vinegar, and sesame oil. 5. To serve, divide the sautéed greens between plates and top with three shrimp balls drizzled with the sauce.
Per serving: Calories: 210; Total fat 9.1g; Sodium 282mg; Total Carbs 3.8g; Fiber 3g; Sugars 8.5g; Protein 22.8g

Green Tea Poached Salmon

Prep time: 10 minutes. | Cooking time: 40 minutes. | Serves: 4

2 cups water
2 tablespoons coconut oil
1 (2-inch) piece fresh ginger, peeled and minced
4 garlic cloves, very sliced
1 teaspoon salt

4 green tea bags
1 pound wild-caught salmon fillet, skinned and cut into 4 equal pieces
¼ cup avocado oil or olive oil

1. In a suitable skillet over medium-high, mix the water, coconut oil, ginger, garlic, and salt. 2. Cook to a boil, cover, reduce its heat to low, and simmer for almost 10 minutes. 3. Remove from the heat, add the tea bags, cover and steep for almost 10 minutes. 4. Remove the tea bags from the liquid and discard. Cover and bring to a simmer over medium-low heat. Carefully place the salmon pieces into the simmering liquid, cover and cook for almost 15 to 18 minutes, until poached through. 5. Using a slotted spoon, remove the salmon pieces from the liquid and serve warm, drizzled with the avocado oil.
Per serving: Calories: 265; Total fat 7.5g; Sodium 163mg; Total Carbs 2.2g; Fiber 3.1g; Sugars 1.4g; Protein 26g

Lemon Pepper Shrimp Zoodles

Prep time: 10 minutes. | Cooking time: 20 minutes. | Serves: 2

¾ pound large shrimp, peeled and deveined
1 lemon, juiced and zested
1 tablespoon fresh parsley, chopped
2 medium zucchinis, spiralized
5 cherry tomatoes, quartered

Essentials
½ teaspoon black pepper, or as needed to taste
½ teaspoon salt, or as needed to taste
1 tablespoon olive oil

1. Mix the shrimp, lemon juice and lemon zest in a mixing bowl and season to taste with black pepper and salt. 2. Ensure that the shrimp is evenly coated with the ingredients. 3. Add the olive oil to a suitable skillet or cast iron pan over a suitable-high heat. 4. Once the oil is hot, add the shrimp and most of the parsley. 5. Stirring often, sauté the shrimp and parsley for almost 5 or 6 minutes, until the shrimp is opaque and cooked through. 6. Add the zoodles (zucchini noodles) and sauté for almost 2-3 minutes or until al dente. 7. Make sure not to overcook. Mix well to get the juices well distributed into the zoodles. 8. Remove this skillet from the heat and stir in half of the remaining parsley. 9. Divide the shrimp and zoodles evenly between four plates and garnish with the remaining fresh parsley along with the quartered cherry tomatoes on top and lemon wedges on the side.
Per serving: Calories: 274; Total fat 6.5g; Sodium 270mg; Total carbs 5.8g; Fiber 0.5g; Sugars 4.5g; Protein 45.3g

Lemon-Dill Salmon with Asparagus

Prep time: 10 minutes. | Cooking time: 20 minutes. | Serves: 2

2 salmon fillets
1 onion, peeled and sliced thin
12 asparagus spears, trimmed
2 garlic cloves, peeled and sliced
6 slices of lemon

1 teaspoon fresh dill, chopped
Essentials
1 tablespoon canola oil (use olive oil for a paleo version)
Salt and black pepper, to taste

1. At 400°F/204°C, preheat your oven. 2. Prepare two big sheets of foil sheet to wrap and bake the fish. 3. Place the asparagus spears in the center of the foil. Top with the salmon fillets. 4. Rub the salmon fillets with black pepper and salt, add the garlic slices and drizzle with canola oil. 5. Place 2 lemon slices and the onion slices over the salmon and fold the foil over to make a packet. 6. Bake the fish in your oven for almost 18-20 minutes. 7. Transfer the salmon and asparagus carefully to serving plates and garnish with the remaining lemon slices and chopped dill. Enjoy!
Per serving: Calories: 201; Total fat 7g; Sodium 321mg; Total Carbs 4g; Fiber 1.4g; Sugars 2.5g; Protein 18.9g

Lemon Baked Cod with Garlic and Tomatoes

Prep time: 10 minutes. | Cooking time: 18 minutes. | Serves: 2

2 cod fillets. for almost 6 ounces
2 garlic cloves, peeled and minced
1 tablespoon fresh lemon juice
2 tablespoons fresh parsley, chopped
4 cherry tomatoes, halved
½ cup baby spinach leaves

Essentials
Salt and ground black pepper, to taste
2 tablespoons coconut oil, for cooking
Nonstick cooking spray (use coconut oil for a paleo version)

1. At 400°F/204°C, preheat your oven. 2. Add the coconut oil to a suitable pot and set over low heat. 3. When the oil begins to sizzle, add the garlic and cook for almost 60 seconds. 3. Stir in the lemon juice and remove the pot from the heat. 4. Coat a glass baking dish with nonstick cooking spray. 5. Add the fish and sprinkle with black pepper and salt. 6. Rub with your hands to coat evenly. 7. Spoon the garlic mixture over the fish, sprinkle with fresh chopped parsley, add the halved tomatoes and bake for almost 14-16 minutes until opaque throughout. 8. Sauté the spinach in some of the juices from the fish for almost 1 minute. Mix well to ensure it receives a good coating of juices. 9. Serve the fish on a bed of baby spinach and drizzle with any remaining juices.
Per serving: Calories: 319; Total fat 12.5g; Sodium 889mg; Total Carbs 9.8g; Fiber 8.6g; Sugars 10g; Protein 36.4g

Pan Seared Tuna Steaks with Pine Nuts

Prep time: 10 minutes. | Cooking time: 10 minutes. | Serves: 2

2 fresh tuna steaks, for almost 3 ounces each
1 teaspoon chili powder
¼ teaspoon dried thyme
½ teaspoon garlic powder
1 tablespoon pine nuts

Handful of arugula or your favorite greens
1 tablespoon olive oil
1 tablespoon butter
Salt and black pepper, to taste

1. Mix all of the seasonings (chili powder, dried thyme, and garlic powder) and add a dash of black pepper and salt. 2. Add a little coating of olive oil to the tuna steaks and sprinkle the seasoning mixture over both sides, distributing it as evenly as possible. 3. Add the olive oil and butter to a suitable skillet and heat over medium-high heat. 4. Once the butter has melted and the oil is hot, add the pine nuts and the tuna steaks and cook for almost 4-5 minutes per side until blackened or cooked to your preference. The pine nuts should be soft and golden brown.
Serve immediately on a bed of arugula.
Per serving: Calories: 504; Total fat 19g; Sodium 1084mg; Total carbs 7.8g; Fiber 0.2g; Sugars 2.4g; Protein 71.2g

Power Poke Bowl

Prep time: 10 minutes. | Cooking time: 0 minutes. | Serves: 2

¼ cup tamari
¼ cup sesame oil
1 tablespoon minced fresh ginger
2 teaspoons red pepper flakes
8 ounces sashimi-grade tuna
¼ cup mayo
2 tablespoons rice vinegar
2 teaspoons sriracha

4 cups mixed greens
¼ cup chopped fresh cilantro
1 avocado, sliced
8 thin cucumber slices
¼ cup sliced scallions, white and green parts
2 teaspoons sesame seeds

1. In a suitable bowl, beat the tamari, sesame oil, ginger, and red pepper flakes. 2. Add the tuna, toss to coat, cover and refrigerate for at least 30 minutes or up to overnight. 3. While the tuna marinates, in a suitable bowl beat the mayo, vinegar, and sriracha. Keep it aside. 4. To prepare the bowls, divide the salad greens and cilantro between bowls. 5. Top with the avocado, cucumber, and scallions. 6. Add half of the marinated tuna mixture and the liquid to each bowl. 7. Drizzle with the spicy mayonnaise mixture and sesame seeds. Serve immediately.
Per serving: Calories: 282; Total fat 21.8g; Sodium 399mg; Total carbs 2.4g; Fiber 1.2g; Sugars 0.7g; Protein 19.1g

Citrus-Marinated Tilapia

Prep time: 10 minutes. | Cooking time: 30 minutes. | Serves: 4

4 tilapia fillets., for almost 4 ounces each
¼ cup lime juice
¼ cup green onions, chopped
1 tablespoon fresh dill, chopped
½ teaspoon garlic powder

Essentials
2 tablespoons coconut oil, for cooking
1 tablespoon water
Salt and black pepper, to taste

1. Mix the coconut oil, green onions, lime juice or lemon juice, dill, garlic powder, and water in a baking dish. Add the fish fillets and toss with your hands to coat. Season with salt. 2. Cover with foil sheet and let marinate in the refrigerator for at least 1 hour. 3. When ready to cook, at 350°F/177°C, preheat your oven, remove the fish from the refrigerator, and bake in your oven for almost 30 minutes until the fillets are cooked through. 4. Place the fillets on a serving plate, season with black pepper and serve. Garnish with dill, if desired.
Per serving: Calories: 403; Total fat 21.8g; Sodium 355mg; Total Carbs 2.3g; Fiber 4.4g; Sugars 4.8g; Protein 43.5g

Swordfish Kebabs with Mint Cream

Prep time: 10 minutes. | Cooking time: 10 minutes. | Serves: 4

1 (13.5-ounce) can full-fat coconut milk	1 pound swordfish steaks, cut into 2-inch cubes
1 cup packed whole fresh mint leaves	1 teaspoon salt
Grated zest and juice of 1 orange	½ teaspoon black pepper, freshly ground
1 teaspoon red pepper flakes	8 cups mixed greens
¼ cup olive oil or avocado oil	

1. In your high-speed blender or food processor, mix the coconut milk, mint, orange zest and juice, and red pepper flakes and blend well. Stream in the oil and blend until smooth. Place the prepared mixture in the refrigerator until ready to serve. 2. Thread the swordfish cubes onto skewers. Sprinkle with black pepper and salt. 3. Heat the grill to medium-high heat. When the grill is very hot, add the skewers and grill for almost 3 to 4 minutes per side, flipping once, until cooked through. 4. To serve, top 2 cups of salad with 1 kebab and drizzle with the mint cream.
Per serving: Calories: 351; Total fat 15.8g; Sodium 271mg; Total Carbs 5.9g; Fiber 2.3g; Sugars 9.1g; Protein 35.7g

Chili Haddock with Vegetables

Prep time: 10 minutes. | Cooking time: 20 minutes. | Serves: 2

1 teaspoon dill weed, chopped	½ medium red chili pepper, chopped
1 small onion, peeled and sliced thin	1 cup vegetables / greens
2 garlic cloves, peeled and minced	2 tablespoons olive oil
2 haddock fillets, for almost 4 ounces	1 tablespoon butter
	Salt and black pepper, to taste
	Lime wedges, for garnish

1. In a suitable bowl, mix the olive oil, butter, dill, garlic, onion, chili, salt, and pepper. 2. Pour the prepared mixture into a suitable skillet set over medium heat. 3. When the oil begins to sizzle, add the fish and cook for almost 7-8 minutes per side. 4. Divide the vegetables or greens between two serving plates, top with the fish fillets, garnish with lime wedges, and enjoy.
Per serving: Calories: 350; Total fat 9.5g; Sodium 523mg; Total Carbs 4g; Fiber 1.5g; Sugars 5g; Protein 50.5g

Nutty Kale Tilapia

Prep time: 10 minutes. | Cooking time: 20 minutes. | Serves: 2

2 tilapia fillets. for almost 4 ounces each	½ cup chicken broth
1 teaspoon seafood seasoning	1 tablespoon canola oil
¼ cup pine nuts	Salt and ground black pepper, to taste
1 bunch of kale, chopped	1 tablespoon butter

1. Add the oil and butter to a suitable skillet and set over medium heat. 2. Rub all the fish pieces with the seafood seasoning and place in the hot pan. 3. Let them cook for almost 4-5 minutes per side until light golden brown. 4. Remove them from this pan and cover. 5. In the same pan, toast the pine nuts for almost 4 minutes. 6. Stir in the kale and chicken broth and cook for almost 3-5 minutes until the kale wilts. 7. Season with black pepper and salt. 8. Place this fish on a serving dish along with kale and enjoy.
Per serving: Calories: 211; Total fat 11.2g; Sodium 523mg; Total Carbs 5.5g; Fiber 0.5g; Sugars 0g; Protein 13.3g

Shrimp and Sausage "Bake"

Prep time: 10 minutes. | Cooking time: 20 minutes. | Serves: 4

2 tablespoons olive oil	½ small sweet onion, chopped
6 ounces chorizo sausage, diced	2 teaspoons minced garlic
½ pound (16 to 20 count) shrimp, peeled and deveined	¼ cup herbed chicken stock
1 red bell pepper, chopped	Pinch red pepper flakes

1. Place a suitable skillet over medium-high heat and add the olive oil. 2. Sauté the sausage until it is warmed through, for almost 6 minutes. 3. Add the shrimp and sauté until it is opaque and just cooked through, for almost 4 minutes. 4. Remove the sausage and shrimp to a bowl and keep it aside. 5. Add the red pepper, onion, and garlic to the skillet and sauté until tender, for almost 4 minutes. 6. Add the chicken stock to the skillet along with the cooked sausage and shrimp. 7. Bring the liquid to a simmer and simmer for almost 3 minutes. Stir in the red pepper flakes and serve.
Per serving: Calories: 412; Total fat 20.8g; Sodium 104mg; Total Carbs 3.5g; Fiber 7.9g; Sugars 13.9g; Protein 17.2g

Herb Butter Scallops

Prep time: 10 minutes. | Cooking time: 10 minutes. | Serves: 4

1 pound sea scallops, cleaned	Juice of 1 lemon
Black pepper, freshly ground	2 teaspoons chopped fresh basil
8 tablespoons butter	1 teaspoon chopped fresh thyme
2 teaspoons minced garlic	

1. Pat the sea scallops dry with paper towels and season them lightly with pepper. 2. Place a suitable skillet over medium heat and add 2 tablespoons of butter. 3. Arrange the scallops in the skillet, evenly spaced but not too close, and sear each side until they are golden brown, for almost 2½ minutes per side. 4. Remove the scallops to a plate and keep it aside. 5. Add the remaining 6 tablespoons of butter to the skillet and sauté the garlic until translucent, for almost 3 minutes. 6. Stir in the lemon juice, basil, and thyme and return the scallops to the skillet, turning to coat them in the sauce. Serve immediately.
Per serving: Calories: 370; Total fat 30.2g; Sodium 185mg; Total carbs 2.6g; Fiber 0.9g; Sugars 0.1g; Protein 22.9g

Pan-Seared Halibut with Citrus Butter Sauce

Prep time: 10 minutes. | Cooking time: 15 minutes. | Serves: 4

4 (5-ounce) halibut fillets, each about 1 inch thick	3 tablespoons dry white wine
Sea salt	1 tablespoon freshly squeezed lemon juice
Black pepper, freshly ground	1 tablespoon freshly squeezed orange juice
¼ cup butter	2 teaspoons chopped fresh parsley
2 teaspoons minced garlic	2 tablespoons olive oil
1 shallot, minced	

1. Pat the halibut fish dry with paper towels and then lightly season the fillets with black pepper and salt. Keep it aside on a paper towel–lined plate. 2. Place a suitable saucepan over medium heat and melt the butter. 3. Sauté the garlic and shallot until tender, for almost 3 minutes. 4. Whisk in the white wine, lemon juice, and orange juice and bring the sauce to a simmer, cooking until it thickens slightly, for almost 2 minutes. 5. Remove the sauce from the heat and stir in the parsley; keep it aside. 6. Place a suitable skillet over medium-high heat and add the olive oil. 7. Panfry the fish until lightly browned and just cooked through, turning them over once, for almost 10 minutes in total. 8. Serve the fish immediately with a spoonful of sauce for each.
Per serving: Calories 384; Total Fat 12.5g; Sodium 621mg; Total Carbs 8.3g; Fiber 4.1g; Sugars 7.2g; Protein 10.1g

Citrus Salmon with Zucchini Noodles

Prep time: 10 minutes. | Cooking time: 25 minutes. | Serves: 2

1 fresh lime, juiced and zested	Salt, to taste
1 garlic clove, peeled and minced	2 tablespoons coconut oil, for cooking
2 large salmon fillets	Optional / Garnish
½ teaspoon dried oregano	Fresh thyme sprig
4 medium zucchinis, spiralized	
Essentials	

1. Heat half of the coconut oil in a pan, add the garlic clove and gradually add half the lime juice to achieve a smooth consistency. Finally, add the dried oregano. 2. Place the salmon into a glass baking dish and add the marinade. 3. Coat each salmon fillet with the marinade and cover the dish. 4. Transfer to the refrigerator and allow the salmon to marinate for almost 3 hours. 5. Use a spiralizer, mandolin, or vegetable peeler to create noodles or strips from the zucchini. 6. Preheat your oven to 450°F/232°C. 7. Take the marinated salmon out of the refrigerator, ensure the salmon is skin-side down and spoon more sauce over the top of the salmon. 8. Place the dish in the center of your oven and bake for almost 11-13 minutes. 9. Sauté the zucchini in the remaining coconut oil and lime juice for almost 3-4 minutes, ensuring the noodles receive a good coating of the juices. 10. Divide the zucchini noodles between two plates or bowls and pour the remaining marinade over the top. Place a salmon fillet on top of each plate or bowl of noodles. Add salt to taste and garnish with a fresh thyme sprig to serve.
Per serving: Calories: 418; Total fat 15.3g; Sodium 427mg; Total carbs 2.4g; Fiber 0.5g; Sugars 1.1g; Protein 64g

Simple Fish Curry

Prep time: 10 minutes. | Cooking time: 25 minutes. | Serves: 4

2 tablespoons coconut oil
1½ tablespoons grated fresh ginger
2 teaspoons minced garlic
1 tablespoon curry powder
½ teaspoon ground cumin

2 cups coconut milk
16 ounces firm white fish, cut into 1-inch chunks
1 cup shredded kale
2 tablespoons chopped cilantro

1. Place a suitable saucepan over medium heat and melt the coconut oil. 2. Sauté the ginger and garlic until lightly browned, for almost 2 minutes. 3. Stir in the curry powder and cumin and sauté until very fragrant. for almost 2 minutes. 4. Stir in the coconut milk and bring the liquid to a boil. 5. Now reduce its heat to low and simmer for almost 5 minutes to infuse the milk with the spices. 6. Add the fish and cook until the fish is cooked through, for almost 10 minutes. 7. Stir in the kale and cilantro and simmer until wilted. for almost 2 minutes. Serve.
Per serving: Calories 339; Total Fat 13.1g; Sodium 211mg; Total Carbs 2.6g; Fiber 0.6g; Sugars 0.8g; Protein 49.

Roasted Salmon with Avocado Salsa

Prep time: 10 minutes. | Cooking time: 12 minutes. | Serves: 4

For the salsa
1 avocado, peeled, pitted, and diced
1 scallion, white and green parts, chopped
½ cup halved cherry tomatoes
Juice of 1 lemon
Zest of 1 lemon
For the fish

1 teaspoon ground cumin
½ teaspoon ground coriander
½ teaspoon onion powder
¼ teaspoon sea salt
Pinch black pepper
Pinch cayenne pepper
4 (4-ounce) boneless, skinless salmon fillets
2 tablespoons olive oil

To make the salsa: In a suitable bowl, stir the avocado, scallion, tomatoes, lemon juice, and lemon zest until mixed. Keep it aside.
To make the fish: 1. At 400°F/204°C, preheat your oven. 2. Layer a suitable baking sheet with foil sheet and keep it aside. 3. In a suitable bowl, stir the cumin, coriander, onion powder, salt, black pepper, and cayenne until well mixed. 4. Rub the salmon fillets with the spice mix and place them on the baking sheet. 5. Drizzle the fillets with the olive oil and roast the fish until it is just cooked through, for almost 15 minutes. 6. Serve the salmon with the avocado salsa.
Per serving: Calories 351; Total Fat 20.6g; Sodium 634mg; Total Carbs 5.4g; Fiber 2.1g; Sugars 2.7g; Protein 35.7g

Thyme Mackerel with Tomato Sauce

Prep time: 10 minutes. | Cooking time: 15 minutes. | Serves: 2

2 mackerel fillets, for almost 4 ounces each
1 green onion, chopped
1 (14 ounces) can chopped tomatoes
1 teaspoon light brown sugar
Small bunch of thyme leaves,

chopped
Fresh cilantro, for serving
1 tablespoon canola oil (use olive oil for a paleo version)
Salt and ground black pepper, to taste

1. Add the oil to a suitable skillet and set over medium heat. 2. Add the onion and sauté for almost 4-5 minutes. 3. Add the salt, pepper, and thyme leaves, stir, and add the tomatoes. 4. When the prepared mixture begins to boil, reduce its heat to low, add the sugar, and let it simmer for almost 5 minutes. 5. Add the mackerel fillets to the sauce, cover, and simmer for almost 10 minutes, until the fish is cooked through. 6. Top with cilantro and serve alongside sautéed or steamed vegetables.
Per serving: Calories: 219; Total fat 7.3g; Sodium 178mg; Total Carbs 7.7g; Fiber 0.3g; Sugars 17.3g; Protein 22.4g

Sole Asiago

Prep time: 10 minutes. | Cooking time: 8 minutes. | Serves: 4

4 (4-ounce) sole fillets
¾ cup ground almonds
¼ cup asiago cheese

2 eggs, beaten
2½ tablespoons melted coconut oil

1. At 350°F/177°C, preheat your oven. Layer a suitable baking sheet with parchment paper and keep it aside. 2. Pat the fish dry with paper towels. 3. Stir the ground almonds and cheese in a suitable bowl. 4. Place the bowl with the beaten eggs in it next to the almond mixture. 5. Dredge a sole fillet in the beaten egg and then hit the fish into the almond mixture so it is completely coated. Place on the baking sheet

and repeat until all the fillets are breaded. 6. Brush both sides of each piece of fish with the coconut oil. 7. Bake the sole until it is cooked through, for almost 8 minutes in total. Serve immediately.
Per serving: Calories 386; Total Fat 3.5g; Sodium 911mg; Total Carbs 5.5g; Fiber 9g; Sugars 4.1g; Protein 41.7g

Baked Coconut Haddock

Prep time: 10 minutes. | Cooking time: 12 minutes. | Serves: 4

4 (5-ounce) boneless haddock fillets
Sea salt
Black pepper, freshly ground

1 cup shredded unsweetened coconut
¼ cup ground hazelnuts
2 tablespoons coconut oil, melted

1. At 400°F/204°C, preheat your oven. 2. Layer a suitable baking sheet with parchment paper and keep it aside. 3. Pat the fillets very dry with paper towels and lightly season them with black pepper and salt. 4. Stir the shredded coconut and hazelnuts in a suitable bowl. 5. Dredge the fish fillets in the coconut mixture so that both sides of each piece are thickly coated. 6. Place this fish on the baking sheet and lightly brush both sides of each piece with the coconut oil. 7. Bake the haddock until the topping is golden and the fish flakes easily with a fork, for almost 12 minutes total. Serve.
Per serving: Calories 460; Total Fat 29.7g; Sodium 536mg; Total Carbs 3.1g; Fiber 6.9g; Sugars 4g; Protein 37.7g

Cheesy Garlic Salmon

Prep time: 10 minutes. | Cooking time: 12 minutes. | Serves: 4

½ cup asiago cheese
2 tablespoons freshly squeezed lemon juice
2 tablespoons butter, at room temperature

2 teaspoons minced garlic
1 teaspoon chopped fresh basil
1 teaspoon chopped fresh oregano
4 (5-ounce) salmon fillets
1 tablespoon olive oil

1. At 350°F/177°C, preheat your oven. Layer a suitable baking sheet with parchment paper and keep it aside. 2. In a suitable bowl, stir the asiago cheese, lemon juice, butter, garlic, basil, and oregano. 3. Pat the salmon pieces dry with paper towels and place the fillets on the baking sheet skin-side down. Divide the topping evenly between the fillets and spread it across the fish using a knife or the back of a spoon. 4. Drizzle the fish with the olive oil and bake until the topping is golden and the fish is just cooked through. for almost 12 minutes. Serve.
Per serving: Calories: 342; Total fat: 30g; Sodium: 40mg; Total Carbs: 13g; sugar: 4g; Fiber: 3g; Protein: 7g

Rosemary-Lemon Snapper Baked in Parchment

Prep time: 10 minutes. | Cooking time: 12 minutes. | Serves: 4

1¼ pounds fresh red snapper fillet, cut into two equal pieces
2 lemons, sliced
6 to 8 sprigs fresh rosemary, stems removed

½ cup olive oil, extra-virgin
6 garlic cloves, sliced
1 teaspoon salt
½ teaspoon black pepper

1. At 425°F/218°C, preheat your oven. 2. Place two large sheets of parchment (about twice the size of each piece of fish) on the counter. 3. Place 1 piece of fish in the center of each sheet. Top the fish pieces with lemon slices and rosemary leaves. 4. In a suitable bowl, mix the olive oil, garlic, salt, and pepper. 5. Drizzle the oil over each piece of fish. Top each piece of fish with a second large sheet of parchment and starting on a long side, fold the paper up to about 1 inch from the fish. 6. Repeat on the remaining sides, going in a clockwise direction. 7. Fold in each corner once to secure. 8. Place both parchment pouches on a suitable baking sheet and bake until the fish is cooked through, 10 to 12 minutes.
Per serving: Calories: 379; Total fat: 14g; Sodium: 308mg; Total Carbs: 17g; sugar: 9g; Fiber: 5g; Protein: 43g

Pan-Fried Scallops

Prep time: 10 minutes. | Cooking time: 5 minutes. | Serves: 1

½ tablespoon avocado oil
1 tablespoon butter or ghee

6 ounces scallops, rinsed with cold water and patted dry

1. In a suitable skillet, heat the oil and butter over high heat until it begins to smoke. 2. Generously season the scallops with black pepper and salt. 3. Gently add the scallops to the skillet, making sure they are not touching. 4. Sear the scallops for almost 90 seconds per side. Serve.
Per serving: Calories 416; Total fat 22.1g; Sodium 642mg; Total Carbs 4.2g; Fiber 0.1g; Sugars 12.4g; Protein 40.6g

Sole with Cucumber Radish Salsa

Prep time: 10 minutes. | Cooking time: 8 minutes. | Serves: 4

½ English cucumber, chopped
½ avocado, diced
4 radishes, finely chopped
½ scallion, white and green parts, finely chopped
⅓ cup avocado oil

Juice of ½ lemon
1 teaspoon chopped fresh thyme
Sea salt
Black pepper, freshly ground
4 (3-ounce) sole fillets
½ cup almond flour

1. In a suitable bowl, mix the cucumber, avocado, radish, scallion, 2 tablespoons oil, lemon juice, and thyme. 2. Season with black pepper and salt and keep it aside. Dredge the sole fillets in almond flour. 3. Heat the remaining oil in a suitable skillet over medium-high heat. 4. Panfry the fish until golden, crispy, and cooked through, turning once, for almost 8 minutes total. Serve immediately with the cucumber salsa.
Per serving: Calories: 418; Total fat: 20g; Sodium: 1121mg; Total Carbs: 15g; sugar: 5g; Fiber: 4g; Protein: 45g

Sole Meunière

Prep time: 10 minutes. | Cooking time: 10 minutes. | Serves: 4

4 (4-ounce) sole fillets
Sea salt
Black pepper, freshly ground
½ cup almond flour

½ cup butter
Juice and zest of 3 lemons
½ cup chopped fresh parsley
1 teaspoon fresh chopped thyme

1. Pat the fish almost dry with paper towels, and season both sides with black pepper and salt. 2. On a suitable plate, dredge the sole in the almond flour. 3. In a suitable skillet over medium-high heat, heat 6 tablespoons of butter. 4. Swirl the skillet until the butter starts to foam and brown flecks appear, for almost 1 minute. 5. Reduce its heat to medium-low, and add the fish fillets to the skillet. 6. Fry the fish until browned on both sides, turning once. for almost 6 minutes in total. 7. Remove this fish from the skillet, and transfer them to plates. 8. Stir in the remaining butter, lemon juice, lemon zest, parsley, and thyme. 9. Whisk over the heat for almost 2 minutes, and then serve the fish with the buttery sauce.
Per serving: Calories: 305; Total fat: 14g; Sodium: 812mg; Total Carbs: 8g; sugar: 2g; Fiber: 2g; Protein: 35g

Swordfish in Tarragon-Citrus Butter

Prep time: 10 minutes. | Cooking time: 20 minutes. | Serves: 4

1 pound swordfish steaks, cut into 2-inch pieces
1 teaspoon salt
¼ teaspoon black pepper
¼ cup olive oil, plus 2 tablespoons

2 tablespoons unsalted butter
Zest and juice of 2 clementines
Zest and juice of 1 lemon
2 tablespoons chopped fresh tarragon

1. In a bowl, toss the swordfish with black pepper and salt. 2. In a suitable skillet, heat ¼ cup olive oil over medium-high heat. 3. Add the swordfish chunks to the hot oil and sear on all sides, 2 to 3 minutes per side. 4. Using a slotted spoon, remove the fish from the skillet and keep warm. 5. Add the remaining olive oil and butter to the oil already in the skillet and return the heat to medium-low. 6. Once the butter has melted, whisk in the clementine and lemon zests and juices, along with the tarragon. 7. Season with salt. Return the fish pieces to this pan and toss to coat in the butter sauce.
Per serving: Calories: 399; Total fat: 22g; saturated fat: 10g; cholesterol: 46mg; carbohydrates: 17g; Fiber: 2g; Protein: 21g

Parmesan-Crusted Tilapia with Sautéed Spinach

Prep time: 10 minutes. | Cooking time: 15 minutes. | Serves: 2

½ cup grated parmesan cheese
2 tablespoons almond flour
1 teaspoon paprika
¼ teaspoon salt
⅛ teaspoon black pepper, freshly ground

2 tilapia fillets
2 tablespoons olive oil
1½ cups spinach
½ teaspoon garlic powder
1 tablespoon chopped fresh parsley

1. At 400°F/204°C, preheat your oven. 2. In a suitable bowl, mix the parmesan cheese, almond flour, paprika, salt, and pepper. 3. Place the tilapia fillets on a plate and drizzle with 1 tablespoon of olive oil. 4. Massage the oil into the fish, and then dredge them in the parmesan mix, coating thoroughly. 5. Layer a baking dish with foil sheet. 6. Place the fillets inside. Put the dish in the preheated oven and bake for almost 10 to 15 minutes, depending on the thickness of the fillets. 7.

While the fillets are cooking, add the remaining tablespoon of olive oil to a suitable skillet and heat over medium-high heat. 8. Add the spinach and sauté until tender, for almost 6 minutes. Add the garlic powder. 9. Cover, and reduce its heat to medium-low. Cook for almost 3 to 5 minutes. 10. Remove the baking dish from your oven. Check the fillets for doneness. 11. Plate the spinach with the fillets on top and serve immediately, garnished with the parsley.
Per serving: Calories: 379; Total fat: 27g; saturated fat: 14g; cholesterol: 107mg; carbohydrates: 18g; Fiber: 5g; Protein: 18g

Brown Butter–Lime Tilapia

Prep time: 10 minutes. | Cooking time: 15 minutes. | Serves: 4

½ cup unsalted butter
¼ cup chopped fresh dill
Juice of 1 lime
4 (4-ounce) tilapia fillets

Sea salt
Black pepper, freshly ground
4 teaspoons coconut oil

1. In a suitable saucepan over medium-high heat, heat the butter until it starts to foam up and fizz. 2. Swirl the saucepan until tiny brown specks form and the butter smells nutty, for almost 1 minute. 3. Remove from the heat, and keep it aside. 4. In your high-speed blender, purée the dill and lime juice until a paste forms. 5. Slowly pour the brown butter into the blender while it is running until an emulsified sauce forms and all the butter is used. 6. Rinse the tilapia fillets, and pat them dry with paper towels. 7. Season this fish lightly with black pepper and salt on both sides. 8. In a suitable skillet over medium-high heat, heat the coconut oil. 9. Brown the fish on both sides, turning once, for almost 10 minutes total. 10. Serve with the brown butter sauce.
Per serving: Calories: 583; Total fat: 50g; saturated fat: 17g; cholesterol: 200mg; carbohydrates: 14g; Fiber: 8g; Protein: 25g

Pan-Fried Tilapia

Prep time: 10 minutes. | Cooking time: 25 minutes. | Serves: 6

6 large tilapia fillets
½ teaspoon salt
½ teaspoon black pepper, freshly ground

2 tablespoons olive oil
½ cup oat fiber or coconut flour
3 tablespoons butter
2 garlic cloves, minced

1. Preheat your oven to 250°F/121°C or its lowest temperature. 2. Layer a suitable baking sheet with paper towels. Season the fillets on both sides with the black pepper and salt. 3. In a suitable skillet over medium-high heat, heat the olive oil. 4. Pour the oat fiber onto a shallow plate. 5. Dredge the fillets in the oat fiber, covering both sides, and shake to remove the excess. 6. Add the fillets to this pan, 1 or 2 at a time so they're not crowded. 7. Pan-fry for almost 3 to 4 minutes per side or until the fish flakes easily with a fork. 8. Use a spatula to transfer the cooked fish to the baking sheet and place in your oven to keep warm while you fry the remaining fillets. 9. Turn the heat under the skillet to low, wipe out any excess oil, and add the butter and garlic. 10. Stir until the butter is melted and the garlic is fragrant, 1 to 2 minutes. 11. Serve the fish with the garlic butter spooned over the top.
Per serving: Calories: 363; Total fat: 17g; saturated fat: 3g; cholesterol: 62mg; carbohydrates: 25g; Fiber: 6g; Protein: 27g

Classic Crab Cakes

Prep time: 10 minutes. | Cooking time: 10 minutes. | Serves: 6

1 large egg, separated
½ cup avocado oil mayonnaise
1 tablespoon Dijon mustard
1 teaspoon old bay seasoning
1 teaspoon dried parsley

1 pound jumbo lump crab meat, picked over for shell pieces
⅓ cup crushed pork rinds
2 tablespoons avocado oil
Lemon wedges, for serving

1. Layer a suitable baking sheet with parchment paper. 2. In a suitable bowl, whisk the egg yolk, mayonnaise, mustard, old bay seasoning, and parsley until well combined. 3. Gently fold in the crabmeat. 4. In a suitable bowl, beat the egg white until soft peaks form. 5. Gently fold the egg whites into the crab mixture, keeping as many large lumps of crab meat as possible. 6. Gently fold in the pork rinds. Divide the prepared crab mixture into 6 equal portions and form into patties. 7. Place the patties on the prepared baking sheet and refrigerate for almost 15 minutes. 8. Heat 1 tablespoon of avocado oil in a suitable skillet over medium heat. 9. Place 3 crab cakes in the skillet and cook for almost 3 to 4 minutes per side, just until golden and cooked through. 10. Repeat with the remaining tablespoon of avocado oil and 3 crab cakes. Serve immediately with lemon wedges (if using).
Per serving: Calories: 255; Total fat: 14g; Sodium: 210mg; Total Carbs: 0g; sugar: 0g; Fiber: 0g; Protein: 33g

Parmesan Baked Tilapia

Prep time: 10 minutes. | Cooking time: 15 minutes. | Serves: 4

¼ cup butter, melted
2 teaspoons garlic salt
1 teaspoon black pepper, freshly ground

4 (4-ounce) tilapia fillets, patted dry
4 ounces grated parmesan cheese
4 ounces crushed pork rinds

1. At 400°F/204°C, preheat your oven. 2. Layer a suitable baking sheet with parchment paper and keep it aside. 3. In a suitable bowl, mix the melted butter, garlic salt, and pepper. 4. Place the tilapia fillets on the prepared baking sheet, then drizzle or brush the butter mixture across each fillet. 5. Sprinkle each fillet with parmesan cheese and crushed pork rinds. 6. Bake for almost 13 minutes, and then turn your oven up to broil and broil for almost 2 more minutes.
Per serving: Calories: 214; Total fat: 15g; saturated fat: 2g; cholesterol: 68mg; carbohydrates: 11g; Fiber: 4g; Protein: 10g

Cream-Poached Trout

Prep time: 10 minutes. | Cooking time: 20 minutes. | Serves: 4

4 (4-ounce) skinless trout fillets
Sea salt
Black pepper, freshly ground
3 tablespoons butter
1 teaspoon chopped fresh parsley, for garnish

1 leek, white and green parts, halved lengthwise, sliced, and thoroughly washed
1 teaspoon minced garlic
1 cup heavy (whipping) cream
Juice of 1 lemon

1. At 400°F/204°C, preheat your oven. 2. Pat the trout fillets dry with paper towels and lightly season with black pepper and salt. 3. Place them in a 9-inch-square baking dish in one layer. Keep it aside. 4. Place a suitable saucepan over medium-high heat and melt the butter. 5. Sauté the leek and garlic until softened, for almost 6 minutes. 6. Add the heavy cream and lemon juice to the saucepan and cook to a boil, whisking. 7. Pour the sauce over the fish and bake until the fish is just cooked through, for 10 to 12 minutes. Serve topped with the parsley.
Per serving: Calories: 383; Total fat: 19g; saturated fat: 3g; cholesterol: 64mg; carbohydrates: 26g; Fiber: 1g; Protein: 21g

Rainbow Trout with Cream Leek Sauce

Prep time: 10 minutes. | Cooking time: 17 minutes. | Serves: 4

2 tablespoons olive oil
2 leeks, white and light green parts, sliced and thoroughly washed
1½ cups canned coconut milk

4 (3-ounce) rainbow trout fillets
2 teaspoons chopped fresh thyme
Sea salt
Black pepper, freshly ground

1. Heat the olive oil in a suitable skillet over medium-high heat. 2. Add the leeks and sauté until they are tender, for almost 7 minutes. 3. Stir in the coconut milk and bring the prepared mixture to a boil. 4. Place the trout in one layer in the liquid and reduce its heat to medium. 5. Simmer until the fish is just cooked through, for almost 10 minutes. 6. Remove the fillets and place onto 4 plates. Mix the thyme into the leek cream sauce. 7. Season the sauce with black pepper and salt. Spoon the leek sauce over the trout and serve.
Per serving: Calories: 279; Total fat: 20g; saturated fat: 15g; cholesterol: 258mg; carbohydrates: 6g; Fiber: 3g; Protein: 19g

Roasted Trout with Swiss Chard

Prep time: 10 minutes. | Cooking time: 15 minutes. | Serves: 4

1 teaspoon salt
½ teaspoon black pepper
4 (8-ounce) trout, cleaned
4 fresh dill sprigs
4 fresh fennel sprigs
2 pounds Swiss chard, cleaned

and leaves separated from stems
¼ cup olive oil
¼ cup butter
1 lemon, quartered
¼ cup dry vermouth, or white wine

1. At 450°F/232°C, preheat your oven. 2. Using ½ teaspoon of salt and ¼ teaspoon of pepper, season the insides of the trout. 3. Place 1 dill sprig and 1 fennel sprig inside each trout. 4. Cut the Swiss chard stems into 2-inch pieces. 5. Cut the leaves crosswise into 1½-inch strips. 6. Cut four large pieces of foil sheet into oval shapes large enough to fit one trout and one-quarter of the Swiss chard, with room enough to be sealed. 7. Using ¾ tablespoon of olive oil, brush the trout. 8. Place one trout in the center of each piece of foil. 9. Top each trout with one-quarter of the Swiss chard. 10. Season the trout with the remaining ½ teaspoon of salt, ¼ teaspoon of pepper, and 3¼ tablespoons of olive oil. 11. Top each trout with 1 tablespoon of butter. 12. Squeeze a lemon quarter over each Swiss chard and trout bundle. 13. Spoon 1 tablespoon of vermouth over each. Close and seal the foil pouches tightly. 14. Place the foil packets on a suitable baking sheet. 15. Bake for almost 10 to 12 minutes, depending on the thickness of the fish. 16. Remove from your oven and allow the packets to cool for almost 1 to 2 minutes before opening. Serve in the foil packet.
Per serving: Calories: 250; Total fat: 9g; saturated fat: 5g; cholesterol: 68mg; carbohydrates: 4g; Fiber: 2g; Protein: 38g

"Spaghetti" with Clams

Prep time: 10 minutes. | Cooking time: 10 minutes. | Serves: 2

1 tablespoon olive oil
1 garlic clove, minced
½ cup chicken broth
2 large zucchinis, spiralized
Salt
Black pepper

1 (6 ounces) can clams, drained and minced
Juice of ½ lemon
2 tablespoons chopped fresh parsley, for garnish

1. In a suitable skillet over medium heat, heat the olive oil. 2. Add garlic and sauté for just under 1 minute. 3. Pour in the chicken stock and bring to a simmer. 4. Add the zucchini noodles and gently toss to combine. 5. Taste and season with black pepper and salt. Stir in the clams and lemon juice. 6. Toss again to mix and cook for almost 2 to 3 minutes to warm through. 7. Serve immediately topped with fresh parsley.
Per serving: Calories: 535; Total fat: 21g; Sodium: 1144mg; Total Carbs: 24g; sugar: 12g; Fiber: 9g; Protein: 62g

Crab Cakes with Green Goddess Dressing

Prep time: 10 minutes. | Cooking time: 17 minutes. | Serves: 4

5 tablespoons avocado oil
½ red bell pepper, finely chopped
1 scallion, white and green parts, finely chopped
¼ jalapeño pepper, finely chopped
¾ pound real crab meat, shredded

¼ cup almond meal
1 egg
1 teaspoon Dijon mustard
Sea salt
Black pepper, freshly ground
½ cup green goddess dressing

1. Heat 2 tablespoons of avocado oil in a suitable skillet over medium-high heat. 2. Sauté the bell pepper, scallion, and jalapeño until softened, for almost 5 minutes. 3. Transfer the cooked vegetables to a suitable bowl and add the crab, almond meal, egg, and mustard, mixing until the ingredients are well combined and hold. 4. Form the crab mixture into 12 patties and place them on a plate, cover with plastic wrap, and chill in the refrigerator to firm for up to 1 hour. 5. Wipe the skillet out and heat the remaining oil over medium-high heat. 6. Panfry the crab cakes until cooked through, for almost 12 minutes per side, turning once. 7. Season with black pepper and salt and top the crab cakes with the dressing and serve.
Per serving: Calories: 345; Total fat: 16g; Sodium: 424mg; Total carbs: 10g; sugar: 3g; Fiber: 1g; Protein: 40g

Crab au Gratin

Prep time: 10 minutes. | Cooking time: 35 minutes. | Serves: 4

½ cup (1 stick) butter
1 (8-ounce) container crab claw meat
2 ounces cream cheese
½ cup heavy (whipping) cream
2 tablespoons freshly squeezed lemon juice
1 tablespoon white wine vinegar

1 teaspoon pink Himalayan sea salt
½ teaspoon black pepper, freshly ground
½ teaspoon onion powder
1 cup shredded cheddar cheese
1 (12-ounce) package cauliflower rice, cooked and drained

1. At 350°F/177°C, preheat your oven. 2. In a suitable sauté pan or skillet, melt the butter over medium heat. 3. Add the crab and cook until warmed through. 4. Add the cream cheese, cream, lemon juice, vinegar, salt, pepper, and onion powder. 5. Keep stirring until the cream cheese fully melts into the sauce. 6. Add ½ cup of cheddar cheese and stir it into the sauce. 7. Spread the cauliflower rice on the bottom of an 8-inch square baking dish. 8. Pour the crab and sauce over, then sprinkle with the remaining ½ cup of cheddar cheese. 9. Bake for almost 25 to 30 minutes, until the sauce is bubbling. Turn the broiler on to high. 10. Broil for an additional 2 to 3 minutes, until the cheese topping is slightly browned. 11. Allow to cool for almost 5 to 10 minutes, then serve.
Per serving: Calories: 338; Total fat 15.7g; Sodium 908mg; Total carbs 8.4g; Fiber 0.8g; Sugars 2.8g; Protein 40.1g

Crab-Stuffed Portabella Mushrooms

Prep time: 10 minutes. | Cooking time: 20 minutes. | Serves: 4

8 portabella mushroom caps	4 scallions, chopped
Nonstick cooking spray	2 tablespoons chopped fresh
4 (6 ounces) cans crabmeat,	parsley
drained	Salt
8 ounces cream cheese	Black pepper, freshly ground
¼ cup sour cream	

1. At 375°F/191°C, preheat your oven. 2. Layer a suitable baking sheet with aluminum sheet. 3. Place the mushrooms on the prepared baking sheet, stem-side up, and coat with cooking spray. 4. Bake for almost 15 minutes. Meanwhile, in a suitable bowl, mix the crab, cream cheese, sour cream, scallions, and parsley. 5. Stir well and season with black pepper and salt to taste. Remove the mushrooms from your oven and pat dry with paper towels. 6. Return to the baking sheet, stem-side up, and divide the crab mixture evenly among them. 7. Return to your oven and bake for almost 5 minutes, or until the crab is warmed through.
Per serving: Calories: 281; Total fat 10.6g; Sodium 929mg; Total carbs 4.3g; Fiber 0.6g; Sugars 0.5g; Protein 40.4g

Sea Scallops with Bacon Cream Sauce

Prep time: 10 minutes. | Cooking time: 20 minutes. | Serves: 4

6 bacon slices, chopped	1 tablespoon olive oil
½ small onion, chopped fine	1 pound sea scallops, washed,
1 teaspoon minced garlic	cleaned, and dried thoroughly
¼ cup dry white wine	Sea salt
1 cup heavy (whipping) cream	Black pepper, freshly ground
1 teaspoon chopped fresh thyme	

1. In a saucepan over medium-high heat, cook the bacon, stirring, until it is crispy, for almost 5 minutes then transfer to a plate. 2. Sauté the onions and garlic in the bacon fat until softened, for almost 3 minutes. 3. Add the white wine, and deglaze the saucepan, stirring to scrape up the browned bits from the bottom. 4. Whisk in the heavy cream and reserved bacon, and bring the prepared mixture to a simmer. 5. Simmer until the sauce thickens, for almost 5 minutes. Remove the sauce from the heat, and stir in the thyme. 6. Keep it aside. In a suitable nonstick skillet over medium-high heat, heat the olive oil. 7. Season the scallops with black pepper and salt. Cook the scallops undisturbed until the bottoms are browned and crisped, for almost 3 minutes. 8. Using tongs, carefully turn the scallops, and sear the other side until they are also browned and crisped, 3 minutes longer. 9. Transfer the seared scallops to a plate, and serve with the sauce.
Per serving: Calories: 499; Total fat 9.5g; Sodium 545mg; Total Carbs 4.2g; Fiber 15.4g; Sugars 2.2g; Protein 41.8g

Pan-Seared Butter Scallops

Prep time: 10 minutes. | Cooking time: 5 minutes. | Serves: 4

¼ cup butter	Black pepper, freshly ground
2 tablespoons olive oil	2 teaspoons chopped garlic
1 pound large scallops	¼ cup chopped fresh parsley
Sea salt	

1. Heat a suitable skillet over high heat. Melt the butter and add the olive oil. 2. Pat the large scallops dry with paper towels and season generously with black pepper and salt. 3. When the butter and oil are hot, place the scallops in this pan, being sure not to crowd them. 4. Tilt this pan slightly and pick up a spoonful of the melted butter. Drizzle this over the scallops as they cook. 5. Sear for almost 2 minutes on the first side. 6. Carefully flip and sear on the second side for almost 2 more minutes, or until the scallops are cooked through and opaque in the center. 7. During the last minute of cooking, add the garlic and parsley, and spoon the flavored oil and butter over the scallops.
Per serving: Calories: 393; Total fat 20g; Sodium 718mg; Total carbs 8g; Fiber 2.2g; Sugars 3.2g; Protein 44.1g

Bacon-Wrapped Scallops and Broccolini

Prep time: 10 minutes. | Cooking time: 15 minutes. | Serves: 3

5 bacon slices	15 broccolini pieces
1 pound scallops (about 10)	1 teaspoon minced garlic
½ teaspoon salt	2 tablespoons dry white wine
¼ teaspoon black pepper	2 teaspoons olive oil
¼ cup (½ stick) butter	

1. Cut the bacon slices in half crosswise, creating 10 small slices. Wrap one slice around each scallop, securing with a toothpick. 2. Season with ¼ teaspoon of salt and ⅛ teaspoon of pepper. 3. Heat a suitable skillet over medium-high heat. Add 3 tablespoons of butter and heat for almost 2 minutes. 4. Add the broccolini, garlic, and wine. Sauté for almost 2 minutes. 5. Cover and reduce its heat to medium-low. Heat a suitable skillet over medium-high heat. 6. Add the remaining tablespoon of butter and the olive oil and heat for almost 2 minutes. 7. Increase the heat under the large skillet to high. Add the scallops. 8. Sear for almost 1½ minutes per side. Roll the scallops onto their sides so the bacon crisps. 9. Cook for almost 1 minute per side. Check the broccolini for doneness. 10. Season with the remaining ¼ teaspoon of salt and ⅛ teaspoon of pepper. 11. Plate immediately with the scallops, saucing with any excess garlic butter from this pan.
Per serving: Calories: 562; Total fat 2.9g; Sodium 19mg; Total carbs 4.7g; Fiber 18.4g; Sugars 8.2g; Protein 19.9g

Sesame-Crusted Tuna with Sweet Chili Vinaigrette

Prep time: 10 minutes. | Cooking time: 5 minutes. | Serves: 4

1 tablespoon Thai chili sauce,	2 tablespoons toasted sesame oil
such as sambal	Sea salt
1 tablespoon rice wine vinegar	Black pepper, freshly ground
¼ cup light olive oil or canola oil	½ cup sesame seeds
4 to 6 drops liquid stevia	4 packed cups mixed spring
4 (6 ounces) ahi tuna steaks	greens

1. In a suitable bowl, mix the chili sauce, vinegar, oil, and stevia. 2. Preheat a suitable skillet over medium-high heat. 3. Pat the tuna dry with paper towels. 4. Coat each side of the steaks with the sesame oil, and season with the black pepper and salt. 5. Spread the sesame seeds in a shallow dish. 6. Press the tuna steaks into the seeds to coat them on both sides. 7. Immediately place the tuna steaks into the hot skillet. 8. Sear per side for almost 1½ minutes for rare. 9. Divide the greens among the serving plates and drizzle each salad with the chili vinaigrette. Transfer the tuna to a cutting board and slice each steak on an angle into ½-inch pieces. It will still be dark and barely warm in the center. Place equal portions of the tuna on each serving plate.
Per serving: Calories: 221; Total fat: 6g; Sodium: 637mg; Total Carbs: 12g; sugar: 3g; Fiber: 2g; Protein: 32g

Crab Cakes with Spicy Tartar Sauce

Prep time: 10 minutes. | Cooking time: 25 minutes. | Serves: 8

For the spicy tartar sauce	lemon juice
½ cup mayonnaise	1 tablespoon whole-grain mustard
1 small garlic clove, grated	1½ teaspoons old bay seasoning
2 teaspoons whole-grain mustard	1 teaspoon gluten-free
1½ teaspoons freshly squeezed	Worcestershire sauce
lemon juice	¼ teaspoon black pepper
1 teaspoon dill relish	2 or 3 dashes hot sauce
½ teaspoon gluten-free	Pinch kosher salt
Worcestershire sauce	1 pound lump crabmeat
¼ teaspoon paprika	3 tablespoons sliced scallion
¼ teaspoon kosher salt	2 tablespoons chopped fresh
2 or 3 dashes hot sauce	parsley
⅛ teaspoon cayenne pepper	1 egg, lightly beaten
For the crab cakes	3½ tablespoons coconut flour
3 tablespoons mayonnaise	¼ cup butter
1 tablespoon freshly squeezed	Lemon wedges, for serving

1. In a suitable bowl, mix the mayonnaise, garlic, mustard, lemon juice, relish, Worcestershire sauce, paprika, salt, and hot sauce. 2. Add cayenne to taste and stir to combine. 3. Refrigerate while preparing the crab cakes. 4. In a suitable bowl, mix the mayonnaise, lemon juice, mustard, old bay seasoning, Worcestershire sauce, black pepper, hot sauce, and salt. 5. Add the crab, scallion, and parsley, and gently toss to coat in the mayonnaise mixture. 6. Gently stir in the egg and coconut flour. Let rest for almost 5 minutes. 7. Divide the crab mixture into 8 portions and form each into a patty about ½-inch thick. 8. In a suitable sauté pan or skillet over medium heat, melt 2 tablespoons of butter. 9. Place 2 or 3 crab cakes in this pan and cook for almost 3 to 4 minutes per side, or until golden. Repeat with the remaining patties. 10. Serve with lemon wedges for squeezing and spicy tartar sauce.
Per Serving: Calories 200; Fat 14.3g; Sodium 657mg; Carbs 4.9g; Fiber 0.9g; Sugar 0.8g; Protein 13g

Seared Tuna with Steamed Turnips, Broccoli, and Green Beans

Prep time: 10 minutes. | Cooking time: 20 minutes. | Serves: 4

1 large turnip, peeled and cut into 1-inch cubes	Black pepper, freshly ground
10 ounces broccoli florets	½ teaspoon onion powder
1 pound green beans, trimmed	½ teaspoon garlic powder
Salt	4 (6 ounces) tuna steaks
	2 tablespoons olive oil

1. Fill a suitable saucepan with about 1 inch of water and place it over medium heat. 2. Insert a steamer basket. Place the turnip in the basket. 3. Place the broccoli on top of the turnip and the green beans on the top of the broccoli. 4. Cover and cook for almost 10 to 15 minutes, until the vegetables are tender. 5. Season with black pepper and salt. Meanwhile, in a suitable dish, mix the onion powder, garlic powder, and 1 teaspoon pepper. 6. Hit the tuna steaks into the spice mixture, coating both sides in a suitable skillet, heat the oil over medium-high heat. 7. Cook the tuna for almost 3 to 4 minutes per side for medium-rare (internal temperature of 115 degrees F, slightly pink in the center) or longer to desired doneness. 8. Transfer the tuna to serving plates with the vegetables.

Per serving: Calories: 450; Total fat: 6g; Sodium: 1251mg; Total Carbs: 51g; sugar: 7g; Fiber: 19g; Protein: 51g

Tuna Casserole

Prep time: 10 minutes. | Cooking time: 40 minutes. | Serves: 6

3 cups zucchini noodles	2 (6-ounces) cans solid white albacore tuna in water, drained
1½ teaspoons salt	½ cup avocado oil mayonnaise
Cooking spray	2 teaspoons Dijon mustard
1 tablespoon avocado oil	1 teaspoon freshly squeezed lemon juice
¼ cup diced white onion	
½ cup sliced baby portabella mushroom caps	½ cup shredded cheddar cheese
1 garlic clove, minced	½ cup shredded mozzarella cheese
¼ teaspoon black pepper	

1. Lay paper towels on top of a suitable baking sheet. 2. Spread the zoodles onto the paper towels, sprinkle with 1 teaspoon salt, and cover with another layer of paper towels. 3. Lightly press down on the zoodles to draw out the water. 4. Allow the zoodles to sit, covered in paper towels, and keep it aside. 5. At 350°F/177°C, preheat your oven. 6. Spray a 9-by-13-inch casserole dish with cooking spray. 7. In a suitable skillet over medium heat, warm the avocado oil. 8. Add the onion and mushrooms and cook, stirring frequently, for almost 4 to 5 minutes or until the onion becomes translucent and the mushrooms begin to brown. 9. Stir in the garlic and cook for almost 1 more minute. 10. Add the zoodles, remaining ½ teaspoon of salt, and the pepper. 11. Cook, stirring frequently, for almost 3 more minutes. The zoodles should be cooked but still al dente. 12. Remove from the heat. In a suitable bowl, use a fork to mix the tuna, mayonnaise, mustard, and lemon juice until well combined. 13. Add the cooked vegetables and stir to coat. Pour the prepared mixture into the prepared dish. 14. Cover with the cheddar and mozzarella. 15. Bake for almost 25 to 30 minutes or until the cheese is golden and bubbly. 16. Let the casserole sit for almost 2 to 3 minutes.

Per serving: Calories: 395; Total fat: 22g; Sodium: 649mg; Total Carbs: 7g; sugar: 0g; Fiber: 3g; Protein: 45g

Tuna Slow-Cooked in Olive Oil

Prep time: 10 minutes. | Cooking time: 45 minutes. | Serves: 4

1 cup olive oil, plus more if needed	2 (2-inch) strips lemon zest
4 (3- to 4-inch) sprigs fresh rosemary	1 teaspoon salt
	½ teaspoon black pepper
8 (3- to 4-inch) sprigs fresh thyme	1 pound fresh tuna steaks (about 1 inch thick)
2 large garlic cloves, sliced	

1. Mix the olive oil, rosemary, thyme, garlic, lemon zest, salt, and pepper over medium-low heat and cook until warm and fragrant, 25 minutes. 2. Remove it from the heat and allow to cool for almost 25 to 30 minutes, until warm but not hot. 3. Add the tuna to the bottom of this pan, adding additional oil if needed so that tuna is fully submerged, and return to medium-low heat. 4. Cook for almost 5 to 10 minutes, or until the oil heats back up and is warm and fragrant but not smoking. 5. Remove this pot from the heat and let the tuna cook in warm oil for almost 4 to 5 minutes, to your desired level of doneness. 6. For a tuna that is rare in the center, cook for almost 2 to 3 minutes. 7. Remove from the oil and serve warm, drizzling 2 to 3 tablespoons

seasoned oil over the tuna. 8. When both have cooled, remove the herb stems with a slotted spoon and pour the cooking oil over the tuna.

Per serving: Calories: 408; Total fat: 16g; Sodium: 858mg; Total Carbs: 7g; sugar: 4g; Fiber: 1g; Protein: 60g

Crab Cakes with Cilantro Crema

Prep time: 10 minutes. | Cooking time: 18 minutes. | Serves: 4

¼ cup almond flour	over for shells
1 egg, whisked	1 tablespoon coconut oil
1 scallion, minced	½ cup sour cream
1 garlic clove, minced	½ cup mayonnaise
½ teaspoon sea salt	1 tablespoon freshly squeezed lime juice
Pinch cayenne pepper	
1 pound lump crabmeat, picked	2 tablespoons minced cilantro

1. At 375°F/191°C, preheat your oven. 2. Layer a suitable baking sheet with parchment paper. 3. In a suitable bowl, whisk the almond flour, egg, scallion, garlic, sea salt, and cayenne pepper. 4. Fold in the crabmeat. Divide the prepared mixture into 8 cakes and place them on the baking sheet. 5. Brush with the oil. Bake for almost 15 to 18 minutes until the cakes are gently browned and set. 6. While the crab cakes bake, whisk the sour cream, mayonnaise, lime juice, and cilantro in a jar to make the cilantro crema. 7. Serve alongside the crab cakes.

Per serving: Calories: 288; Total fat: 14g; Sodium: 692mg; Total Carbs: 8g; sugar: 1g; Fiber: 2g; Protein: 34g

Spicy Crab Cakes

Prep time: 10 minutes. | Cooking time: 20 minutes. | Serves: 4

1 pound crab	1 teaspoon Dijon mustard
½ cup almond flour, plus additional for dusting	1 teaspoon Worcestershire sauce
½ red bell pepper, minced	1 teaspoon chopped fresh dill
¼ cup mayonnaise	Splash tabasco sauce
3 tablespoons minced red onion	3 tablespoons olive oil, extra-virgin

1. In a suitable bowl, mix the crab, almond flour, red pepper, mayonnaise, red onion, Dijon mustard, Worcestershire sauce, dill, and tabasco sauce until the prepared mixture holds when pressed. 2. Form the crab mixture into 12 patties, and refrigerate them on a plate, covered, for almost 1 hour. 3. Dust with additional almond flour. In a suitable skillet over medium-high heat, heat the olive oil. 4. Cook the crab cakes in batches, until golden brown and heated through. for almost 10 minutes per side. Serve.

Per serving: Calories: 396; Total fat: 16g; Sodium: 395mg; Total Carbs: 36g; sugar: 4g; Fiber: 6g; Protein: 30g

Crab Cakes with Garlic Aioli

Prep time: 10 minutes. | Cooking time: 15 minutes. | Serves: 4

For the crab cakes	¼ teaspoon salt
½ pound jumbo lump crabmeat	¼ teaspoon black pepper
½ pound lump crabmeat	1 cup shredded parmesan cheese
¼ cup mayonnaise	3 tablespoons butter
1 large egg, beaten	For the aioli
¼ cup coconut flour	2 teaspoons minced garlic
1 teaspoon mustard	1 tablespoon freshly squeezed lemon juice
1 teaspoon seafood seasoning	
¼ teaspoon paprika	1 large egg
1 teaspoon minced garlic	½ teaspoon salt
¼ cup finely chopped onion	⅛ teaspoon black pepper, freshly ground
¼ cup finely chopped bell pepper	
1 tablespoon finely chopped fresh parsley	½ cup olive oil

1. In a suitable bowl, mix the jumbo lump crabmeat, lump crabmeat, mayonnaise, egg, coconut flour, mustard, seafood seasoning, paprika, garlic, onion, bell pepper, parsley, salt, and pepper. 2. Mix well. Mix in the parmesan cheese. Divide the crabmeat mixture into six equal portions. 3. Form each into a patty. Refrigerate to firm up while making the aioli. 4. In a food processor, mix the garlic and lemon juice until smooth. 5. Add the egg, salt, and pepper. Purée, while slowly adding the olive oil until the aioli forms. 6. Heat a suitable skillet over medium-high heat. Add the butter. 7. Cook for almost 1 minute. Gently add the crab cakes to this pan. 8. Cook for almost 7 minutes, being careful not to burn the butter. 9. Reduce its heat to medium. Flip the cakes. Cook for almost 5 to 7 minutes more, or until done. 10. Transfer the crab cakes to paper towels to drain. 11. Serve immediately with half of the aioli.

Per serving: Calories: 385; Total fat: 19g; Sodium: 762mg; Total Carbs: 20g; sugar: 17g; Fiber: 3g; Protein: 35g

Coconut Saffron Mussels

Prep time: 10 minutes. | Cooking time: 12 minutes. | Serves: 4

¼ cup low-sodium vegetable or chicken stock
Pinch saffron
3 tablespoons coconut oil
1 scallion, white and green parts, sliced
2 teaspoons minced garlic
1 teaspoon peeled, grated fresh ginger
1 cup canned coconut milk
Juice and zest of 1 lime
1½ pounds fresh mussels, scrubbed and debearded
2 tablespoons chopped fresh cilantro

1. Put the stock in a suitable bowl and sprinkle in the saffron. Keep it aside for almost 15 minutes. 2. Heat the oil in a suitable skillet and sauté the scallions, garlic, and ginger until softened, for almost 3 minutes. 3. Stir in the coconut milk, saffron and liquid, lime juice, and lime zest and cook to a boil. 4. Toss in the mussels, cover, and steam until the shells are open. for almost 8 minutes. 5. Discard any unopened shells and take the skillet off the heat. Stir in the cilantro. Serve immediately with the sauce.
Per serving: Calories: 474; Total fat 25.6g; Sodium 430mg; Total carbs 1.5g; Fiber 0.5g; Sugars 0.3g; Protein 61.1g

Spicy Italian Sausage and Mussels

Prep time: 10 minutes. | Cooking time: 20 minutes. | Serves: 4

2 tablespoons olive oil, extra-virgin
8 ounces spicy Italian sausage, casings removed
1 medium onion, halved and sliced
4 garlic cloves, smashed
½ cup dry red wine
2 tablespoons tomato paste
1 cup chicken bone broth or low-sodium chicken broth
2 pounds fresh mussels, scrubbed and debearded
Sea salt
Black pepper, freshly ground
2 tablespoons cold butter, cut into pieces

1. Preheat the oil in a suitable pot over medium heat. 2. Cook the sausage and onion for almost 7 to 8 minutes, until the sausage is gently browned and the onion begins to soften. 3. Add the garlic and cook for almost 30 seconds. 4. Add the wine and tomato paste and scrape this pan with a wooden spoon to remove the bits stuck to the bottom. Simmer for almost 2 minutes to burn off some of the alcohol. 5. Add the chicken broth and the mussels to the pot. Season with black pepper and salt. 6. Toss well, cover, and steam for almost 8 to 10 minutes. 7. Remove cooked mussels, vegetables, and sausage to a serving dish. 8. Return the pot to the stove and simmer the cooking liquid until reduced to about 1 cup. 9. Whisk in the butter 1 tablespoon at a time. 10. Pour the broth over the mussels, vegetables, and sausage.
Per serving: Calories: 304; Total fat 5.9g; Sodium 619mg; Total carbs 7.4g; Fiber 0g; Sugars 0g; Protein 52.3g

Steamed Mussels with Garlic and Thyme

Prep time: 10 minutes. | Cooking time: 20 minutes. | Serves: 8

4 pounds mussels, cleaned, scrubbed, and debearded
½ cup butter
3 tablespoons olive oil
½ cup diced onion
4 garlic cloves, minced
½ cup diced tomato
1 tablespoon fresh thyme
½ cup white wine
1 cup chicken or seafood broth
2 tablespoons freshly squeezed lemon juice
½ teaspoon salt
¼ teaspoon black pepper, freshly ground

1. Place the cleaned mussels in a suitable bowl. Cover with cool water. Keep it aside. 2. In a suitable, heavy pot over medium heat, heat the butter and olive oil for almost 1 minute. 3. Add the onions. Cook for almost 3 to 5 minutes, until translucent. 4. Add the garlic and cook for almost 1 to 2 minutes more. 5. Add the tomato, thyme, white wine, broth, lemon juice, salt, and pepper. 6. Increase the heat and bring the prepared mixture to a boil. Add the mussels and cover the pot. 7. Cook for almost 8 to 10 minutes, shaking the pot at various intervals to allow the mussels to cook evenly. 8. Pour the steaming mussels into a bowl. Discard any that are unopened. Serve immediately.
Per serving: Calories: 454; Total fat 22.8g; Sodium 373mg; Total carbs 2.2g; Fiber 1.2g; Sugars 1.1g; Protein 61.8g

Sea Scallops with Curry Sauce

Prep time: 10 minutes. | Cooking time: 18 minutes. | Serves: 4

¾ pound sea scallops, washed, cleaned, and thoroughly dried
Sea salt
Black pepper, freshly ground
3 tablespoons olive oil
1 tablespoon peeled, grated fresh ginger
1 to 1½ tablespoons Thai red
curry paste
1½ cups canned coconut milk
1 tablespoon chopped fresh cilantro
Zest and juice of 1 lime

1. Season the scallops with black pepper and salt. 2. Heat the olive oil in a suitable skillet over medium-high heat. 3. Pan sear the scallops until browned. for almost 3 minutes; turn and brown the other side for almost 3 minutes. 4. Transfer the scallops to a plate, cover loosely with foil, and keep it aside. 5. Return the skillet to the heat and sauté the ginger until softened. for almost 2 minutes. 6. Stir in the curry paste, coconut milk, cilantro, lime juice, and lime zest and bring to a simmer for almost 10 minutes. 7. Reduce its heat to low and return the scallops to the skillet, along with any juices on the plate. 8. Turn the scallops with tongs to coat in the sauce and serve.
Per serving: Calories: 222; Total fat 14.2g; Sodium 288mg; Total carbs 2.6g; Fiber 0.9g; Sugars 1.8g; Protein 22.6g

Crab Fried Rice

Prep time: 10 minutes. | Cooking time: 12 minutes. | Serves: 4

¼ cup avocado oil
½ yellow onion, diced
4 garlic cloves, minced
2 large eggs, beaten
6 cups cauliflower rice
¼ cup coconut aminos
1 tablespoon sesame oil
1 (8-ounce) container lump
crabmeat, drained
8 cherry tomatoes, halved
Pink Himalayan salt
Black pepper
Fresh chopped cilantro, for garnish
Sliced scallions, for garnish
Sesame seeds, for garnish

1. In a suitable sauté pan or skillet, heat the avocado oil over medium-high heat. 2. Add the onions and garlic and cook for almost 3 to 4 minutes, or until soft. 3. Push the onions and garlic to one side of the skillet and pour the eggs into the other side. 4. Let the eggs set for almost 30 seconds or so. 5. Add the cauliflower rice, coconut aminos, and sesame oil, tossing everything and breaking up the eggs. 6. Cook the cauliflower rice for almost 5 minutes, stirring frequently until the cauliflower softens. 7. Add in the crab and tomatoes and season with black pepper and salt. 8. Cook for almost 2 more minutes and top with cilantro, scallions, and sesame seeds.
Per serving: Calories: 293; Total fat 11g; Sodium 1510mg; Total Carbs 5g; Fiber 10.1g; Sugars 19g; Protein 16g

Crispy Wings

Prep time: 15 minutes| Cook time: 60 minutes| Serves: 4

1 pound chicken wing sections
2 large eggs, beaten
¼ cup heavy whipping cream
2 ounces ground pork rinds
⅛ teaspoon chili powder
¼ teaspoon salt
⅛ teaspoon ground black pepper

1. Preheat oven to 375°F/191°C. Prepare a baking sheet with parchment paper. 2. Mix all ingredients except wings and pork rinds in a large bowl. Stir in wings until coated. 3. Spread pork rinds on a large plate. Shake excess batter off wing sections and dredge both sides in rinds. 4. Evenly space wings on the prepared baking sheet so they are not touching. Bake for 60 minutes, gently flipping halfway through. Serve warm.
Per Serving: Calories 328; Fat 22g; Sodium 355mg; Carbs 0g; Fiber 0g; Sugar 0g; Protein 29g

Avocado Chips

Prep time: 10 minutes| Cook time: 24 minutes| Serves: 4

2 medium avocados, peeled, pitted, and mashed
1½ cups shredded Swiss cheese
⅛ teaspoon ground black pepper
½ teaspoon paprika
2 teaspoons 100% lemon juice
½ teaspoon garlic powder
½ teaspoon Italian seasoning
⅛ teaspoon salt

1. Preheat oven to 350°F/177°C. Prepare a baking sheet with parchment paper. 2. In a bowl, stir all ingredients except paprika. Scoop teaspoon-sized mounds of the mixture onto the prepared baking sheet, spaced out at least ½" to prevent touching after they are flattened. 3. Spray the back of a serving spoon with nonstick cooking spray and press it into the mounds to flatten each into an irregular shape. Sprinkle "chips" with even amounts of paprika. 4. Bake for 21–24 minutes until crispy and starting to brown. 5. Remove from oven, distribute into four small bowls, and serve immediately.
Per Serving: Calories 269; Fat 20g; Sodium 106mg; Carbs 9g; Fiber 5g; Sugar 1g; Protein 12g

Popcorns

Prep time: 5 minutes| Cook time: 40 minutes| Serves: 4

1 head cauliflower, cut it bite-sized florets
1 tablespoon butter-flavored salt,
divided
¼ cup butter-flavored coconut oil, melted

1. Add cauliflower to a large bowl and top with oil and ½ tablespoon butter-flavored salt. Stir to coat. 2. Add ¼ of the florets to an air fryer crisper tray, spaced out as much as possible. Cook for 10 minutes at 400°F/205°C, shaking the basket halfway through. 3. Repeat the process until all "popcorn" is cooked. 4. Top with remaining butter-flavored salt. Serve warm.
Per Serving: Calories 182; Fat 14g; Sodium 1806mg; Carbs 10g; Fiber 4g; Sugar 4g; Protein 4g

Taquitos

Prep time: 15 minutes| Cook time: 11 minutes| Serves: 4

4 (1-ounce) deli slices Cheddar cheese
¼ teaspoon garlic powder
⅛ teaspoon ground black pepper
1 large black olive, sliced
2 ounces full-fat cream cheese,
softened
1 (5-ounce) can white meat chicken, drained and shredded
2 tablespoons finely chopped green onion, divided

1. Preheat oven to 360°F/182°C. Prepare a baking sheet by lining parchment paper. 2. Place cheese slices on the baking sheet. 3. Bake the cheese for 8–10 minutes until edges start to brown. 4. Microwave cream cheese along with chicken, garlic powder, 1 tablespoon green onion, and pepper for 1 minute. 5. Mix well until blend. 6. Place equal amounts of chicken mixture on each cheese square. 7. Roll the cheese slice like a little burrito and make tiny taquitos. Then garnish the taquitos with sliced olive. 8. Place rolls onto a plate, sprinkle with the remaining tablespoon green onion, and serve warm.
Per Serving: Calories 193; Fat 13g; Sodium 406mg; Carbs 1g; Fiber 0g; Sugar 1g; Protein 14 g

Bake Kale Chips

Prep time: 10 minutes| Cook time: 20 minutes| Serves: 8

2 tablespoons olive oil
¼ teaspoon garlic powder
¼ teaspoon Italian seasoning
¼ teaspoon salt
⅛ teaspoon ground black pepper
2 medium bunches kale, stems and ribs removed
¼ cup grated Parmesan cheese

1. Chop the kale into bite-size pieces. 2. Preheat oven to 300°F/149°C. Prepare a baking sheet with parchment paper. 3. In a bowl, whisk all ingredients except kale and Parmesan. Place the chopped kale in a large bowl and top with seasoning mixture. Toss until all leaves are coated. 4. Evenly spread the kale on the baking pan and cook for 10 minutes. Turn leaves and bake for another 10 minutes until crispy. 5. Let cool slightly, sprinkle evenly with cheese, and serve.
Per Serving: Calories 46; Fat 4g; Sodium 131mg; Carbs 1g; Fiber 0g; Sugar 0g; Protein 1g

Ants On a Log

Prep time: 10 minutes| Cook time: 0 minutes| Serves: 4

2 (5-ounce) cans tuna packed in oil, drained
4 medium stalks celery, cut into 3"–4" sections
¼ cup sliced black olives
¼ cup full-fat mayonnaise
1 tablespoon 100% lemon juice
¼ teaspoon salt

1. Stir to combine all ingredients except celery and olives in a medium bowl. 2. Evenly spread tuna mixture on celery, filling the grooves of each stalk. 3. Place several olive slices in a line along with the tuna mixture on each stalk. Serve immediately.
Per Serving: Calories 222; Fat 16g; Sodium 590mg; Carbs 3g; Fiber 1g; Sugar 1g; Protein 16g

Cheese Ball

Prep time: 10 minutes plus 1 hour for chilling| Cook time: 0 minutes| Serves: 8

8 ounces full-fat cream cheese, softened
1 cup shredded Italian cheese blend
½ teaspoon garlic powder
½ teaspoon salt
⅛ teaspoon ground black pepper
½ cup no-sugar-added bacon bits
½ cup finely chopped green onion, divided
¼ cup sun-dried tomatoes, diced

1. In a large mixing bowl, add cheeses, ¼ cup green onion, tomatoes, garlic powder, salt, and pepper and mix until smooth. 2. Spread the cling film on the counter and scoop out the cheese mixture into a mound on top. Form the plastic wrap around the mixture and shape into a ball. Let cool in refrigerator for 1 hour. Set aside the remaining ingredients. 3. Before serving, spread bacon and remaining green onion on parchment paper. Roll the unwrapped ball on the mixture until evenly coated. Serve on a fancy holiday plate.
Per Serving: Calories 181; Fat 14g; Sodium 513mg; Carbs 3g; Fiber 0g; Sugar 1g; Protein 9g

Dragon Tail Poppahs

Prep time: 15 minutes| Cook time: 19 minutes| Serves: 8

8 (2") jalapeños, halved, seeded, and deveined
1 (1-ounce) package ranch powder seasoning mix
½ cup shredded Cheddar cheese
4 ounces full-fat cream cheese, softened
¼ cup full-fat mayonnaise

1. Preheat oven to 375°F/191°C. Prepare a baking sheet with parchment paper. 2. In a medium microwave-safe bowl, microwave peppers with ¼ cup water for 3 minutes to soften. Drain and let cool. 3. Line up peppers on baking sheet, cut-side up. 4. Add cream cheese, mayonnaise, ranch powder, and shredded cheese in a separate medium microwave-safe bowl. Microwave for 30 seconds and stir. Microwave another 15 seconds and stir. 5. Carefully scoop mixture into sandwich-sized bag. 6. Using makeshift pastry bag, fill jalapeño halves evenly with mixture. 7. Bake for 15 minutes until peppers are fully softened and cheese is golden brown.
Per Serving: Calories 153; Fat 12g; Sodium 173mg; Carbs 2g; Fiber 1g; Sugar 1g; Protein 7g

Tofu Fries

Prep time: 25 minutes| Cook time: 20 minutes| Serves: 4

1 (12-ounce) package extra-firm tofu
⅛ teaspoon salt, divided
⅛ teaspoon black pepper, divided
2 tablespoons sesame oil
⅛ teaspoon creole seasoning, divided

1. Wrap tofu in a paper towel for 20 minutes to remove excess water. 2. Once water has drained out, cut it into the small cubes. Heat oil over medium heat in a cooking pan. 3. In a bowl, mix salt, pepper, and creole seasoning. Sprinkle one-third of spice mixture evenly into pan and add tofu evenly. 4. Sprinkle one-third of spices on top and let fry for 5 minutes on each side, flipping three times (for the four sides), browning all four sides. 5. Dust tofu with remaining spice mixture. 6. Remove from heat. Enjoy while hot!
Per Serving: Calories 119; Fat 10g; Sodium 126mg; Carbs 1g; Fiber 1g; Sugar 1g; Protein 7g

Crackers

Prep time: 15 minutes| Cook time: 40 minutes| Serves: 10

1 cup blanched almond flour
2 tablespoons psyllium husk powder
2 tablespoons chia seeds
2 tablespoons hemp hearts
2 tablespoons flaxseed meal
2 tablespoons shelled pumpkin
seeds
2 tablespoons Everything and More seasoning
½ tablespoon salt
1½ cups water
1 squirt liquid stevia

1. Preheat oven to 350°F/177°C. 2. In a mixing bowl, combine dry ingredients. Add water and liquid stevia and mix until a thick dough is formed. 3. Place dough between two pieces of parchment paper and roll out to desired cracker thickness. 4. Remove top of parchment sheet and use a pizza cutter to cut dough into desired cracker shapes. While cracker shapes are still on bottom piece of parchment paper, put on a baking sheet and into oven. 5. Bake for 30–40 minutes until centers of the crackers are hard. 6. Let cool for 5 minutes, then serve.
Per Serving: Calories 111; Fat 6g; Sodium 541mg; Carbs 7g; Fiber 2g; Sugar 1g; Protein 5g

Ranch Dorito Crackers

Prep time: 15 minutes| Cook time: 37 minutes| Serves: 7

2 cups riced cauliflower, uncooked
⅛ teaspoon salt
⅛ teaspoon black pepper
1½ cups grated Parmesan cheese
2 teaspoons ranch seasoning powder

1. Preheat oven to 375°F/191°C. 2. In a medium microwave-safe bowl, microwave riced cauliflower for 1 minute. Stir and microwave for 1 more minute. 3. Let cool and scoop cauliflower onto a clean dish towel. Squeeze out excess water. 4. Return to bowl and add Parmesan, ranch seasoning, salt, and pepper. Mix thoroughly until a moist dough is formed. 5. Place the dough on parchment paper. Then place the second piece of parchment paper on top of the dough. Use a rolling pin to flatten the dough to the thickness of a Dorito. 6. After the dough is rolled to the desired thickness, remove the top parchment sheet and cut it into triangle shapes roughly the size of Doritos. 7. Place the parchment paper with crackers to a baking sheet. Leave enough space between each cracker to cook evenly and won't stick to nearby crackers during baking. 8. Bake for 25–35 minutes until golden brown. 9. Let cool and serve.
Per Serving: Calories 98; Fat 5g; Sodium 510mg; Carbs 5g; Fiber 1g; Sugar 1g; Protein 7g

Creamy Chipped Artichokes

Prep time: 5 minutes| Cook time: 35 minutes| Serves: 4

½ teaspoon salt, divided
½ cup full-fat mayonnaise
2 large artichokes, trimmed
2 tablespoons lemon juice

1. In a large pot, prepare 1" water with ¼ teaspoon salt. 2. Put artichokes in a steamer basket inside the pot, stem-side up, and cover pot. When boiling starts, lower heat and leave untouched for 25 minutes. 3. Test to see if done by pulling off outer leaf using tongs. If it doesn't come off easily, add additional water to pot and steam for 5–10 more minutes. Let cool. 4. Serve with dip, combining lemon juice, mayonnaise, and remaining salt.
Per Serving: Calories 219; Fat 20g; Sodium 497mg; Carbs 8g; Fiber

5g; Sugar 1g; Protein 2g

Red Pepper Edamame

Prep time: 18 minutes| Cook time: 1 minutes| Serves: 4

2 cups frozen raw edamame in the shell
2 cloves garlic, peeled and minced
1 tablespoon peanut oil
⅛ teaspoon salt
½ teaspoon red pepper flakes

1. In a medium microwave-safe bowl with ½ cup water, microwave edamame for 4–5 minutes. 2. In a medium saucepan over medium heat, add peanut oil. Add minced garlic and salt. Stir 3–5 minutes to soften the garlic. 3. Add edamame and stir 2–3 minutes until well heated and coated. Turn off heat and cover saucepan to steam edamame for 5 additional minutes. 4. Add red pepper flakes and toss well to coat evenly. Serve immediately for best results.
Per Serving: Calories 131; Fat 7g; Sodium 87mg; Carbs 9g; Fiber 6g; Sugar 1g; Protein 10g

Jalapeño Chips

Prep time: 10 minutes| Cook time: 13 minutes| Serves: 6

1½ cups shredded Parmesan cheese
6 strips no-sugar-added bacon, cooked and crumbled
1½ cups shredded Cheddar cheese
2 medium jalapeños, thinly sliced in rings

1. Preheat oven to 380°F/193°C. Prepare a baking sheet with parchment paper. 2. Put 1-tablespoon-sized mounds of Parmesan on the baking sheet, 1" apart, until all Parmesan is distributed. 3. Top each with an equal amount of Cheddar and press down to form compact circles no more than 2" across. 4. Place a jalapeño ring centered on top of each circle. Cover evenly with bacon bits. 5. Bake for 10–13 minutes until firm and starting to brown. Serve warm.
Per Serving: Calories 252; Fat 17g; Sodium 714mg; Carbs 2g; Fiber 0g; Sugar 0g; Protein 18g

Radish Chips

Prep time: 10 minutes| Cook time: 13 minutes| Serves: 1

⅛ teaspoon salt
⅛ teaspoon ground black pepper
1 cup thinly sliced (⅛" thick) radishes
½ teaspoon garlic powder
1 teaspoon finely chopped fresh parsley
1 tablespoon olive oil
1 tablespoon white vinegar

1. Add all ingredients except parsley in a medium bowl and stir until all radish slices are coated with seasonings. 2. Place in an air fryer and cook at 380°F/193°C for 12–13 minutes. Shake the basket to turn chips halfway through. 3. Cool slightly, sprinkle with parsley, and serve.
Per Serving: Calories 145; Fat 13g; Sodium 335mg; Carbs 5g; Fiber 2g; Sugar 2g; Protein 1g

Bacon-Stuffed Mushrooms

Prep time: 15 minutes| Cook time: 23 minutes| Serves: 4

12 large whole mushrooms, approximately 2" wide
2 tablespoons unsalted butter
1 medium green onion, finely chopped
1 teaspoon paprika
⅛ teaspoon salt
⅛ teaspoon black pepper
8 ounces cooked no-sugar-added bacon, crumbled
7 ounces full-fat cream cheese, softened
½ cup full-fat mayonnaise

1. Preheat oven to 400°F/204°C. Prepare a baking sheet with parchment paper. 2. Remove mushroom stems from caps, being very careful not to break edges of cap, and scrape out the black gills if the mushroom is mature enough for the gills to be visible. Chop the trimmed stem pieces finely. 3. In a frying pan, fry mushroom trimmings with butter for 3 minutes until soft over medium heat. Place caps on baking sheet, rounded-side down. 4. In a medium bowl, combine fried mushroom trimmings with the remaining ingredients. Scoop the mixture evenly into the caps. 5. Bake for 20 minutes until filling bubbles and turns golden brown.
Per Serving: Calories 690; Fat 59g; Sodium 1387mg; Carbs 6g; Fiber 1g; Sugar 3g; Protein 25g

Bacon Asparagus

Prep time: 20 minutes| Cook time: 25 minutes| Serves: 6

6 strips no-sugar-added bacon, uncooked
24 asparagus spears
2 tablespoons olive oil
⅛ teaspoon salt

1. Line up asparagus and cut entire bunch at the "snapping" point, making all of your stalk's uniform in length. 2. On a microwave-safe plate, microwave asparagus for 2 minutes to soften. Let cool for 5 minutes. 3. Lay strip of bacon on a cutting board at a 45-degree angle. Lay four asparagus spears centered on bacon in an "up and down" position. 4. Pick up bacon and asparagus where they meet and wrap two ends of bacon around the asparagus in opposite. 5. Wrap bacon tightly and secure, pinning bacon to asparagus at ends with toothpicks. Don't worry if bacon doesn't cover entire spears. 6. Grease asparagus with olive oil and sprinkle with salt. Heat a medium nonstick pan over medium heat. Cook asparagus/bacon for 3–5 minutes per side while turning to cook thoroughly. Continue flipping until bacon is brown and crispy.
Per Serving: Calories 106; Fat 8g; Sodium 243mg; Carbs 3g; Fiber 1g; Sugar 1g; Protein 5g

Cucumber Salsa

Prep time: 10 minutes| Cook time: 0 minutes| Serves: 8

2 medium cucumbers
2 medium tomatoes
1 clove garlic, peeled and minced
2 tablespoons lime juice
4 medium jalapeño peppers, deveined, seeded, and finely chopped
½ medium red onion, peeled and chopped
2 teaspoons dried parsley
2 teaspoons finely chopped cilantro
½ teaspoon salt

1. Finely chop or pulse cucumbers and tomatoes separately in a food processor to desired consistency. 2. Add to a mixing bowl along with rest of the ingredients and mix thoroughly. Serve.
Per Serving: Calories 23; Fat 0g; Sodium 149mg; Carbs 6g; Fiber 1g; Sugar 3g; Protein 1g

Buffalo Chicken Thighs

Prep time: 15 minutes| Cook time: 30 minutes| Serves: 10

2 (4.2-ounce) chicken breasts from cooked rotisserie chicken
1 (8-ounce) package full-fat cream cheese, softened
½ cup finely chopped green onion
¼ cup buffalo wing sauce
1 teaspoon garlic powder
½ pound no-sugar-added bacon,
cooked and crumbled
2 cups shredded whole milk mozzarella cheese
1 cup shredded Cheddar cheese
1 (1-ounce) package ranch powder seasoning mix
1 cup full-fat mayonnaise
1 cup full-fat sour cream

1. Preheat oven to 350°F/177°C. Grease a 2-quart (8" × 8") baking dish. 2. In a small bowl, finely shred chicken. In the baking dish, combine chicken with remaining ingredients, except bacon, to mix well. 3. Bake for 25–30 minutes; stop when bubbling and browned on top. 4. Top with the crumbled bacon. Serve immediately.
Per Serving: Calories 538; Fat 43g; Sodium 1236mg; Carbs 5g; Fiber 0g; Sugar 2g; Protein 25g

Traditional El Presidente Guac

Prep time: 10 minutes| Cook time: 0 minutes| Serves: 4

2 large avocados, peeled and pitted
1 tablespoon garlic powder
1 tablespoon onion powder
⅛ teaspoon salt
⅛ teaspoon chili powder
4 tablespoons finely chopped cilantro
1 Roma tomato, finely chopped
4 teaspoons lime juice

1. In a medium bowl, mash avocados and combine with dry spices. 2. Add cilantro, tomato, and lime juice and mix again. Serve.
Per Serving: Calories 131; Fat 9g; Sodium 83mg; Carbs 10g; Fiber 5g; Sugar 1g; Protein 2g

Hot Chili-Garlic Wings

Prep time: 15 minutes| Cook time: 60 minutes| Serves: 4

3 tablespoons Thai chili-garlic sauce
12 chicken wings, separated at the joint
½ teaspoon salt
½ teaspoon freshly ground black pepper
2 tablespoons avocado oil
2 teaspoons onion powder
1 garlic clove, minced
2 scallions, for garnish

1. Preheat the oven to 375°F/191°C. Set aside a rimmed baking sheet lined with parchment paper or aluminum foil. 2. Combine the chili-garlic sauce, oil, onion powder, and garlic in a resealable bag. Add the wings to the bag, seal, and shake until well coated. 3. Arrange the wings on the baking sheet in a single layer and sprinkle with the salt and pepper. 4. Bake for 1 hour until crispy and fully cooked, turning once halfway through. Remove from the oven and serve garnished with the sliced scallions.
Per Serving: Calories 685; Fat 49g; Sodium 645mg; Carbs 2g; Fiber 1g; Sugar 0g; Protein 56g

Steak Bites with Pepper Sauce

Prep time: 15 minutes| Cook time: 5 minutes| Serves: 4

For the steak
1-pound sirloin steak, cut into 1-inch cubes
2 tablespoons unsalted butter, divided
¼ teaspoon salt
¼ teaspoon freshly ground black pepper
For the sauce
12-ounce jar roasted red bell
peppers, drained
½ cup extra-virgin olive oil
2 tablespoons freshly squeezed lemon juice
1 garlic clove, peeled
½ teaspoon dried basil
¼ teaspoon salt
¼ teaspoon freshly ground black pepper

To make the steak: 1. Season the steak cubes with the salt and pepper. 2. In a large pan, melt 1 tablespoon of butter over medium-high heat. Once the butter begins to brown, working in batches, add the steak to the pan in a single layer. Cook without stirring or flipping for 30 to 45 seconds, then flip the pieces over with a spatula and cook for 30 to 45 seconds. This will brown the outside but keep the inside medium-rare. 3. Transfer to the plate and repeat the process with the remaining butter and steak cubes.
To make the sauce: 1. In a blender, puree the roasted peppers, oil, lemon juice, garlic, basil, salt, and pepper until smooth. Transfer the sauce to four small bowls for dipping. Serve immediately with the steak bites.
Per Serving: Calories 528; Fat 46g; Sodium 866mg; Carbs 5g; Fiber 1g; Sugar 3g; Protein 23g

Classy Crudités with Dip

Prep time: 15 minutes| Cook time: 0 minutes| Serves: 8

Vegetables
1 cup green beans, trimmed
2 cups broccoli florets
2 cups cauliflower florets
1 cup whole cherry tomatoes
1 bunch asparagus, trimmed
1 green bell pepper, seeded and chopped
Sour Cream Dip
2 cups full-fat sour cream
½ teaspoon garlic powder
⅛ teaspoon salt
⅛ teaspoon black pepper
3 tablespoons dry chives
1 tablespoon lemon juice
½ cup dried parsley

1. Cut vegetables into bite-sized uniform pieces. Arrange in like groups around the outside edge of a large serving platter, leaving room in the middle for dip. 2. Make dip by combining dip ingredients in a medium-sized decorative bowl and mixing well. 3. Place dip bowl in the center of platter and serve.
Per Serving: Calories 146; Fat 10g; Sodium 88mg; Carbs 9g; Fiber 3g; Sugar 5g; Protein 4g

Delicious Devil Eggs

Prep time: 10 minutes| Cook time: 9 minutes| Serves: 6

6 large eggs
3 tablespoons full-fat mayonnaise
⅛ teaspoon salt
⅛ teaspoon black pepper
⅛ teaspoon ground cayenne
⅛ teaspoon paprika
1 teaspoon plain white vinegar
1 teaspoon spicy mustard

1. Hard-boil eggs using a steamer basket in the Instant Pot on high pressure for 9 minutes. Release pressure and remove eggs. 2. Peel eggs and slice in half lengthwise—place yolks in a medium bowl. Mash and mix yolks with mayonnaise, vinegar, mustard, salt, and black pepper. 3. Scrape the mixture into a sandwich-sized plastic bag and snip off one corner, making a hole about the width of a pencil. Use a makeshift pastry bag to fill egg white halves with yolk mixture. 4. Garnish Devilish Eggs with cayenne and paprika (mostly for color) and serve.
Per Serving: Calories 125; Fat 9g; Sodium 164mg; Carbs 1g; Fiber 0g; Sugar 1g; Protein 6g

Cheesy Hangover Homies

Prep time: 10 minutes| Cook time: 15 minutes| Serves: 2

1 tablespoon avocado oil
1 large turnip, peeled and diced
1 tablespoon minced onion
4 large eggs, lightly beaten
¼ cup sour cream
¼ cup shredded cheddar cheese

½ avocado, peeled, pitted, and sliced
Pinch salt
Pinch freshly ground black pepper
1 scallion, both green and white parts, chopped

1. In a pan, heat the oil over medium-high flame. Add the turnip and onion and cook, stirring frequently, until tender, for 12 to 15 minutes. 2. Meanwhile, warm a nonstick pan over medium heat. Pour in the eggs and pull them from side to side with a spatula as they cook to form soft curds. Evenly divide the cooked eggs between two plates. 3. When the turnip mixture is done, add it to the eggs, dividing evenly. 4. Mix the sour cream and cheddar in a small bowl, then add to the eggs and turnips. 5. Divide the avocado between the plates and season with salt and pepper. Garnish with the scallion. Serve immediately.
Per Serving: Calories 439; Fat 34g; Sodium 457mg; Carbs 15g; Fiber 6g; Sugar 7g; Protein 19g

Bacon and Cheese Stuffed Jalapeños

Prep time: 15 minutes| Cook time: 15 minutes| Serves: 12

6 bacon slices
8 ounces cream cheese, at room temperature
½ cup crumbled blue cheese
1 teaspoon onion powder

1 teaspoon garlic powder
Pinch salt
Pinch freshly ground black pepper
12 jalapeño peppers, halved lengthwise and seeded

1. Preheat the oven to 400°F/204°C. Set aside a rimmed baking sheet lined with parchment paper or aluminum foil. 2. In a pan, cook the bacon over medium-high heat until the fat renders, for about 10 minutes. Transfer to a lined plate with paper towels to cool, then crumble. Transfer to a lined plate with paper towels; mix the bacon, cream cheese, blue cheese, garlic, onion powder, salt, and pepper. Fill the hollow of each jalapeño half with the bacon and cheese mixture and arrange cut-side up on the baking sheet. Bake for 15 minutes, rotating the sheet halfway through. 3. Serve hot.
Per Serving: Calories 75; Fat 7g; Sodium 874mg; Carbs 1g; Fiber 0g; Sugar 1g; Protein 3g

Tropical Shrimp Dippers

Prep time: 15 minutes| Cook time: 15 minutes| Serves: 6

For the shrimp
Coconut oil cooking spray
½ cup coconut flour
1 teaspoon freshly ground black pepper
2 large eggs
½ cup unsweetened coconut flakes
⅓ cup crushed pork rinds
30 large shrimp, peeled and

deveined, tails left on
For the sauce
½ cup unsweetened peanut butter or almond butter
½ cup tamari or coconut aminos
¼ cup water
1 tablespoon red curry paste
1 teaspoon Thai chili-garlic sauce (optional)

To make the shrimp: 1. Preheat the oven to 425°F. Mist a rimmed baking sheet with coconut oil and set aside. 2. Prepare three shallow bowls for dredging: Combine the coconut flour and pepper in the first bowl. In the second bowl, beat the eggs. In the third bowl, mix the coconut flakes and crushed pork rinds. Line the bowls up in the same order, with the prepped baking sheet at the end. Dip each shrimp into the flour mixture, the egg, and the coconut flake mixture. Place the coated shrimp on the baking sheet. Continue until all the shrimp are dredged, then mist the tops of the shrimp with coconut oil. 3. Bake the shrimp for 10 minutes, then flip and continue baking for 5 to 6 minutes, until the shrimp are fully cooked.
To make the sauce: 1. In a bowl, stir the peanut butter, tamari, water, curry paste, and chili-garlic sauce (if using) until smooth. Transfer to a group serving bowl or individually portioned dishes. 2. Serve the shrimp with the dipping sauce.
Per Serving: Calories 317; Fat 17g; Sodium 376mg; Carbs 13g; Fiber 7g; Sugar 4g; Protein 28g

Loaded Chayote Fries

Prep time: 10 minutes| Cook time: 30 minutes| Serves: 4

4 bacon slices
4 chayote squash
1 tablespoon avocado oil, extra-

virgin
½ teaspoon salt
⅛ teaspoon freshly ground black

pepper
½ cup shredded cheddar cheese

4 scallions, sliced

1. Preheat the oven to 425°F/218°C. Set aside a rimmed baking sheet lined with parchment paper or aluminum foil. 2. In a pan, cook the bacon over medium-high heat until the fat renders, about 10 minutes. Transfer to a lined plate with paper towels to cool, then crumble. 3. Peel off the skin from the chayote squash. Rinse the sticky coating from the peeled squash. Spiralize the chayote into curly shapes. Or, if you don't have a spiralizer, cut the squash into ¼-inch-thick fry-style wedges. Discard any remnants of the center seeds. Toss the chayote with the oil, salt, and pepper then spread on the baking sheet in a single layer. 4. Roast for 15 minutes for curly fries or 20 minutes for wedges, or until tender and browned. 5. Remove the chayote fries from the oven and set the temperature to broil. Sprinkle the cheddar evenly over the top and return to the oven. Broil the fries for 1 - 2 minutes until the cheese melted. 6. Sprinkle the bacon and scallions over the top. Serve immediately.
Per Serving: Calories 175; Fat 12g; Sodium 421mg; Carbs 11g; Fiber 4g; Sugar 4g; Protein 8g

Bacon-Wrapped Pickles

Prep time: 5 minutes| Cook time: 20 minutes| Serves: 4

6 strips uncooked no-sugar-added bacon, cut in half lengthwise

3 large pickles
¼ cup ranch dressing

1. Preheat oven to 425°F/218°C. Prepare a baking sheet with foil. 2. Quarter each pickle lengthwise (yielding twelve spears). 3. Wrap each pickles with a strip of bacon. Place on a baking sheet. Bake for 20 minutes or until crispy, flipping at the midpoint. 4. Serve your crispy bacon-wrapped pickles while still hot with a side of the ranch dipping sauce.
Per Serving: Calories 96; Fat 6g; Sodium 1117mg; Carbs 3g; Fiber 1g; Sugar 1g; Protein 6g

Zucchini Chips

Prep time: 20 minutes plus 2 hours to marinate| Cook time: 120 minutes| Serves: 4

2 large zucchinis, thinly sliced crosswise
½ cup apple cider vinegar

1 tablespoon extra-virgin olive oil
1 teaspoon sea salt

1. Place the sliced zucchini in a shallow glass dish and cover with the vinegar. Let it marinate in the refrigerator for 2 hours or overnight. 2. Once marinated, lay out sheets of paper towel and place the drained zucchini on them in a single layer. Cover with additional paper towels and set a weighted baking sheet on top to remove excess moisture. 3. Preheat the oven to 235°F/113°C. Prepare two rimmed baking trays by lining them with parchment paper and lightly brushing each with some oil. 4. Arrange the zucchini slices closely on the baking sheets but in a single layer. Grease the rest of the oil and sprinkle with the salt. 5. Bake for 2 hours, without flipping, until crisp and golden. If some zucchini slices cook faster than others, remove the crisp slices and allow the damp ones to bake longer. Transfer the finished zucchini to cool the pans to fresh, dry paper towels. Serve.
Per Serving: Calories 64; Fat 4g; Sodium 475mg; Carbs 5g; Fiber 2g; Sugar 3g; Protein 2g

Stuffed Mushrooms with Burrata

Prep time: 15 minutes| Cook time: 15 minutes| Serves: 10

20 cremini mushroom caps, cleaned
1 tablespoon extra-virgin olive oil
¼ cup chopped arugula, divided
6 ounces fresh burrata cheese or fresh mozzarella, at room

temperature, cut or torn into 20 even-size chunks
5 cherry tomatoes, quartered
¼ teaspoon flaky sea salt
¼ teaspoon freshly ground black pepper

1. Preheat the oven to 425°F/218°C. Prepare a rimmed baking tray by lining it with parchment paper or aluminum foil. 2. Tossing the mushroom caps in the oil on the prepared baking sheet and place them gill-side up. Distribute half of the arugula evenly among the mushrooms. Place a burrata chunk in each cap, followed by a cherry tomato quarter. Sprinkle the salt, pepper, and remaining arugula over the tops of the stuffed mushrooms. 3. Bake the mushrooms for 15 to 20 minutes, until the mushrooms are tender. Transfer to a platter and serve immediately.
Per Serving: Calories 73; Fat 5g; Sodium 74mg; Carbs 2g; Fiber 1g; Sugar 1g; Protein 5g

Cheesy Buffalo Chicken Quesadillas

Prep time: 15 minutes| Cook time: 35 minutes| Serves: 4

For the tortillas
2 large eggs
10½ tablespoons unsweetened coconut milk beverage or unsweetened almond milk, divided
8 teaspoons coconut flour
1 teaspoon unflavored gelatin powder or psyllium husk powder

Extra-virgin olive oil, for greasing the pan
For the filling
2 tablespoons extra-virgin olive oil
1 large boneless, skinless chicken breast
1 cup shredded cheddar cheese
¼ cup Buffalo hot sauce

To make the tortillas: 1. In a large bowl, whisk the eggs, 6½ tablespoons of coconut milk, and the coconut flour until the batter is smooth. 2. In a bowl, combine the remaining coconut milk and gelatin powder and let sit for 5 minutes. Whisk the gelatin mixture until smooth, without clumps, then pour into the coconut flour batter and whisk to combine. The batter should be a liquid, pourable consistency. If it's too thick, add additional coconut milk, 1 tablespoon at a time, until the batter is thin enough to pour and easily spread over the pan. 3. Lightly coat a medium nonstick pan with oil and warm over medium heat. Pour one-quarter of the batter (about ¼ cup) into the hot pan and swirl to distribute the mixture and coat the bottom of the pan as you would when be making omelets or crepes. Cover and cook for 2 minutes. Flip the tortilla, cover, and cook for an additional 2 minutes. Transfer to a clean plate. Repeat to make a total of 4 tortillas.
To make the filling: 1. In a large pan, heat the oil over medium-high heat. Add the chicken breast and cook for 4 to 5 minutes per side, turning once, until no longer pink. Remove from the heat. When cool enough, shred or dice. Combine the cooked chicken, cheddar, and Buffalo hot sauce in a large bowl. 2. Set the nonstick pan over medium-low heat. Lay one of the tortillas in the pan. Spread one-quarter of the chicken mixture (about ½ cup) on half of the tortilla, then fold the other side over the top. 3. Cover and cook for 1 minute, then flip, cover, and cook for another minute, or until the cheese has melted. Remove from the heat. Repeat the steps for all four quesadillas. Cut into triangle wedges and serve immediately.
Per Serving: Calories 267; Fat 17g; Sodium 666mg; Carbs 9g; Fiber 2g; Sugar 2g; Protein 20g

Glazed Meatballs

Prep time: 10 minutes| Cook time: 35 minutes| Serves: 6

8 ounces ground pork
8 ounces ground beef
½ cup shredded zucchini, drained
1 large egg
1 garlic clove, minced
1¼ teaspoons salt, divided

¼ teaspoon freshly ground black pepper, divided
1 (6-ounce) can tomato paste
¼ cup crystallized allulose or sweetener of choice
2 tablespoons apple cider vinegar

1. Preheat the oven to 325°F/163°C. Prepare a rimmed baking tray by lining it with aluminum foil and place a wire rack on top. 2. In a large bowl, combine the pork, beef, zucchini, egg, garlic, ¾ teaspoon of salt, and ⅛ teaspoon of pepper. Pull off tablespoon-size portions and roll into balls. Set on the rack. Bake for 20 minutes. 3. In a large saucepan, combine the tomato paste, allulose, vinegar, remaining ½ teaspoon of salt, and remaining ⅛ teaspoon of pepper. Simmer them over medium heat and simmer for 5 minutes. Reduce the heat to low. 4. Add the parbaked meatballs to the pan and cook for 10 minutes, gently stirring to coat the meatballs thoroughly. 5. Serve hot immediately.
Per Serving: Calories 234; Fat 16g; Sodium 589mg; Carbs 6g; Fiber 1g; Sugar 4g; Protein 15g

Mac 'N' Cheese Balls

Prep time: 30 minutes| Cook time: 20 minutes| Serves: 6

1 tablespoon extra-virgin olive oil
1 head cauliflower, cut into ½-inch pieces
2 tablespoons cubed cream cheese
½ cup heavy cream
¼ teaspoon xanthan gum
1 cup shredded cheddar cheese

½ teaspoon salt
¼ teaspoon smoked paprika
1 cup avocado oil
½ cup finely crushed pork rinds
½ cup almond flour
1 large egg

1. In a pan, set the heat to medium and then heat the olive oil. Add the cauliflower and sauté for 10 minutes or until tender. 2. In a medium saucepan, melt the cream cheese over medium-low heat. Gradually adjust the heat to medium, whisk in the heavy cream and xanthan gum, and bring to a boil. Eliminate from the heat and whisk in the cheddar until smooth. Stir in the salt and smoked paprika. 3. Pour the cheese mixture over the cauliflower pieces and stir well. Allow to cool, then chill in the refrigerator for 3 hours, or until firm. 4. In a large cast-iron pan or small Dutch oven, heat the avocado oil over medium-high heat until hot enough to sizzle a crumb of bread dropped in it. 5. Set up a dredging station: Combine the pork rinds and almond flour in one bowl. Beat the egg in a second bowl. Scoop the cheesy cauliflower mixture into 1-inch balls. Dip them into the egg, and dredge in the pork-rind mixture until fully coated. 6. Working in batches, place the balls in the hot oil and cook for 2 to 3 minutes, until crispy. Serve immediately.
Per Serving: Calories 156; Fat 15g; Sodium 458mg; Carbs 3g; Fiber 1g; Sugar 1g; Protein 5g

Pretzel Bites with Sauce

Prep time: 25 minutes| Cook time: 10 minutes| Serves: 6

For the pretzels
1 tablespoon warm water
1 teaspoon active dry yeast
½ cup almond flour
1 large egg
1 cup shredded low-moisture mozzarella cheese
2 tablespoons cream cheese
1 tablespoon unsalted butter, melted

¼ teaspoon coarse salt
For the cheese sauce
1 tablespoon unsalted butter
¼ cup heavy cream
¼ cup shredded cheddar cheese
½ teaspoon mustard powder
¼ teaspoon freshly ground black pepper
⅛ teaspoon fine salt

To make the pretzels: 1. Preheat the oven to 400°F/204°C. Prepare a rimmed baking tray by lining it with parchment paper or a silicone baking mat and set aside. 2. In a bowl, mix the water with the yeast and let rest for 5 to 10 minutes, until the yeast rehydrates. Add the almond flour and egg and whisk to combine. 3. In a microwave-safe bowl, microwave the mozzarella and cream cheese in 30-second intervals, stirring with a fork, until the cheese is soft, pliable, and fully melted. Transfer the melted cheese to the bowl with the yeast mixture and use a fork to mix until thoroughly combined. 4. Divide the dough into four equal portions. Spread sheet of parchment paper on the work surface. Wet your hands with warm water and roll one dough portion into a long rope about 1 inch in diameter. Cut the dough into 1-inch lengths and place them on the baking sheet. Repeat with the remaining dough. 5. Brush the dough pieces with the melted butter and sprinkle with the salt. Bake for 10 to 12 minutes, until golden brown.
To make the cheese sauce: 1. In a saucepan, melt the butter. Whisk cream in and bring the butter cream mix to boil, and then remove from the heat. Stir in the cheddar, mustard powder, pepper, and salt until smooth and thoroughly combined. Transfer to a serving dish. 2. Serve the pretzel bites with the cheese sauce for dipping.
Per Serving: Calories 221; Fat 19g; Sodium 478mg; Carbs 4g; Fiber 1g; Sugar 1g; Protein 9g

Roasted Greek Cauliflower

Prep time: 10 minutes. | Cooking time: 35 minutes. | Serves: 6

6 cups cauliflower florets
½ cup olive oil
1 teaspoon dried oregano
½ teaspoon salt
¼ teaspoon black pepper, freshly ground
10 pitted Kalamata olives, coarsely chopped

2 cups baby spinach leaves, coarsely chopped
¼ cup fresh parsley leaves, coarsely chopped
8 ounces crumbled feta cheese
4 ounces goat cheese
½ cup heavy cream

1. At 425°F/218°C, preheat your oven. 2. In a suitable bowl, mix the cauliflower florets, ¼ cup of olive oil, oregano, salt, and pepper and toss to coat well. Transfer to a 9-by-13-inch glass baking dish, reserving the oiled bowl. Roast the cauliflower for almost 15 to 20 minutes, or until just starting to turn golden brown. 3. Meanwhile, in the same suitable bowl, mix the olives, spinach, parsley, half the feta, the goat cheese, and the remaining ¼ cup of olive oil. Stir to mix well and incorporate the goat cheese into the prepared mixture. 4. Transfer the hot cauliflower to the suitable bowl with the olive-and-cheese mixture and toss to coat well. Add the heavy cream and toss again. Transfer back to the baking dish and sprinkle the remaining 4 ounces of feta on top of the vegetables. Return to your oven and roast until bubbly, 10 to 12 minutes. Serve warm.
Per serving: Calories: 197; Total fat 17g; Sodium 426mg; Total Carbs 2.5g; Fiber 3g; Sugars 4.8g; Protein 1.9g

Crostini

Prep time: 15 minutes| Cook time: 35 minutes| Serves: 6

For the crostini
6 egg whites, large size
½ teaspoon baking powder
½ teaspoon xanthan gum
1 (30-gram) scoop unsweetened, unflavored whey protein powder
2 tablespoons extra-virgin olive oil
⅛ teaspoon salt
For the tapenade
1 cup Kalamata olives or mixed

olive varieties, pitted
¼ cup fresh basil leaves
2 tablespoons extra-virgin olive oil
2 tablespoons capers
1 tablespoon freshly squeezed lemon juice
1 garlic clove, peeled
Pinch salt
Pinch freshly ground black pepper

Preheat the oven to 350°F/177°C. Prepare a rimmed baking tray with parchment paper or a silicone baking mat and set aside.
To make the crostini: 1. In a bowl, mix the egg whites, baking powder, and xanthan gum and beat on medium until stiff peaks form. Gently fold the protein powder into the egg white mixture. Scoop the mixture onto the baking sheet into 2 long, thin log-shaped mounds (like baguettes). Bake the crostini for 20 to 25 minutes, until crisp and golden brown. Remove from the oven. Increase the temperature to 375°F/191°C. 2.. When the baguettes are cool, use a serrated knife to cut each loaf crosswise into ¼-inch-thick slices. 3. Lightly grease both sides of each piece with the oil and lay the slices flat on the baking sheet. Sprinkle the tops with the salt. Bake for 5 minutes, then flip the crostini and bake for an additional 5 minutes. Remove from the oven and transfer to a rack to cool.
To make the tapenade: In a food processor, combine the olives, basil leaves, oil, capers, lemon juice, garlic, salt, and pepper and pulse until the desired consistency. Scrape down the sides between pulses. Several pulses yield a relish-like texture, while more pulsing creates a spreadable sauce.
Spoon the tapenade onto the prepared crostini and serve immediately.
Per Serving: Calories 141; Fat 11g; Sodium 669mg; Carbs 4g; Fiber 1g; Sugar 0g; Protein 7g

Creamy Salami Pinwheels

Prep time: 15 minutes| Cook time: 0 minutes| Serves: 8

1 (8-ounce) block cream cheese
8 ounces deli-style hard salami, thinly sliced

1 tablespoon chopped arugula
2 scallions, chopped

1. Spread a plastic wrap on a work surface and smooth out any wrinkles. Place the cream cheese in the center. Cover with another sheet of wrap and, using a rolling pin, roll it into a thin (about ¼ inch thick) rectangle. Remove the upper plastic wrap and cover the cheese with a layer of overlapping salami slices, in a fashion similar to roof tiling. Place a fresh layer of plastic wrap over the top when the cream cheese is fully covered and no longer visible. Flip the wrapped salami and cheese so that the cream cheese side is facing up. Remove the top piece of plastic wrap and sprinkle the arugula and scallions evenly over the cream cheese. 2. Tightly roll the salami up and over the cream cheese (as you would a jelly roll) until you meet the other long side to form a log with the salami surface on the outside. Wrap the log tightly with plastic wrap, securing each end by twisting the wrap. Roll the wrapped log over the work surface to smooth out any trapped air pockets within the log. Cool until ready to serve. 3. To serve, remove the plastic wrap and use a very sharp knife to cut crosswise into ¼-inch-thick slices. Place on a platter and serve.
Per Serving: Calories 205; Fat 19g; Sodium 698mg; Carbs 2g; Fiber 0g; Sugar 1g; Protein 7g

Cheeseburgers

Prep time: 15 minutes| Cook time: 20 minutes| Serves: 4

For the buns
6 egg whites, large size
½ teaspoon baking powder
½ teaspoon xanthan gum
1 (30-gram) scoop unsweetened unflavored whey protein powder
1 tablespoon ground flaxseed
¼ teaspoon sesame seeds
For the burgers
1 pound ground beef

¼ teaspoon salt
¼ teaspoon freshly ground black pepper
1 tablespoon unsalted butter
4 cheddar cheese slices
For assembly
1 tablespoon mayonnaise
1 tablespoon yellow mustard
1 dill pickle, sliced

Preheat the oven to 350°F/177°C. Prepare a rimmed baking tray with parchment paper or a silicone baking mat and set aside.
To make the buns: 1. In a bowl, beat the egg whites, baking powder, and xanthan gum on medium for 7 to 8 minutes, until stiff peaks form. Mix the protein powder and ground flaxseed together in a small bowl, then gently fold into the egg white mixture. Scoop four separate mounds of the mixture onto the baking sheet. Sprinkle the sesame seeds over the top. 2. Bake them for 15-20 minutes until golden brown. Remove from the oven to cool, then slice the rolls in half horizontally.
To make the burgers: Combine the ground beef, salt, and pepper in a large bowl. Divide the meat into four portions and form into 1-inch-thick patties with the palms of your hand or a burger press. In a pan, melt the butter. Place the patties in the hot pan without crowding them. Cook patties for 3 to 4 minutes, then flip and top with the cheddar slices. Cook again 3 to 4 minutes, until the burgers reach your preferred doneness.
To assemble: Dress the buns with a thin layer of mayonnaise and mustard. Place the cheesy patties on the bottom half of the buns and top with pickle slices. Top with the buns and serve immediately.
Per Serving: Calories 508; Fat 38g; Sodium 478mg; Carbs 3g; Fiber 0g; Sugar 1g; Protein 36g

Delicious Caprese Skewers

Prep time: 15 minutes| Cook time: 0 minutes| Serves: 6

48 fresh basil leaves
18 cherry tomatoes, halved
24 small fresh mozzarella balls

1 tablespoon balsamic vinegar
⅛ teaspoon salt

1. Onto each of 12 wooden skewers, thread 4 basil leaves, 3 cherry tomato halves, and 2 mozzarella balls, alternating as you go. 2. Lay the skewers flat on a serving tray and drizzle the balsamic vinegar in a zigzag pattern over the top. Sprinkle salt over them and serve immediately or store refrigerated in an airtight container for up to 1 day.
Per Serving: Calories 41; Fat 2g; Sodium 378mg; Carbs 3g; Fiber 1g; Sugar 2g; Protein 3g

Salmon Cucumber Bites with Tzatziki

Prep time: 30 minutes| Cook time: 0 minutes| Serves: 6

2½ large cucumbers, divided
½ cup plain Greek yogurt
1½ tablespoons chopped fresh dill, divided
1½ teaspoons freshly squeezed lemon juice

1 garlic clove, minced
Pinch salt
Pinch freshly ground black pepper
4 ounces smoked thin strips salmon

1. Trim the ends from the 2 whole cucumbers and cut into about 24 (¾-inch-thick) discs. Use a melon baller or spoon to scoop out a ½-inch-deep well in the center of each disc. Pat dry cucumbers to drain excess moisture. 2. Finely grate the half cucumber onto a paper towel. Wrap the cucumber in the towel and squeeze out excess moisture. Place the grated cucumber in a large bowl. Add the yogurt, 1 tablespoon of dill, lemon juice, garlic, salt, and pepper, and mix. 3. Fill each cucumber cup with the tzatziki sauce. Top each cucumber with a strip of smoked salmon and garnish all the cups with the remaining ½ tablespoon of dill. Serve immediately.
Per Serving: Calories 54; Fat 2g; Sodium 1023mg; Carbs 6g; Fiber 1g; Sugar 3g; Protein 5g

Traditional Spinach-Artichoke Dip

Prep time: 10 minutes| Cook time: 15 minutes| Serves: 6

1 tablespoon extra-virgin olive oil
¼ medium onion, diced
1 package frozen spinach, thawed and drained
1 can artichoke hearts
1 garlic clove, minced
8 ounces cream cheese, at room

temperature
¼ cup grated Parmesan cheese
1 cup Greek yogurt
¼ cup mayonnaise
Pinch salt
Pinch freshly ground black pepper

1. In a pan, heat the oil and cook the onion until translucent, about 10 minutes. Add the spinach, artichokes, and garlic and sauté for 3 to 5 minutes, until the spinach and artichokes are tender. 2. Lower the heat and add in the cream cheese and Parmesan until melted. Eliminate from the heat and stir in the yogurt and mayonnaise until thoroughly combined—season with salt and pepper. 3. Serve as a dip or a spread.
Per Serving: Calories 341; Fat 31g; Sodium 847mg; Carbs 10g; Fiber 4g; Sugar 3g; Protein 8g

The Best Deviled Eggs

Prep time: 10 minutes. | Cooking time: 15 minutes. | Serves: 4

1 tablespoon mayonnaise
1 tablespoon olive oil
1 teaspoon Dijon mustard
1 teaspoon anchovy paste
¼ teaspoon black pepper, freshly ground

4 large hard-boiled eggs, shelled
8 pitted green olives, chopped
1 tablespoon red onion, minced
1 tablespoon fresh parsley, minced

1. In a suitable bowl, beat the mayonnaise, olive oil, mustard, anchovy paste, and pepper. Keep it aside. 2. Slice the hard-boiled eggs in half lengthwise, remove the yolks, and place the yolks in a suitable bowl. Reserve the egg white halves and keep it aside. 3. Smash the yolks well with a fork and stir in the mayonnaise mixture. Add the olives, onion, and parsley and stir to combine. 4. Spoon the filling into each egg white half. Cover and chill for almost 30 minutes or up to 24 hours before serving cold.
Per serving: Calories: 382; Total fat 21g; Sodium 1176mg; Total Carbs 9.5g; Fiber 7.2g; Sugars 8.9g; Protein 2.8g

Brussels Sprouts with Pancetta and Walnuts

Prep time: 10 minutes. | Cooking time: 40 minutes. | Serves: 4

½ cup walnuts
1 pound Brussels sprouts, trimmed and halved
6 tablespoons olive oil
½ teaspoon salt

½ teaspoon garlic powder
¼ teaspoon black pepper
4 ounces pancetta, cut into ½-inch strips
2 tablespoons balsamic vinegar

1. At 425°F/218°C, preheat your oven. Place the walnuts on a suitable baking sheet lined with foil sheet. 2. Toast the walnuts until just browned and fragrant, but not burned, 3 to 4 minutes. Remove from your oven, chop, and keep it aside, reserving the foil on the baking sheet. 3. In a suitable bowl, mix the Brussels sprouts, 4 tablespoons of olive oil, the salt, garlic powder, and pepper and toss to coat well. 4. Transfer the Brussels sprouts to the prepared baking sheet. Do not rinse the bowl. Roast the sprouts for almost 20 minutes. Remove from your oven, sprinkle with this pancetta, and toss to blend. Return to your oven and roast until the sprouts are golden brown and pancetta is crispy, another 10 to 15 minutes. Remove from your oven and return to the reserved bowl. 5. Add the chopped toasted walnuts to the warm Brussels sprouts and pancetta, and toss to coat. In a suitable bowl, beat the remaining 2 tablespoons of olive oil and the vinegar and drizzle over the prepared mixture. Toss to coat and serve warm.
Per serving: Calories: 111; Total fat 5.4g; Sodium 1357mg; Total carbs 8.7g; Fiber 2g; Sugars 3.9g; Protein 9.1g

Garlicky Creamed Spinach

Prep time: 10 minutes. | Cooking time: 15 minutes. | Serves: 4

4 tablespoons unsalted butter
½ small onion, minced
4 cloves garlic, minced
1 (16 ounces) package frozen spinach (about 4 cups), thawed and drained of excess water
4 ounces cream cheese, room

temperature
½ cup heavy cream
1 teaspoon salt
¼ teaspoon black pepper, freshly ground
¼ teaspoon nutmeg

1. Heat the butter in a suitable skillet over low heat. Add the onion and sauté for almost 3 to 4 minutes, or until starting to turn golden. Add the garlic and sauté for another 1 to 2 minutes, or until fragrant. 2. Add the spinach and sauté for almost 1 to 2 minutes, or until the water has released. 3. Stir in the cream cheese and cook over low heat until melted and well incorporated with the spinach, 2 to 3 minutes. 4. Whisk in the heavy cream, salt, pepper, and nutmeg (if using). Increase heat to medium and cook, whisking constantly, until smooth and creamy, 3 to 4 minutes. Serve warm.
Per serving: Calories: 229; Total fat 12.6g; Sodium 875mg; Total Carbs 6.2g; Fiber 4.6g; Sugars 8.9g; Protein 5.4g

Roasted Delicata Squash and Kale Salad

Prep time: 10 minutes. | Cooking time: 20 minutes. | Serves: 8

1 cup slivered delicata squash half-moons. for almost ¼ inch thick
6 tablespoons olive oil
1 teaspoon salt
4 cups baby kale or baby spinach

leaves
¼ cup roasted pumpkin seeds
1 tablespoon balsamic vinegar
¼ teaspoon black pepper
4 ounces goat cheese, crumbled

1. At 400°F/204°C, preheat your oven and layer a rimmed baking sheet with foil sheet. 2. In a suitable bowl, toss the squash, 2 tablespoons of olive oil, and ½ teaspoon of salt. Spread the squash in a single layer on the prepared baking sheet, reserving the bowl, and roast until golden and tender, for 15 to 20 minutes. 3. Meanwhile, place the kale in the reserved bowl. Add the pumpkin seeds. Keep it aside. 4. In a suitable bowl, beat the remaining 4 tablespoons of olive oil, the remaining ½ teaspoon of salt, the vinegar, and pepper and keep it aside. 5. When the squash has cooked, remove from your oven and add the warm squash to the greens. Drizzle with the dressing and toss to coat well. Top with goat cheese and serve warm.
Per serving: Calories: 350; Total fat 34.4g; Sodium 1079mg; Total carbs 7.8g; Fiber 2.3g; Sugars 3.1g; Protein 4.9g

Sausage Balls

Prep time: 10 minutes. | Cooking time: 25 minutes. | Serves: 12

1 pound bulk Italian sausage (not sweet)
1 cup almond flour
1½ cups finely shredded cheddar cheese

1 large egg
2 teaspoons baking powder
1 teaspoon onion powder
1 teaspoon fennel seed
½ teaspoon cayenne pepper

1. At 350°F/177°C, preheat your oven and layer a rimmed baking sheet with foil sheet. 2. In a suitable bowl, mix all the recipe ingredients. Use a fork to mix until well blended. 3. Form the sausage mixture into 1½-inch balls and place 1 inch apart on the prepared baking sheet. 4. Bake for almost 20 to 25 minutes, or until browned and cooked through.
Per serving: Calories: 307; Total fat 3.8g; Sodium 789mg; Total Carbs 7.2g; Fiber 22.6g; Sugars 3.3g; Protein 21.2g

Bacon-Studded Pimento Cheese

Prep time: 10 minutes. | Cooking time: 5 minutes. | Serves: 6

2 ounces bacon (about 4 thick slices)
4 ounces cream cheese, room temperature
¼ cup mayonnaise
¼ teaspoon onion powder

¼ teaspoon cayenne pepper
1 cup thick-shredded extra-sharp cheddar cheese
2 ounces jarred diced pimentos, drained

1. Chop the raw bacon into ½-inch-thick pieces. Cook in a suitable skillet over medium heat until crispy, 3 to 4 minutes. 2. Use a slotted spoon and transfer the bacon onto a layer of paper towels. Reserve the rendered fat. 3. In a suitable bowl, mix the cream cheese, mayonnaise, onion powder, and cayenne (if using), and mix with an electric mixer or by hand until smooth and creamy. 4. Add the rendered bacon fat, cheddar cheese, and pimentos and mix until well combined. 5. Refrigerate for 30 minutes before serving to allow flavors to blend. 6. Serve cold with raw veggies such as celery, cucumber, or radish.
Per serving: Calories: 277; Total fat 21g; Sodium 925mg; Total Carbs 0.1g; Fiber 4.8g; Sugars 8.1g; Protein 6.7g

Crunchy Granola Bars

Prep time: 10 minutes. | Cooking time: 15 minutes. | Serves: 16

½ cup unsweetened almond butter
2 tablespoons coconut oil
2 to 4 tablespoons granulated swerve sweetener
1 egg white
1 teaspoon ground cinnamon
1 teaspoon vanilla extract

¼ teaspoon salt
2 tablespoons almond flour
1 cup unsweetened coconut flakes
1 cup slivered almonds
1 cup chopped roasted unsalted pecans
1 cup shelled pumpkin seeds

1. At 350°F/177°C, preheat your oven. 2. Line an 8-inch square glass baking dish with parchment paper, letting the paper hang over the sides. 3. In a suitable glass bowl, mix the almond butter, coconut oil, and sweetener and microwave for almost 30 seconds, or until the coconut oil is melted. 4. Whisk in the egg white, cinnamon, vanilla extract, and salt until smooth and creamy. 5. Stir in the almond flour, coconut flakes, almonds, pecans, and pumpkin seeds until thoroughly combined. 6. Transfer the prepared mixture into the prepared dish and press down firmly with a spatula to cover the bottom evenly. 7. Bake for almost 15 minutes, or until crispy and slightly browned around the edges. 8. Allow to cool completely before cutting into 16 bars. Bars can be stored tightly wrapped in the freezer for up to 3 months.
Per serving: Calories: 186; Total fat 1.3g; Sodium 526mg; Total Carbs 6.2g; Fiber 2.5g; Sugars 4.2g; Protein 6.8g

Pecan Sandy Fat Bombs

Prep time: 10 minutes. | Cooking time: 0 minutes. | Serves: 8

½ cup (1 stick) unsalted butter, room temperature
¼ cup granulated swerve sweetener
½ teaspoon vanilla extract
1 cup almond flour
¾ cup chopped roasted unsalted pecans

1. In a suitable bowl, use an electric mixer on medium speed to cream the butter and sweetener until smooth. Add the vanilla and beat well. 2. Add the almond flour and ½ cup of chopped pecans, and stir until well incorporated. Place the prepared mixture in the refrigerator for almost 30 minutes, or until slightly hardened. Meanwhile, very finely chop the remaining ¼ cup of pecans. 3. Using a spoon or your hands, form the chilled mixture into 8 (1-inch) round balls and place on a suitable baking sheet lined with parchment paper. 4. Roll each ball in the finely chopped pecans, and refrigerate for at least 30 minutes before serving.
Per serving: Calories: 228; Total fat 17.8g; Sodium 168mg; Total Carbs 1.9g; Fiber 1.7g; Sugars 4.9g; Protein 9.1g

Almond and Chocolate Chia Pudding

Prep time: 10 minutes. | Cooking time: 0 minutes. | Serves: 4

1 (14-ounce) can full-fat coconut milk
⅓ cup chia seeds
1 tablespoon unsweetened cocoa powder
2 tablespoons unsweetened
almond butter
2 to 3 teaspoons granulated swerve sweetener
½ teaspoon vanilla extract
½ teaspoon almond extract

1. Mix all the recipe ingredients in a suitable bowl, whisking well to fully incorporate the almond butter. 2. Divide the prepared mixture between four ramekins or small glass jars. 3. Cover and refrigerate for at least 6 hours, preferably overnight. Serve cold.
Per serving: Calories: 235; Total fat 17.6g; Sodium 24mg; Total Carbs 5.8g; Fiber 3.8g; Sugars 7.2g; Protein 8.1g

Broccoli and Carrot Bites

Prep time: 10 minutes. | Cooking time: 12 minutes. | Serves: 20

1 (10-ounce) steamer bag broccoli, cooked according to package instructions
½ cup shredded sharp cheddar cheese
2 tablespoons peeled and grated
carrot
½ cup blanched finely ground almond flour
1 large egg, whisked
¼ teaspoon salt
¼ teaspoon ground black pepper

1. Let cooked broccoli cool 5 minutes, then wring out excess moisture with a kitchen towel. In a suitable bowl, mix broccoli with cheddar, carrot, flour, egg, salt, and pepper. Scoop 2 tablespoons of the prepared mixture into a ball, then roll into a bite-sized piece. Repeat with remaining mixture to form twenty bites. 2. Cut a piece of parchment to fit into the bottom of air fryer basket. Place bites into a single layer on ungreased parchment. Set the temperature to 320°F/160°C and set the timer for almost 12 minutes, turning bites halfway through cooking. Bites will be golden brown when done. Serve warm.
Per serving: Calories: 490; Total fat 17.2g; Sodium 33mg; Total Carbs 6.2g; Fiber 19.1g; Sugars 11.6g; Protein 21.7g

Bacon-Wrapped Jalapeño Poppers

Prep time: 10 minutes. | Cooking time: 12 minutes. | Serves: 12

3 ounces cream cheese, softened
⅓ cup shredded mild cheddar cheese
¼ teaspoon garlic powder
6 jalapeños (approximately 4" long), tops removed, sliced in half lengthwise and seeded
12 slices sugar-free bacon

1. Place cream cheese, cheddar, and garlic powder in a suitable microwave-safe bowl. 2. Microwave 30 seconds on high, then stir. Spoon cheese mixture evenly into hollowed jalapeños. 3. Wrap 1 slice bacon around each jalapeño half, completely covering jalapeño, and secure with a toothpick. Place jalapeños into ungreased air fryer basket. Set the temperature to 400°F/204°C and set the timer for almost 12 minutes, turning jalapeños halfway through cooking. Bacon will be crispy when done. Serve warm.
Per serving: Calories: 197; Total fat 16.8g; Sodium 0mg; Total carbs 9.1g; Fiber 3.9g; Sugars 3.3g; Protein 6g

Spicy Cheese-Stuffed Mushrooms

Prep time: 10 minutes. | Cooking time: 8 minutes. | Serves: 10

4 ounces cream cheese, softened
6 tablespoons shredded pepper jack cheese
2 tablespoons chopped pickled jalapeños
20 medium button mushrooms, stems removed
2 tablespoons olive oil
¼ teaspoon salt
⅛ teaspoon ground black pepper

1. In a suitable bowl, mix cream cheese, pepper jack cheese, and jalapeños. 2. Drizzle mushrooms with olive oil, then sprinkle with black pepper and salt. Spoon 2 tablespoons cheese mixture into each mushroom and place in a single layer into ungreased air fryer basket. Set the temperature to 370°F/188°C and set the timer for almost 8 minutes, checking halfway through cooking to ensure even cooking, rearranging if some are darker than others. When they're golden and cheese is bubbling, mushrooms will be done. Serve warm.
Per serving: Calories: 82; Total fat 7.4g; Sodium 158mg; Total Carbs 1.7g; Fiber 0.4g; Sugars 1.2g; Protein 3g

Pepperoni Chips

Prep time: 10 minutes. | Cooking time: 8 minutes. | Serves: 2

14 slices pepperoni

1. Place pepperoni slices into ungreased air fryer basket. 2. Set the temperature to 350°F/177°C and set the timer for almost 8 minutes. 3. Pepperoni will be browned and crispy when done. 4. Let cool 5 minutes before serving. Serve.
Per serving: Calories: 134; Total fat 10.8g; Sodium 129mg; Total carbs 8.6g; Fiber 3.1g; Sugars 1.6g; Protein 3.6g

Bacon-Wrapped Onion Rings

Prep time: 10 minutes. | Cooking time: 10 minutes. | Serves: 8

1 large white onion, peeled and cut into 16 (¼"-thick) slices
8 slices sugar-free bacon

1. Stack 2 slices onion and wrap with 1 slice bacon. Secure with a toothpick. Repeat with remaining onion slices and bacon. 2. Place onion rings into ungreased air fryer basket. Set the temperature to 350°F/177°C and set the timer for almost 10 minutes, turning rings halfway through cooking. Bacon will be crispy when done. Serve warm.
Per serving: Calories: 113; Total fat 10.2g; Sodium 123mg; Total carbs 2g; Fiber 0.3g; Sugars 1g; Protein 3.5g

Three Cheese Dip

Prep time: 10 minutes. | Cooking time: 12 minutes. | Serves: 8

8 ounces cream cheese, softened
½ cup mayonnaise
¼ cup sour cream
½ cup shredded sharp cheddar
cheese
¼ cup shredded Monterey jack cheese

1. In a suitable bowl, mix all the recipe ingredients. Scoop mixture into an ungreased 4-cup nonstick baking dish and place into air fryer basket. 2. Set the temperature to 375°F/191°C and set the timer for almost 12 minutes. Dip will be browned on top and bubbling when done. Serve warm.
Per serving: Calories: 155; Total fat 7.3g; Sodium 242mg; Total Carbs 2.3g; Fiber 3.5g; Sugars 0.4g; Protein 1.3g

Buffalo Chicken Dip

Prep time: 10 minutes. | Cooking time: 12 minutes. | Serves: 8

8 ounces cream cheese, softened
2 cups chopped cooked chicken thighs
½ cup buffalo sauce
1 cup shredded mild cheddar cheese

1. In a suitable bowl, mix cream cheese, chicken, buffalo sauce, and ½ cup cheddar. Scoop dip into an ungreased 4-cup nonstick baking dish and top with remaining cheddar. 2. Place dish into air fryer basket. Set the temperature to 375°F/191°C and set the timer for almost 12 minutes. 3. Dip will be browned on top and bubbling when done. Serve warm.
Per serving: Calories: 285; Total fat 6.4g; Sodium 297mg; Total Carbs 1.8g; Fiber 2.8g; Sugars 2.1g; Protein 5.5g

Pepperoni Rolls

Prep time: 10 minutes. | Cooking time: 8 minutes. | Serves: 6

2½ cups shredded mozzarella cheese
2 ounces cream cheese, softened
1 cup blanched finely ground

almond flour
48 slices pepperoni
2 teaspoons Italian seasoning

1. In a suitable microwave-safe bowl, mix mozzarella, cream cheese, and flour. Microwave on high 90 seconds until cheese is melted. 2. Using a wooden spoon, mix melted mixture 2 minutes until a dough forms. 3. Once dough is cool enough to work with your hands. For almost 2 minutes, spread it out into a 12" × 4" rectangle on ungreased parchment paper. Line dough with pepperoni into four even rows. Sprinkle Italian seasoning evenly over pepperoni. 4. Starting at the long end of the prepared dough, roll up until a log is formed. Slice the log into twelve even pieces. 5. Place pizza rolls in an ungreased 6" nonstick baking dish. Set the temperature to 375°F/191°C and set the timer for almost 8 minutes. Rolls will be golden and firm when done. Allow cooked rolls to cool 10 minutes before serving.
Per serving: Calories: 319; Total fat 22.4g; Sodium 746mg; Total Carbs 7g; Fiber 3.4g; Sugars 2.3g; Protein 24.5g

Bean Free "Hummus"

Prep time: 10 minutes. | Cooking time: 2 minutes. | Serves: 4

1 zucchini, seeded and chopped
3 cups cauliflower florets
4 tablespoons tahini
3 tablespoons lemon juice
2 cloves garlic

1 teaspoon smoked paprika
3 tablespoons olive oil
¼ cup heavy cream
1 tablespoon butter
Black pepper and salt to taste

1. Heat the butter in a saucepan and add the cauliflower. Sauté until tender. 2. Place the cooked cauliflower and all of the remaining ingredients in your high-speed blender or food processor and blend on high about 2 minutes, until smooth and creamy. 3. If the prepared mixture is too thick, add a bit of water until desired consistency is reached. 4. Transfer to a serving bowl, cover and refrigerate for at least 30 minutes. 5. Serve alongside fresh vegetables such as carrots, celery and broccoli.
Per serving: Calories: 277; Total fat 21g; Sodium 925mg; Total Carbs 0.1g; Fiber 4.8g; Sugars 8.1g; Protein 6.7g

Bacon and Avocado Deviled Eggs

Prep time: 10 minutes. | Cooking time: 0 minutes. | Serves: 4

1 ripe avocado
4 large eggs, hard-boiled
4 slices bacon, cooked and crumbled (use organic nitrate-free bacon for a paleo version)

1 red chili pepper, seeded and minced
1 garlic clove, minced
2 tablespoons lemon juice
Black pepper and salt to taste

1. Peel the eggs, halve them lengthwise and transfer the yolks to a mixing bowl. 2. Add the avocado, chili pepper, garlic and lemon juice to the bowl. 3. Mash with a fork until well combined. Season with black pepper and salt. 4. Scoop the prepared mixture into the egg whites and top with the crumbled bacon. 5. Refrigerate until cold or serve right away!
Per serving: Calories: 361; Total fat 10.3g; Sodium 1557mg; Total Carbs 2.2g; Fiber 5.7g; Sugars 3.6g; Protein 16.7g

Carrot Fries with Herb Sauce

Prep time: 10 minutes. | Cooking time: 30 minutes. | Serves: 6

Fries
5 carrots
1 tablespoon butter, melted
3 tablespoons olive oil
Black pepper and salt to taste
Herb sauce
5 tablespoons sour cream
5 tablespoons heavy cream
1 tablespoon fresh thyme,

chopped
1 teaspoon fresh oregano, chopped
¼ teaspoon fresh rosemary, chopped
4 tablespoons Parmesan cheese, grated
Black pepper and salt to taste

1. At 350°F/177°C, preheat your oven. Prepare a suitable baking sheet with parchment paper or non-stick cooking spray. 2. Cut the carrots into even pieces about the size of French fries. 3. Place in a suitable mixing bowl and toss with the olive oil, melted butter, black pepper and salt. 4. Transfer to the prepared baking sheet and bake for almost 30 minutes, flipping halfway through. 5. While the carrots bake,

prepare the herb sauce by combining the sour cream with the heavy cream, cheese and fresh herbs. Season with black pepper and salt. Mix until smooth.
Remove the fries from your oven and serve alongside the herb sauce.
Per serving: Calories: 134; Total fat 10.8g; Sodium 129mg; Total carbs 8.6g; Fiber 3.1g; Sugars 1.6g; Protein 3.6g

Zesty Onion Rings

Prep time: 10 minutes. | Cooking time: 10 minutes. | Serves: 2

1 large onion, sliced into rings
½ cup almond flour
1 egg
½ teaspoon garlic powder

1 teaspoon paprika
1 teaspoon cayenne pepper
1 teaspoon salt

1. At 400°F/204°C, preheat your oven and lining a suitable baking sheet with parchment paper. 2. Add the egg to a mixing bowl and then add the almond flour and seasoning to another bowl. Mix the almond flour mixture well. 3. Dip the sliced onions into the egg mixture, followed by the almond flour mix, covering both sides of the sliced onions. 4. Add the onion rings to the baking sheet and bake for almost 10 minutes per side or until crispy.
Per serving: Calories: 134; Total fat 10.8g; Sodium 129mg; Total carbs 8.6g; Fiber 3.1g; Sugars 1.6g; Protein 3.6g

Ranch Chicken Bites

Prep time: 10 minutes. | Cooking time: 15 minutes. | Serves: 6

2 (6 ounces) boneless, skinless chicken breasts, cut into 1" cubes
1 tablespoon coconut oil
½ teaspoon salt
¼ teaspoon ground black pepper

⅓ cup ranch dressing
½ cup shredded Colby cheese
4 slices cooked sugar-free bacon, crumbled

1. Drizzle chicken with coconut oil. Sprinkle with black pepper and salt, and place into an ungreased 6" round nonstick baking dish. 2. Place dish into air fryer basket. 3. Set the temperature to 370°F/188°C and set the timer for almost 10 minutes, stirring chicken halfway through cooking. 4. When the pot beeps, drizzle ranch dressing over chicken and top with Colby and bacon. 5. Set the temperature to 400°F/204°C and set the timer for almost 5 minutes. 6. When done, chicken will be browned and have an internal temperature of at least 165°F/74°C. Serve warm.
Per serving: Calories: 448; Total fat 8.5g; Sodium 247mg; Total Carbs 7.7g; Fiber 32.5g; Sugars 6g; Protein 27g

Bacon-Wrapped Mozzarella Sticks

Prep time: 10 minutes. | Cooking time: 12 minutes. | Serves: 6

6 sticks mozzarella string cheese   6 slices sugar-free bacon

1. Place mozzarella sticks on a suitable plate, cover, and place into freezer 1 hour until frozen solid. 2. Wrap each mozzarella stick in 1 piece of bacon and secure with a toothpick. 3. Place into ungreased air fryer basket. Set the temperature to 400°F/204°C and set the timer for almost 12 minutes, turning sticks once during cooking. 4. Bacon will be crispy when done. Serve warm.
Per serving: Calories: 373; Total fat 12g; Sodium 1364mg; Total Carbs 3.3g; Fiber 31.3g; Sugars 6.4g; Protein 19.1g

Buffalo Cauliflower Bites

Prep time: 10 minutes. | Cooking time: 15 minutes. | Serves: 6

1 medium head cauliflower, leaves and core removed, cut into bite-sized pieces
4 tablespoons salted butter,

melted
¼ cup dry ranch seasoning
⅓ cup buffalo sauce

1. Place cauliflower pieces into a suitable bowl. 2. Pour butter over cauliflower and toss to coat. Sprinkle in ranch seasoning and toss to coat. 3. Place cauliflower into ungreased air fryer basket. 4. Set the temperature to 350°F/177°C and set the timer for almost 12 minutes, shaking the basket three times during cooking. 5. When the pot beeps, place cooked cauliflower in a clean suitable bowl. 6. Toss with buffalo sauce, then return to air fryer basket to cook another 3 minutes. 7. Cauliflower bites will be darkened at the edges and tender when done. Serve warm.
Per serving: Calories: 495; Total fat 13g; Sodium 334mg; Total Carbs 3.7g; Fiber 20.7g; Sugars 12.9g; Protein 24.6g

Charcuterie Board

Prep time: 15 minutes| Cook time: 0 minutes| Serves: 10

½ cup small fresh mozzarella balls
½ cup halved strawberries
½ cup raspberries
½ cup green olives or olives of choice, pitted
¼ cup whole almonds
½ cup cheddar cheese cubes
4 ounces pepper Jack cheese, thinly sliced
4 ounces Swiss cheese, thinly sliced
4 ounces prosciutto, thinly sliced
4 ounces hard salami, thinly sliced
6 bacon slices, cooked and halved
4 ounces turkey, thinly sliced

1. Choose a large flat serving platter that can comfortably hold all the ingredients in your desired arrangement. Place the mozzarella, strawberries, raspberries, olives, and almonds in small separate bowls. Set the containers on the platter spaced apart. 2. Begin arranging the remaining meats and cheeses around the bowls, adjusting aesthetics as you fill the space. Start near the dishes, working out and away from the bowl to tightly fill the empty space on the platter in a single layer. If necessary, stack the upward. Tuck in open spaces, fan-out, roll, and fold items if necessary. Serve hot.
Per Serving: Calories 263; Fat 19g; Sodium 741mg; Carbs 4g; Fiber 1g; Sugar 1g; Protein 18g

Crudités Platter

Prep time: 30 minutes| Cook time: 0 minutes| Serves: 10

1 cup mayonnaise
1 cup sour cream
1 teaspoon onion powder
Generous pinch salt
Generous pinch freshly ground black pepper
½ cup cucumber slices, cut at an angle
½ cup celery sticks (4 inches long)
½ cup quartered radishes
½ cup cherry tomatoes
½ cup broccoli florets
½ cup cauliflower florets
½ cup snap peas
½ cup orange bell pepper strips
2 Belgian endives, leaves separated
1 cup Kalamata olives or mixed olive varieties, pitted
½ cup whole pickled banana peppers

1. Choose one or two large flat serving platters that can comfortably hold several cups of cut vegetables and dips in your desired arrangement. 2. Combine the mayonnaise, sour cream, onion powder, salt, and pepper in a small bowl. Transfer the dip to one or two clean serving bowls (depending on the number of platters) and swirl the top. Place a bowl near the center of each serving platter. 3. Begin arranging the vegetables, and adjusting for aesthetics as you fill the space. Start near the dip(s), working out and away from the bowl to tightly fill the space on the platter with the vegetables. Tuck into empty spaces and fan out items as necessary. Serve immediately.
Per Serving: Calories 227; Fat 23g; Sodium 689mg; Carbs 5g; Fiber 2g; Sugar 2g; Protein 2g

Crispy Deviled Eggs

Prep time: 10 minutes. | Cooking time: 25 minutes. | Serves: 12

7 large eggs
1 ounce plain pork rinds, finely crushed
2 tablespoons mayonnaise
¼ teaspoon salt
¼ teaspoon ground black pepper

1. Place 6 whole eggs into ungreased air fryer basket. Set the temperature to 220°F/104°C and set the timer for almost 20 minutes. When done, place eggs into a bowl of ice water to cool 5 minutes. 2. Peel cold eggs, then cut in half lengthwise. Remove yolks and place aside in a suitable bowl. 3. In a separate suitable bowl, whisk remaining raw egg. Place pork rinds in a separate suitable bowl. Dip each egg white into whisked egg, then gently coat with pork rinds. Spritz with cooking spray and place into ungreased air fryer basket. Set the temperature to 400°F/204°C and set the timer for almost 5 minutes, turning eggs halfway through cooking. Eggs will be golden when done. 4. Mash yolks in bowl with mayonnaise until smooth. Sprinkle with black pepper and salt and mix. 5. Spoon 2 tablespoons yolk mixture into each fried egg white. Serve warm.
Per serving: Calories: 153; Total fat 13g; Sodium 82mg; Total carbs 7.9g; Fiber 0.7g; Sugars 1.2g; Protein 3.6g

Hard-Boiled Eggs in the Air Fryer

Prep time: 10 minutes. | Cooking time: 12 minutes. | Serves: 6

3 tablespoons sriracha hot chili   sauce

1 medium head cabbage, cored and diced
2 tablespoons coconut oil, melted
½ teaspoon salt
12 slices sugar-free bacon
½ cup mayonnaise
¼ teaspoon garlic powder

1. Evenly brush 2 tablespoons sriracha onto cabbage pieces. Drizzle evenly with coconut oil, then sprinkle with salt. 2. Wrap each cabbage piece with bacon and secure with a toothpick. Place into ungreased air fryer basket. Set the temperature to 375°F/191°C and set the timer for almost 12 minutes, turning cabbage halfway through cooking. Bacon will be cooked and crispy when done. 3. In a suitable bowl, beat mayonnaise, garlic powder, and remaining sriracha. Use as a dipping sauce for cabbage bites.
Per serving: Calories: 346; Total fat 31.5g; Sodium 620mg; Total carbs 8.4g; Fiber 2.3g; Sugars 4.4g; Protein 9.2g

Cauliflower Buns

Prep time: 10 minutes. | Cooking time: 12 minutes. | Serves: 8

1 (12-ounce) steamer bag cauliflower, cooked according to package instructions
½ cup shredded mozzarella cheese
¼ cup shredded mild cheddar
cheese
¼ cup blanched finely ground almond flour
1 large egg
½ teaspoon salt

1. Let cooked cauliflower cool about 10 minutes. Use a kitchen towel to wring out excess moisture, then place cauliflower in a food processor. 2. Add mozzarella, cheddar, flour, egg, and salt to the food processor and pulse twenty times until mixture is combined. It will resemble a soft, wet dough. 3. Divide mixture into eight piles. Wet your hands with water to prevent sticking, then press each pile into a flat bun shape. for almost ½" thick. 4. Cut a sheet of parchment to fit air fryer basket. Working in batches if needed, place the formed dough onto ungreased parchment in air fryer basket. Set the temperature to 350°F/177°C and set the timer for almost 12 minutes, turning buns halfway through cooking. 5. Let buns cool 10 minutes before serving. Serve warm.
Per serving: Calories: 178; Total fat 15.4g; Sodium 39mg; Total carbs 7.7g; Fiber 3.4; Sugars 2.8g; Protein 5.2g

Mini Greek Meatballs

Prep time: 10 minutes. | Cooking time: 10 minutes. | Serves: 9

1 cup fresh spinach leaves
¼ cup peeled and diced red onion
½ cup crumbled feta cheese
1 pound 85/15 ground turkey
½ teaspoon salt
½ teaspoon ground cumin
¼ teaspoon ground black pepper

1. Place spinach, onion, and feta in a food processor, and pulse ten times until spinach is chopped. Scoop into a suitable bowl. 2. Add turkey to bowl and sprinkle with salt, cumin, and pepper. Mix until fully combined. Roll mixture into thirty-six meatballs (about 1 tablespoon each). 3. Place meatballs into ungreased air fryer basket, working in batches if needed. Set the temperature to 350°F/177°C and set the timer for almost 10 minutes, shaking basket twice during cooking. Meatballs will be browned and have an internal temperature of at least 165°F/74°C when done. Serve warm.
Per serving: Calories: 268; Total fat 24g; Sodium 231mg; Total Carbs 1g; Fiber 0.2g; Sugars 0.6g; Protein 11g

Sweet and Spicy Beef Jerky

Prep time: 10 minutes. | Cooking time: 4 hours. | Serves: 6

1 pound eye of round beef, fat trimmed, sliced into ¼"-thick strips
¼ cup soy sauce
2 tablespoons sriracha hot chili
sauce
½ teaspoon ground black pepper
2 tablespoons granular brown erythritol

1. Place beef in a suitable sealable bowl or bag. Pour soy sauce and sriracha into bowl or bag, then sprinkle in pepper and erythritol. Shake or stir to mix ingredients and coat steak. Cover and place in refrigerator to marinate at least 2 hours up to overnight. 2. Once marinated, remove strips from marinade and pat dry. Place into ungreased air fryer basket in a single layer, working in batches if needed. Set the temperature to 180°F/82°C and set the timer for almost 4 hours. Jerky will be chewy and dark brown when done. Store in airtight container in a cool, dry place up to 2 weeks.
Per serving: Calories: 100; Total fat 2.6g; Sodium 416mg; Total Carbs 3.1g; Fiber 0.2g; Sugars 1.3g; Protein 16.3g

Sausage-Stuffed Mushrooms

Prep time: 10 minutes. | Cooking time: 20 minutes. | Serves: 6

½ pound ground pork sausage	½ ounce plain pork rinds, finely
¼ teaspoon salt	crushed
¼ teaspoon garlic powder	1 pound cremini mushrooms,
2 medium scallions, trimmed and	stems removed
chopped	

1. In a suitable bowl, mix sausage, salt, garlic powder, scallions, and pork rinds. Scoop 1 tablespoon mixture into center of each mushroom cap. 2. Place mushrooms into ungreased air fryer basket. Set the temperature to 375°F/191°C and set the timer for almost 20 minutes. Pork will be fully cooked to at least 145°F/63°C in the center and browned when done. Serve warm.
Per serving: Calories: 354; Total fat 11.5g; Sodium 417mg; Total Carbs 58g; Fiber 8.8g; Sugars 2.2g; Protein 14.7g

Spicy Turkey Meatballs

Prep time: 10 minutes. | Cooking time: 15 minutes. | Serves: 6

1 pound 85/15 ground turkey	½ teaspoon salt
1 large egg, whisked	½ teaspoon paprika
¼ cup sriracha hot chili sauce	¼ teaspoon ground black pepper

1. Mix all the recipe ingredients in a suitable bowl. Roll mixture into eighteen meatballs, for almost 3 tablespoons each. 2. Place meatballs into ungreased air fryer basket. Set the temperature to 375°F/191°C and set the timer for almost 15 minutes, shaking the basket three times during cooking. Meatballs will be done when browned and internal temperature is at least 165°F/74°C. Serve warm.
Per serving: Calories: 380; Total fat 34.5g; Sodium 242mg; Total Carbs 0.7g; Fiber 0.2g; Sugars 0.4g; Protein 15.6g

Crispy Salami Roll-Ups

Prep time: 10 minutes. | Cooking time: 4 minutes. | Serves: 4

4 ounces cream cheese, broken	16 (0.5-ounce) deli slices genoa
into 16 equal pieces	salami

1. Place a piece of cream cheese at the edge of a slice of salami and roll to close. 2. Secure with a toothpick. Repeat with remaining cream cheese pieces and salami. 3. Place roll-ups in an ungreased 6" round nonstick baking dish and place into air fryer basket. 4. Set the temperature to 350°F/177°C and set the timer for almost 4 minutes. Serve.
Per serving: Calories: 408; Total fat 8.8g; Sodium 1064mg; Total Carbs 8.8g; Fiber 3.5g; Sugars 7g; Protein 11.9g

Parmesan Zucchini Fries

Prep time: 10 minutes. | Cooking time: 10 minutes. | Serves: 8

2 medium zucchini, ends	½ cup blanched finely ground
removed, quartered lengthwise,	almond flour
and sliced into 3"-long fries	¾ cup grated parmesan cheese
½ teaspoon salt	1 teaspoon Italian seasoning
⅓ cup heavy whipping cream	

1. Sprinkle zucchini with salt and wrap in a kitchen towel to draw out excess moisture. 2. Let sit 2 hours. 3. Pour cream into a suitable bowl. In a separate suitable bowl, beat flour, parmesan, and Italian seasoning. 4. Place each zucchini fry into cream, then gently shake off excess. 5. Press each fry into dry mixture, coating each side, then place into ungreased air fryer basket. 6. Set the temperature to 400°F/204°C and set the timer for almost 10 minutes, turning fries halfway through cooking. Fries will be golden and crispy when done. 7. Place on clean parchment sheet to cool 5 minutes before serving.
Per serving: Calories: 112; Total fat 9.2g; Sodium 344mg; Total Carbs 3.4g; Fiber 1g; Sugars 0.6g; Protein 4.8g

Fried Ranch Pickles

Prep time: 10 minutes. | Cooking time: 10 minutes. | Serves: 4

4 dill pickle spears, halved	almond flour
lengthwise	½ cup grated parmesan cheese
¼ cup ranch dressing	2 tablespoons dry ranch seasoning
½ cup blanched finely ground	

1. Wrap spears in a kitchen towel 30 minutes to soak up excess pickle juice. 2. Pour ranch dressing into a suitable bowl and add pickle spears. 3. In a separate suitable bowl, mix flour, parmesan, and dry ranch seasoning. 4. Remove each spear from ranch dressing and shake off excess. 5. Press gently into dry mixture to coat all sides. 6. Place spears into ungreased air fryer basket. 7. Set the temperature to 400°F/204°C and set the timer for almost 10 minutes, turning spears three times during cooking. Serve warm.
Per serving: Calories: 263; Total fat 19.5g; Sodium 1249mg; Total Carbs 5.3g; Fiber 4.7g; Sugars 5.2g; Protein 10.6g

Bacon and Mozzarella Dates

Prep time: 10 minutes. | Cooking time: 14 minutes. | Serves: 5

5 medjool dates, pitted and	5 slices bacon
chopped	1½ cups mozzarella cheese, sliced

1. At 375°F/191°C, preheat your oven and grease a suitable baking sheet. 2. Heat a suitable skillet over medium heat. 3. Cook the bacon for almost 2 minutes per side, until almost cooked through but still pliable. 4. Wrap some chopped dates in a cheese slice then wrap with half a slice of bacon. 5. Secure them with a toothpick and place on the baking sheet. 6. Repeat until all of the ingredients are used. 7. Bake for almost 10 minutes, until the bacon is crisp. Serve immediately!
Per serving: Calories: 397; Total fat 20g; Sodium 483mg; Total Carbs 5.8g; Fiber 4.5g; Sugars 8.8g; Protein 6.6g

Chipotle Lime Kale Chips

Prep time: 10 minutes. | Cooking time: 30 minutes. | Serves: 6

1 large bunch of kale, stems	1 teaspoon chipotle powder
removed	3 tablespoons olive oil
2 teaspoons lime juice	Black pepper and salt to taste
1 teaspoon lime zest	

1. At 325°F/163°C, preheat your oven. 2. Prepare two baking sheets with parchment paper. 3. In a suitable bowl, mix the kale leaves with the lime juice, zest and olive oil. 4. Toss until the leaves are well coated. 5. Spread the kale leaves onto the baking sheets in an even layer. 6. Sprinkle with the chipotle powder, pepper and salt. 7. Bake for almost 30 minutes or until crisp.
Per serving: Calories: 142; Total fat 7.9g; Sodium 2mg; Total Carbs 9.2g; Fiber 3.4g; Sugars 15.8g; Protein 2.3g

Avocado Fries

Prep time: 10 minutes. | Cooking time: 6 minutes. | Serves: 6

1 large egg	2 medium avocados, peeled,
¼ cup coconut flour	pitted, and sliced into ¼"-thick
2 ounces plain pork rinds, finely	fries
crushed	

1. Whisk egg in a suitable bowl. Place coconut flour and pork rinds in two separate suitable bowls. Dip 1 avocado slice into egg, then coat in coconut flour. 2. Dip in egg once more, then press gently into pork rinds to coat on both sides. Repeat with remaining avocado slices. 3. Place slices into ungreased air fryer basket. Set the temperature to 400°F/204°C and set the timer for almost 6 minutes, turning "fries" halfway through. Fries will be crispy on the outside and soft inside when done. Let cool before serving.
Per serving: Calories: 172; Total fat 13.6g; Sodium 199mg; Total Carbs 6g; Fiber 4.6g; Sugars 0.7g; Protein 8.3g

Bacon Cauliflower Skewers

Prep time: 10 minutes. | Cooking time: 12 minutes. | Serves: 4

4 slices sugar-free bacon, cut into	florets
thirds	1½ tablespoons olive oil
¼ medium yellow onion, peeled	¼ teaspoon salt
and cut into 1" pieces	¼ teaspoon garlic powder
4 ounces (about 8) cauliflower	

1. Place 1 piece bacon and 2 pieces onion on a 6" skewer. Add a second piece bacon, and 2 cauliflower florets, followed by another piece of bacon onto skewer. Repeat with remaining ingredients and three additional skewers to make four total skewers. 2. Drizzle skewers with olive oil, then sprinkle with salt and garlic powder. Place skewers into ungreased air fryer basket. Set the temperature to 375°F/191°C and set the timer for almost 12 minutes, turning the skewers halfway through cooking. When done, vegetables will be tender and bacon will be crispy. Serve warm.
Per serving: Calories: 154; Total fat 9.1g; Sodium 15mg; Total Carbs 5.9g; Fiber 2.4g; Sugars 9.4g; Protein 4.5g

Chapter 7 Vegetables and Sides

Cheesy Basil Mozzarella Zoodles

Prep time: 10 minutes| Cook time: 10 minutes| Serves: 2

3 medium zucchinis, spiralized
Small bunch of basil leaves
½ teaspoon garlic powder
1 tablespoon pine nuts, toasted
2 tablespoons fresh lemon juice

¼ cup shredded mozzarella cheese
1 tablespoon canola oil
Salt and ground black pepper, to taste

1. Heat canola oil and sauté zoodles for a few minutes until lightly golden and al dente. Spice with salt, garlic powder, and pepper. 2. Add the basil leaves with pine nuts, and lemon juice on low heat. Simmer the zoodles for 2-4 minutes. When sauce thickens sprinkle with mozzarella cheese on it and remove from heat. 3. Serve warm.
Per Serving: Calories 101; Fat 7g; Sodium 304mg; Carbs 5g; Fiber 1g; Sugar 3g; Protein 6g

Provolone Citrus Salad

Prep time: 15 minutes| Cook time: 6 minutes| Serves: 2

2 cups arugula
2 clementines, peeled and segmented
3 ounces provolone cheese
5 cherry tomatoes, halved

½ pomegranate, deseeded
1 teaspoon lemon juice
Sea salt, to taste
2 teaspoons olive oil

1. Slice the provolone cheese into bite-size slices. 2. Place the cheese chunks on a preheated grill for about 3 minutes. Grill marks should appear on the cheese. 3. In a bowl, place the arugula and toss with the clementines, cherry tomatoes along with pomegranate seeds. Top the delicious salad with the grilled provolone slices. 4. Mix the olive oil, lemon juice, and salt in a small bowl. 5. Drizzle this mixture over the salad.
Per Serving: Calories 256; Fat 17g; Sodium 456mg; Carbs 14g; Fiber 5g; Sugar 6g; Protein 13g

Avocado Salad

Prep time: 5 minutes| Cook time: 0 minutes| Serves: 2

1 large avocado, pitted and flesh removed
3 Roma tomatoes
½ cup crushed walnuts
1 cup feta cheese, crumbled
2 garlic cloves, peeled and

minced
2 cups fresh basil leaves or baby spinach
2 tablespoons olive oil
1 tablespoon lemon juice
Salt and pepper to taste

1. Chop the avocado into about ½ inch chunks. Transfer to a serving bowl. 2. Add tomatoes slices to the bowl with the walnuts. Whisk the olive oil, lemon juice, and garlic together in a small bowl. 3. Crumble the feta cheese into the bowl, drizzle with the dressing, and toss until everything is well combined. 4. Serve on a bed of basil leaves or baby spinach.5. Season with salt and black pepper to taste.
Per Serving: Calories 371; Fat 32g; Sodium 506mg; Carbs 9g; Fiber 9g; Sugar 2g; Protein 7g

Spaghetti Squash Noodles

Prep time: 15 minutes| Cook time: 50 minutes| Serves: 2

1 medium spaghetti squash
¼ cup feta cheese, crumbled
3 tablespoons heavy cream
Juice of ½ a lemon
Small bunch of fresh basil, chopped

2 tablespoons olive oil
Salt and ground black pepper, to taste
Italian seasoning
Garlic powder
1 tablespoon butter

1. Preheat oven to 375°F/191°C. Slice the spaghetti squash in two lengthwise pieces and remove the seeds. 2. Grease the inside of each half with olive oil, place on a baking tray and bake for about 40 minutes. 3. With fork pull the flesh into strands. 4. Transfer the squash strands into a serving bowl. 5. Whisk the heavy cream, lemon juice with chopped basil in a small bowl. 6. Top the feta cheese to the squash noodles, spiced with salt and pepper, and mix well.7. Drizzle the noodles with the heavy cream mixture. 8. Fully coat the noodles with sauce. 9. If desired, divide between two plates, top with a pat of butter, and serve.
Per Serving: Calories 339; Fat 33g; Sodium 647mg; Carbs 9g; Fiber

3g; Sugar 4g; Protein 5g

Greens and Tofu Scramble

Prep time: 20 minutes| Cook time: 20 minutes| Serves: 2

½ large head cabbage, thinly sliced
½ red onion, peeled and sliced
2 large handfuls baby spinach
2 garlic cloves, peeled and minced

8 ounces extra-firm tofu
12 Kalamata olives
2 tablespoons olive oil
Salt and ground black pepper, to taste

1. Wrap the tofu in cheesecloth and press the excess liquid out. 2. Combine the cabbage, onion, garlic, and olive oil. 2. Spiced with salt and pepper well to coat. 3. Heat olive oil. Add the cabbage mixture to the pan and sauté it for 5-7 minutes until slightly tender. 4. Add the spinach in cabbage and reduce heat to low. 5. Crumble the tofu into the pan. 6. Add the olives and mix well to combine. 7. Cook for 10-12 minutes until the tofu is cooked and the spinach and cabbage is tender. 8. Spice with salt and pepper, divide between two plates, and serve.
Per Serving: Calories 260; Fat 23g; Sodium 431mg; Carbs 5g; Fiber 1g; Sugar 2g; Protein 12g

Cheesy Veggie Casserole

Prep time: 30 minutes| Cook time: 45 minutes| Serves: 2

2 small eggplants, sliced about ¼-inch thick
½ red bell pepper, seeded and diced
¼ cup gluten-free bran flakes or gluten-free breadcrumbs
½ cup shredded mozzarella

cheese
1 cup kale, chopped
1 egg, beaten
¼ cup olive oil
Salt and ground black pepper to taste

1. Preheat oven to 350°F/177°C. 2. Coat an 8-in by 8-inch baking dish with oil. 3. Place the bell pepper, sliced eggplant, cheese, bran flakes, and kale in a bowl. 4. Season with spices and drizzle oil on it. Toss well to coat oil and spices evenly and place in baking tray. 5. Bake in oven for 40 minutes until the vegetables are tender and the top is golden brown. Serve immediately.
Per Serving: Calories 311; Fat 14g; Sodium 523mg; Carbs 11g; Fiber 10g; Sugar 1g; Protein 16g

Bacon Brussels Sprouts

Prep time: 5 minutes| Cook time: 30 minutes| Serves: 6

6 strips no-sugar-added bacon, halved

12 large Brussels sprouts

1. Preheat the oven to 380°F/193°C. Prepare a baking sheet by lining it with parchment paper. 2. Spread bacon on the prepared baking sheet and roll up a Brussels sprout in each strip. 3. Bake the rolled sprouts for 25–30 minutes, flipping halfway until bacon is crisp and sprouts are softened. Remove from baking sheet and serve warm.
Per Serving: Calories 70; Fat 4g; Sodium 203mg; Carbs 4g; Fiber 1g; Sugar 1g; Protein 5g

Tofu Stir-Fry

Prep time: 20 minutes| Cook time: 15 minutes| Serves: 2

8 ounces extra firm tofu, pressed dry
1 teaspoon minced fresh ginger
1 cup kale, chopped
½ teaspoon garlic powder

2-3 tablespoons gluten-free soy sauce, to taste
2 tablespoons toasted sesame seeds
1 tablespoon sesame oil

1. Cut the tofu into small cubes, about ½ inch. 2. Add the sesame oil to a large pan and place over medium-high heat. 3. Add the tofu and sauté until golden on all sides. 4. Add the fresh ginger, garlic powder, kale, and desired amount of soy sauce. Cook for 3-5 minutes, frequently stirring, until the kale wilts. 5. Remove from heat and divide into 2 serving bowls. Top with sesame seeds and serve.
Per Serving: Calories 226; Fat 17g; Sodium 441mg; Carbs 7g; Fiber 2g; Sugar 3g; Protein 15g

Cauliflower Risotto

Prep time: 10 minutes| Cook time: 15 minutes| Serves: 2

2 cups cauliflower
8 medium white button mushrooms, trimmed
3 garlic cloves, peeled and minced
1 cup vegetable broth
½ cup cream cheese
½ cup mozzarella cheese
2 tablespoons olive oil
Salt and ground black pepper, to taste
1 teaspoon dried oregano

1. Thoroughly wash the cauliflower, cut cauliflower into florets and pulse until it resembles white rice in a food processor. 2. Heat the olive oil and cook the garlic and mushrooms for about 2 minutes. 3. Stir in the "cauliflower rice". 4. Pour in the vegetable broth in cauliflower rice. 5. Simmer on low heat for tenderness. When the cauliflower is al dente, cook it for another 7-10 minutes until all the liquid has been absorbed. 6. Stir in the mozzarella cheese and cream cheese and spiced with salt, pepper, and oregano. 7. When cheese melted, transfer to a serving bowl and serve warm.
Per Serving: Calories 423; Fat 34g; Sodium 356mg; Carbs 8g; Fiber 4g; Sugar 2g; Protein 18g

Feta Skewers

Prep time: 10 minutes| Cook time: 0 minutes| Serves: 2

2 cups cherry tomatoes
1 cup fresh basil leaves
2 cups baby mozzarella cheese balls
1 tablespoon oregano
1-2 tablespoons extra-virgin olive oil
1 cup yellow bell pepper

1. Wash and clean the vegetables. Chop the peppers in small squares. 2. Combine the olive oil and oregano and rub the herbed oil to the mozzarella balls. 3. Assemble the spiced ingredients on skewers in the following order: tomatoes, mozzarella, bell pepper chunks, and basil leaves and serve.
Per Serving: Calories 280; Fat 22g; Sodium 369mg; Carbs 7g; Fiber 2g; Sugar 9g; Protein 13g

Asparagus with Cherry Tomatoes and Cheese

Prep time: 5 minutes| Cook time: 12 minutes| Serves: 2

1 small bunch fresh asparagus, trimmed
¼ cup Romano cheese, grated
1 onion, peeled and sliced thin
2 garlic cloves, peeled and
minced
10 cherry tomatoes, halved
¼ cup extra-virgin olive oil
⅔ cup water

1. Add the water and asparagus to a large pan and set over medium heat. 2. Cook for about 10 minutes until the asparagus softens. Drain water from the pan and return to the stove over low heat. 3. Add the olive oil, onion, garlic, and tomatoes to the asparagus and mix well to combine. Top with grated cheese and cook for another 1-2 minutes until the cheese is melted.
Per Serving: Calories 193; Fat 15g; Sodium 421mg; Carbs 7g; Fiber 2g; Sugar 3g; Protein 5g

Citrus-Dijon Beans

Prep time: 10 minutes| Cook time: 10 minutes| Serves: 2

½ pound French green beans, trimmed
1 lime, juiced
1 tablespoon Dijon mustard
2 garlic cloves, peeled and minced
2 tablespoons heavy cream
1 tablespoon butter

1. Boil the beans until crisp tender and drain them. 2. Melt the butter and cook garlic for a minute. Stir in the heavy cream and mustard. Cook for another 3-4 minutes. 3. Add the beans and mix to the mustard mixture. 4. Add the lime juice and stir well to combine. 5. Serve immediately—the mustard flavor pairs well with a red meat dish.
Per Serving: Calories 159; Fat 12g; Sodium 412mg; Carbs 12g; Fiber 4g; Sugar 2g; Protein 3g

Gruyere-Stuffed Peppers

Prep time: 10 minutes| Cook time: 20 minutes| Serves: 2

2 small bell peppers, any color
1 cup shredded Gruyere cheese
2 tablespoons fresh parsley,
minced
1 clove garlic, peeled and minced
2 green onions, chopped

10 green olives, pitted and chopped
Salt and ground black pepper, to
taste
2 tablespoons olive oil
¼ cup whole leaf basil

1. Preheat oven to 375°F/191°C. 2. Chop off the bell pepper's tops and remove the core and seeds. Rub the pepper with olive oil, place on a roasting pan, and roast for about 20 minutes. Allow cooling slightly. 3. Combine the minced garlic, green onion, parsley, and olives in a small bowl. Add the shredded Gruyere and mix well. 4. Stuff each pepper with the cheese mixture. 5. Place back to the oven and cook for 5 minutes. Transfer to a serving plate, garnish with basil, and enjoy.
Per Serving: Calories 461; Fat 37g; Sodium 411mg; Carbs 8g; Fiber 3g; Sugar 2g; Protein 22g

Trot Mushroom Salad

Prep time: 15 minutes plus 2 hours for marinating| Cook time: 15 minutes| Serves: 6

3 tablespoons apple cider vinegar
1 tablespoon olive oil
½ tablespoon garlic powder
¼ teaspoon salt
⅛ teaspoon ground black pepper
2 pounds Portobello mushrooms,
chopped into bite-sized pieces
½ cup seeded and thinly sliced red bell pepper
1 tablespoon finely chopped green onion

1. Whisk to combine vinegar, oil, garlic powder, salt, and black pepper in a medium mixing bowl. 2. Pour vinegar marinade into a 2-gallon resealable bag along with mushrooms and bell pepper. Seal after all the air is squeezed out. Knead the bag until all the vegetables are thoroughly coated with the marinade. 3. Let marinate in the refrigerator for at least 2 hours, preferably overnight. 4. Add contents of bag to a large pan over medium heat. Cook covered for 15 minutes, stirring regularly. 5. Let cool and serve warm topped with green onion as a garnish.
Per Serving: Calories 61; Fat 2g; Sodium 111mg; Carbs 7g; Fiber 2g; Sugar 4g; Protein 3g

Tangy Pickles

Prep time: 5 minutes| Cook time: 10 minutes| Serves: 10

5 medium cucumbers, trimmed and quartered lengthwise
¾ cup apple cider vinegar
¾ cup water
1½ tablespoons salt
1 tablespoon minced garlic
1 tablespoon finely chopped fresh dill

1. Place twenty cucumber spears in a large jar. 2. In a medium saucepan over medium heat, combine the remaining ingredients except for dill. Cook for 10 minutes, stirring regularly to dissolve salt. Let cool. 3. Stir in dill. Transfer mixture to the jar, covering the spears until jar is almost full, and tighten the lid. 4. Refrigerate overnight. Serve chilled.
Per Serving: Calories 22; Fat 0g; Sodium 107mg; Carbs 6g; Fiber 1g; Sugar 3g; Protein 1g

Fried Green Tomatoes

Prep time: 20 minutes| Cook time: 1 hour 20 minutes| Serves: 8

2 pounds green tomatoes
1 cup superfine blanched almond flour
1 teaspoon paprika
½ teaspoon salt
¼ teaspoon ground black pepper
3 large eggs
3 tablespoons heavy whipping cream
1 cup textured vegetable protein

1. Trim ends off tomatoes and slice into discs ¼"–⅜" thick, cutting through the center axes of tomatoes. 2. Set out two dinner plates and one medium bowl. On one plate, combine flour, paprika, salt, and pepper. In the bowl, whisk together eggs and cream—Spread TVP on a remaining plate. 3. Coat both sides of tomato slice first in flour dredge. Then dip in egg wash and shake off extra. Finally, press both sides of each piece into TVP. 4. Arrange coated slices on an air fryer crisper tray, ensuring they are not touching. Air-fry it for 10 minutes at 400°F/204°C, flip, and cook for another 10 minutes at the same temperature. Repeat in small batches until done. Serve warm.
Per Serving: Calories 103; Fat 5g; Sodium 99mg; Carbs 8g; Fiber 3g; Sugar 2g; Protein 7g

Regular Italian Frittata

Prep time: 10 minutes| Cook time: 10 minutes| Serves: 2

1½ cups fresh cauliflower florets
1 bell pepper, seeded and julienned
1 teaspoon garlic powder
4 cherry tomatoes, halved
1 tablespoon goat cheese,
crumbled
4 medium eggs
1 tablespoon canola oil
Salt and pepper, to taste
⅔ teaspoon thyme
½ cup milk

1. Preheat oven to 350°F/177°C with the temperature setting. 2. Boil cauliflower until crisp-tender. Transfer to a colander and drain. 3. In a pan, heat the oil. Sauté the julienned peppers for 3-4 minutes. 4. Add the cauliflower with garlic powder to the pan. 5. Spice with thyme, salt, and pepper, and cook further for 1-2 minutes. 6. Cook in the tomatoes until heated through. 7. Beat the eggs with milk until frothy. 8. Pour the egg mixture evenly in the pan. Cook for about 2 minutes. 9. Sprinkle the goat cheese over the frittata. 10. Place the frittata in the oven for 6-8 minutes. 11. Slice frittata wedges and serve warm.
Per Serving: Calories 258; Fat 18g; Sodium 374mg; Carbs 7g; Fiber 5g; Sugar 3g; Protein 16g

Tropical Broccoli

Prep time: 5 minutes| Cook time: 18 minutes| Serves: 2

¼ cup coconut oil, melted
½ teaspoon salt
2 cups broccoli florets

1. In a small bowl, whisk oil and salt together until salt dissolves. 2. Dip the top of each floret in the oil mixture and place half the florets on the slotted crisper tray of an air fryer. Spread out to ensure even cooking. 3. Cook at 400°F/204°C for 9 minutes in the air fryer, stopping to shake the basket halfway through. Repeat until all broccoli is cooked. Serve immediately.
Per Serving: Calories 265; Fat 26g; Sodium 611mg; Carbs 6g; Fiber 2g; Sugar 2g; Protein 3g

Cheesy Cabbage Cribbage

Prep time: 10 minutes| Cook time: 40 minutes| Serves: 4

3 tablespoons unsalted butter, melted
¼ teaspoon garlic powder
¼ teaspoon salt
⅛ teaspoon ground black pepper
½ large cabbage, cut through the stem into 4 wedges
1 cup grated Parmesan cheese, divided

1. Preheat oven to 375°F/191°C. Prepare a baking sheet with parchment paper. 2. Whisk to combine butter, garlic powder, salt, and pepper in a small bowl. Brush mixture onto both cut sides of each cabbage wedge. 3. Sprinkle ¾ cup Parmesan evenly onto both cut sides of each wedge. 4. Bake for 40 minutes, flipping wedges halfway through, until they start to brown. 5. Sprinkle with remaining cheese and serve warm.
Per Serving: Calories 220; Fat 14g; Sodium 625mg; Carbs 13g; Fiber 4g; Sugar 5g; Protein 9g

Asparagus Fries

Prep time: 10 minutes| Cook time: 20 minutes| Serves: 6

3 large eggs
1 teaspoon heavy whipping cream
1 cup superfine blanched almond flour
1 cup grated Parmesan cheese
¼ teaspoon baking powder
¼ teaspoon cayenne pepper
¼ teaspoon garlic powder
¼ teaspoon salt
⅛ teaspoon ground black pepper
2 pounds asparagus, trimmed

1. Whisk together eggs and cream in a shallow 9" × 9" baking dish. In a second baking dish of similar size, stir to combine flour, Parmesan, baking powder, cayenne pepper, garlic powder, salt, and black pepper. 2. Coat asparagus spears in egg wash and shake off any extra. Next, roll and press spears into dry mixture until thoroughly coated. 3. Evenly spread half the asparagus on the crisper tray of an air fryer and cook for 8–10 minutes at 400°F/204°C, turning asparagus over halfway through cooking time. 4. Repeat with remaining half of asparagus until all spears are cooked. Serve warm.
Per Serving: Calories 131; Fat 8g; Sodium 228mg; Carbs 7g; Fiber 3g; Sugar 2g; Protein 8g

Garlic Spinach Stir-Fry

Prep time: 5 minutes| Cook time: 5 minutes| Serves: 2

2 cups spinach, chopped
1 teaspoon toasted sesame seeds
2 garlic cloves, peeled and minced
½ tablespoon coconut aminos
½ teaspoon rice vinegar
½ teaspoon raw honey
1 tablespoon peanut oil
Ground black pepper, to taste

1. Place the spinach in a large saucepan of boiling water and cook for 3-4 minutes until the greens wilt. 2. Add the cooked spinach to a bowl and rinse with cold water. Drain and squeeze with hands to remove as much water as possible—place in a salad bowl. 3. To prepare the dressing: Combine the coconut aminos, peanut oil, rice vinegar, sesame seeds, garlic, honey, and pepper in a small bowl. Whisk until well combined. 4. Pour over the dressing to the spinach and toss to coat. 5. Refrigerate for at least 1 hour before serving.
Per Serving: Calories 101; Fat 8g; Sodium 632mg; Carbs 5g; Fiber 1g; Sugar 6g; Protein 2g

Balsamic Broccoli Stir-Fry

Prep time: 15 minutes| Cook time: 15 minutes| Serves: 2

1 large head of broccoli, cut into florets
2 tablespoons balsamic vinegar
2 garlic cloves, peeled and minced
½ red onion, peeled and diced
2 tablespoons sesame oil
Salt and ground black pepper, to taste

1. Preheat oven to 450°F/232°C. 2. In a bowl, combine the broccoli with sesame oil. Season with salt and pepper to taste and mix well to coat. 3. Transfer the greased broccoli to a large baking dish lined with parchment and roast in the oven for 18-20 minutes until golden brown. Cool the broccoli and transfer to a salad bowl. 4. Whisk the balsamic vinegar, onion, and garlic in a small bowl, season with salt and pepper, and pour over the roasted broccoli. Mix well to coat and enjoy.
Per Serving: Calories 159; Fat 14g; Sodium 245mg; Carbs 8g; Fiber 1g; Sugar 3g; Protein 1g

Sushi

Prep time: 10 minutes| Cook time: 0 minutes| Serves: 4

8 strips thick-cut turkey bacon, cooked but pliable enough to curl into a circle
4 tablespoons full-fat cream cheese, softened, divided
½ medium cucumber, cut into
thin, 1"-long sticks
½ green bell pepper, cut into 1"-long strips
2 baby carrots, cut into thin, 1"-long sticks

1. Lay bacon strips flat and evenly spread 3 tablespoons cream cheese on top side. 2. Evenly place cucumber, bell pepper, and carrots in a tight, organized manner on cream cheese. Only cover the first 4"–5" of each strip, leaving the end bare for overlap. 3. Starting from the vegetable-covered end, tightly roll bacon strips into a sushi-like circle. Secure with the remaining 1 tablespoon cream cheese (or a toothpick if the bacon is stubborn). 4. Transfer rolls to a serving plate, placed on their side. Serve immediately.
Per Serving: Calories 274; Fat 20g; Sodium 832mg; Carbs 4g; Fiber 1g; Sugar 2g; Protein 17g

Veggie Casserole

Prep time: 10 minutes| Cook time: 55 minutes| Serves: 8

1 tablespoon olive oil
2 cups drained, sliced canned mushrooms
1 cup full-fat sour cream
1½ cups shredded Swiss cheese
1 teaspoon garlic powder
½ teaspoon salt
¼ teaspoon ground black pepper
8 cups broccoli and cauliflower floret mix

1. Preheat oven to 350°F/177°C. Grease a 9" × 12" × 2" baking dish. 2. Heat oil in a large soup pot. Add mushrooms and sauté for 5 minutes. Add sour cream, cheese, garlic powder, salt, and pepper and simmer for 5 minutes. 3. Add broccoli and cauliflower mixture to a large microwave-safe bowl, then microwave for 5 minutes to soften partially. 4. Stir florets into pot with the mushroom mixture until coated. 5. Bake it covered for 35–40 minutes. Serve warm.
Per Serving: Calories 191; Fat 12g; Sodium 378mg; Carbs 10g; Fiber 3g; Sugar 3g; Protein 10g

Stuffed Mushrooms

Prep time: 10 minutes| Cook time: 20 minutes| Serves: 8

½ teaspoon salt, divided
6 ounces full-fat cream cheese, softened
⅓ cup grated Parmesan cheese
¼ teaspoon onion powder
¼ teaspoon dried oregano
¼ teaspoon garlic powder
⅛ teaspoon ground black pepper
24 medium (width of 1"–2") mushroom caps, cleaned
2 tablespoons olive oil

1. Preheat the oven to 390°F/199°C. Place a wire rack on a parchment paper-lined baking sheet. 2. Stir to combine ¼ teaspoon salt, cream cheese, Parmesan, onion powder, oregano, garlic powder, and pepper in a medium bowl. 3. Evenly stuff each mushroom cap with cheese mixture. 4. Pour oil into a small bowl. Dip the bottoms of each mushroom cap into oil, then sprinkle with the remaining ¼ teaspoon of salt. 5. Place caps on the wire rack, so they are not touching and bake for 17–20 minutes until caps soften and the cheese mixture starts to brown. Serve warm.
Per Serving: Calories 132; Fat 11g; Sodium 300mg; Carbs 3g; Fiber 1g; Sugar 2g; Protein 4g

Green Beans

Prep time: 10 minutes| Cook time: 24 minutes| Serves: 4

1 pound fresh green beans, trimmed
2 tablespoons olive oil
½ tablespoon soy sauce
½ teaspoon garlic powder
⅛ teaspoon ground black pepper
1 tablespoon sesame seeds

1. Use tongs to toss green beans with oil, soy sauce, garlic powder, and pepper in a large bowl. 2. Evenly spread half the beans on the crisper tray of an air fryer and sprinkle with half the sesame seeds. 3. Bake for 12 minutes at 400°F/204°C, removing the tray to shake the beans halfway through cooking. 4. Transfer cooked beans to a plate and repeat with remaining green beans. Serve warm.
Per Serving: Calories 105; Fat 8g; Sodium 115mg; Carbs 8g; Fiber 3g; Sugar 3g; Protein 2g

Zucchini Boats

Prep time: 10 minutes| Cook time: 30 minutes| Serves: 4

2 medium zucchinis
½ cup grated cheddar cheese
2 ounces full-fat cream cheese, softened
¼ cup diced onion
¼ cup full-fat sour cream
2 tablespoons melted unsalted
butter
¼ teaspoon salt
4 strips no-sugar-added bacon, cooked and crumbled
1 medium jalapeño pepper, deveined, seeded, and finely chopped

1. Preheat the oven to 350°F/177°C. 2. Cut the zucchinis in half lengthwise. Cut in half at the midpoint to create eight "boats" 3" to 4" long to be hollowed out. 3. With a spoon, scoop out each boat; try to get the most out but leave enough so the sides aren't too thin (about ¼" max). Chop the removed flesh finely and put in a medium bowl. 4. Place eight scooped-out boats in a large greased baking dish. 5. Add remaining ingredients except bacon and jalapeños to the bowl with zucchini flesh and mix well. Divide the mixture evenly and scoop it into the boats. 6. Top with crumbled bacon and jalapeño. 7. Bake it for 30 minutes until filling bubbles up, and zucchini boats are softened. Remove from oven and let cool for 5 minutes. Serve.
Per Serving: Calories 259; Fat 20g; Sodium 496mg; Carbs 6g; Fiber 1g; Sugar 4g; Protein 10g

Zucchini Fries

Prep time: 10 minutes| Cook time: 23 minutes| Serves: 4

2 medium zucchinis
¼ teaspoon salt
¼ teaspoon black pepper
¼ teaspoon garlic powder
¾ cup grated Parmesan cheese
1 large egg, beaten

1. Preheat the oven to 425°F/218°C. Prepare a baking sheet with foil. Place a rack onto a baking sheet. 2. Slice zucchini in half, lengthwise, until you have created eight long sticks of similar size. Then cut bars in half across the middle, making sixteen pieces (per zucchini). 3. Mix salt, pepper, garlic powder, and cheese in a medium bowl. 4. In a separate bowl, beat egg. 5. First, dip stick in the egg. Second, press each side into the spices. 6. Place spaced apart on the rack in a layer. 7. Bake the chips for 20 minutes, flipping fries and rotating pan halfway through until browned and crispy. 8. Then broil fries for 2–3 minutes

until dark golden.
Per Serving: Calories 113; Fat 6g; Sodium 509mg; Carbs 6g; Fiber 1g; Sugar 3g; Protein 8g

Radish Potatoes

Prep time: 5 minutes| Cook time: 50 minutes| Serves: 4

20 medium radishes, trimmed and halved
2 tablespoons olive oil
2 teaspoons Italian seasoning,
divided
¼ teaspoon salt
¼ teaspoon black pepper
¼ cup grated Parmesan cheese

1. Preheat the oven to 400°F/204°C. Grease a baking pan with olive oil. Add halved radishes to the baking dish, brush with olive oil, and dust with half of the Italian seasoning, salt, and pepper. 2. Bake for 45 minutes until light brown and crisp. Toss and re-season halfway through. 3. Add Parmesan on top and bake for 5 more minutes. Remove from the oven and your golden radishes are ready to serve.
Per Serving: Calories 89; Fat 8g; Sodium 266mg; Carbs 2g; Fiber 0g; Sugar 0g; Protein 2g

Smashed Cauliflower

Prep time: 10 minutes| Cook time: 18 minutes| Serves: 6

1 pound cauliflower florets
3 tablespoons unsalted butter
¼ teaspoon garlic powder
½ cup fat-free sour cream
2 tablespoons chopped green
onion, divided
1 cup shredded cheddar cheese, divided
¼ teaspoon salt

1. Steam florets for 10–15 minutes until very soft. Remove from heat and let sit in a metal colander for 10–15 minutes to release water. 2. Pulse florets in a food processor for 2–3 minutes until fluffy. Add butter, garlic powder, and sour cream and process for 2–3 more minutes until it resembles mashed potatoes. 3. Scoop cauliflower into a medium microwave-safe bowl and mix in two-thirds of the green onion and ½ cup cheese and salt. Microwave for 2–3 minutes. 4. Serve and sprinkle remaining cheese and green onion on top.
Per Serving: Calories 183; Fat 14g; Sodium 250mg; Carbs 5g; Fiber 2g; Sugar 2g; Protein 6g

Baked Jalapeño and Cheese Cauliflower Mash

Prep time: 10 minutes. | Cooking time: 15 minutes. | Serves: 6

1 (12-ounce) steamer bag cauliflower florets, cooked according to package instructions
2 tablespoons salted butter, softened
2 ounces cream cheese, softened
½ cup shredded sharp cheddar cheese
¼ cup pickled jalapeños
½ teaspoon salt
¼ teaspoon ground black pepper

1. Place cooked cauliflower into a food processor with remaining ingredients. Pulse twenty times until cauliflower is smooth and all the recipe ingredients are combined. 2. Spoon mash into an ungreased 6" round nonstick baking dish. Place dish into air fryer basket. Set the temperature to 380 degrees F and set the timer for almost 15 minutes. The top will be golden brown when done. Serve warm.
Per serving: Calories: 393; Total fat 8.9g; Sodium 124mg; Total Carbs 4.7g; Fiber 8.1g; Sugars 2.6g; Protein 14.7g

Burger Bun for One

Prep time: 10 minutes. | Cooking time: 5 minutes. | Serves: 1

2 tablespoons salted butter, melted
¼ cup blanched finely ground almond flour
¼ teaspoon baking powder
⅛ teaspoon apple cider vinegar
1 large egg, whisked

1. Pour butter into an ungreased 4" ramekin. Add flour, baking powder, and vinegar to ramekin and stir until well-mixed. Add egg and stir until batter is mostly smooth. 2. Place ramekin into air fryer basket. Set the temperature to 350°F/177°C and set the timer for almost 5 minutes. When done, the center will be firm and the top slightly browned. Let cool. For almost 5 minutes, then remove from ramekin and slice in half. Serve.
Per serving: Calories: 162; Total fat 9.8g; Sodium 359mg; Total Carbs 7.7g; Fiber 5.1g; Sugars 6.1g; Protein 6.3g

Creamed Spinach

Prep time: 5 minutes| Cook time: 15 minutes| Serves: 6

20 ounces fresh spinach, finely chopped
⅓ cup grated Parmesan cheese
6 ounces full-fat cream cheese, softened
4 tablespoons full-fat sour cream
½ teaspoon garlic powder
½ teaspoon onion powder
¼ teaspoon salt
¼ teaspoon black pepper

1. In a nonstick pan, add spinach. Cook for 3–5 minutes while stirring until wilted and excess water is removed. 2. Add remaining ingredients and stir for 5–10 minutes until cheeses are melted and are blended. Serve.
Per Serving: Calories 158; Fat 11g; Sodium 378mg; Carbs 6g; Fiber 2g; Sugar 2g; Protein 6g

Oven-Safe Baking Dishes

Prep time: 10 minutes. | Cooking time: 12 minutes. | Serves: 4

2 cups trimmed and halved fresh Brussels sprouts
2 tablespoons olive oil
¼ teaspoon salt
¼ teaspoon ground black pepper
2 tablespoons balsamic vinegar
2 slices cooked sugar-free bacon, crumbled

1. In a suitable bowl, toss Brussels sprouts in olive oil, then sprinkle with black pepper and salt. 2. Place into ungreased air fryer basket. Set the temperature to 375°F/191°C and set the timer for almost 12 minutes, shaking the basket halfway through cooking. Brussels sprouts will be tender and browned when done. 3. Place sprouts in a suitable serving dish and drizzle with balsamic vinegar. Sprinkle bacon over top. Serve warm.
Per serving: Calories: 393; Total fat 8.9g; Sodium 124mg; Total Carbs 4.7g; Fiber 8.1g; Sugars 2.6g; Protein 14.7g

Roasted Asparagus

Prep time: 10 minutes. | Cooking time: 12 minutes. | Serves: 4

1 tablespoon olive oil
1 pound asparagus spears, ends trimmed
¼ teaspoon salt
¼ teaspoon ground black pepper
1 tablespoon salted butter, melted

1. In a suitable bowl, drizzle olive oil over asparagus spears and sprinkle with black pepper and salt. 2. Place spears into ungreased air fryer basket. Set the temperature to 375°F/191°C and set the timer for almost 12 minutes, shaking the basket halfway through cooking. Asparagus will be lightly browned and tender when done. 3. Transfer to a suitable dish and drizzle with butter. Serve warm.
Per serving: Calories: 121; Total fat 9.5g; Sodium 266mg; Total carbs 5.4g; Fiber 1.8g; Sugars 1.7g; Protein 5.9g

Cheesy Baked Asparagus

Prep time: 10 minutes. | Cooking time: 18 minutes. | Serves: 4

½ cup heavy whipping cream
½ cup grated parmesan cheese
2 ounces cream cheese, softened
1 pound asparagus, ends trimmed,
chopped into 1" pieces
¼ teaspoon salt
¼ teaspoon ground black pepper

1. In a suitable bowl, beat heavy cream, parmesan, and cream cheese until well-mixed. 2. Place asparagus into an ungreased 6" round nonstick baking dish. Pour cheese mixture over top and sprinkle with black pepper and salt. 3. Place dish into air fryer basket. Set the temperature to 350°F/177°C and set the timer for almost 18 minutes. Asparagus will be tender when done. Serve warm.
Per serving: Calories: 144; Total fat 10.6g; Sodium 528mg; Total Carbs 1.8g; Fiber 1.2g; Sugars 4.9g; Protein 4.3g

Dijon Roast Cabbage

Prep time: 10 minutes. | Cooking time: 10 minutes. | Serves: 4

1 small head cabbage, cored and sliced into 1"-thick slices
2 tablespoons olive oil
½ teaspoon salt
1 tablespoon Dijon mustard
1 teaspoon apple cider vinegar
1 teaspoon granular erythritol

1. Drizzle each cabbage slice with 1 tablespoon olive oil, then sprinkle with salt. Place slices into ungreased air fryer basket, working in batches if needed. Set the temperature to 350°F/177°C and set the timer for almost 10 minutes. Cabbage will be tender and edges will begin to brown when done. 2. In a suitable bowl, whisk remaining olive oil with mustard, vinegar, and erythritol. Drizzle over cabbage in a suitable serving dish. Serve warm.
Per serving: Calories: 196; Total fat 13.9g; Sodium 479mg; Total carbs 7g; Fiber 0.6g; Sugars 2.9g; Protein 11.7g

Garlic Parmesan–Roasted Cauliflower

Prep time: 10 minutes. | Cooking time: 15 minutes. | Serves: 6

1 medium head cauliflower, leaves and core removed, cut into florets
2 tablespoons salted butter, melted
½ tablespoon salt
2 cloves garlic, peeled and finely minced
½ cup grated parmesan cheese

1. Toss cauliflower in a suitable bowl with butter. Sprinkle with salt, garlic, and ¼ cup parmesan. Place florets into ungreased air fryer basket. Set the temperature to 350°F/177°C and set the timer for almost 15 minutes, shaking basket halfway through cooking. Cauliflower will be browned at the edges and tender when done. 2. Transfer florets to a suitable serving dish and sprinkle with remaining parmesan. Serve warm.
Per serving: Calories: 207; Total fat 15.9g; Sodium 366mg; Total carbs 5.4g; Fiber 1.3g; Sugars 2.4g; Protein 12.1g

Cauliflower Rice Balls

Prep time: 10 minutes. | Cooking time: 8 minutes. | Serves: 4

1 (10-ounce) steamer bag cauliflower rice, cooked according to package instructions
½ cup shredded mozzarella cheese
1 large egg
2 ounces plain pork rinds, finely crushed
¼ teaspoon salt
½ teaspoon Italian seasoning

1. Place cauliflower into a suitable bowl and mix with mozzarella. 2. Whisk egg in a separate suitable bowl. Place pork rinds into another suitable bowl with salt and Italian seasoning. 3. Separate cauliflower mixture into four equal sections and form each into a ball. Carefully dip a ball into whisked egg, then roll in pork rinds. Repeat with remaining balls. 4. Place cauliflower balls into ungreased air fryer basket. Set the temperature to 400°F/204°C and set the timer for almost 8 minutes. Rice balls will be golden when done. 5. Use a spatula to carefully move cauliflower balls to a suitable dish for serving. Serve warm.
Per serving: Calories: 259; Total fat 14.9g; Sodium 325mg; Total Carbs 6.2g; Fiber 4.9g; Sugars 7.4g; Protein 8.5g

Cheesy Loaded Broccoli

Prep time: 10 minutes. | Cooking time: 10 minutes. | Serves: 2

3 cups fresh broccoli florets
1 tablespoon coconut oil
¼ teaspoon salt
½ cup shredded sharp cheddar cheese
¼ cup sour cream
4 slices cooked sugar-free bacon, crumbled
1 medium scallion, trimmed and sliced

1. Place broccoli into ungreased air fryer basket, drizzle with coconut oil, and sprinkle with salt. 2. Set the temperature to 350°F/177°C and set the timer for almost 8 minutes. Shake basket three times during cooking to avoid burned spots. 3. When the pot beeps, sprinkle broccoli with cheddar and set the timer for almost 2 additional minutes. When done, cheese will be melted and broccoli will be tender. 4. Serve warm in a suitable serving dish, topped with sour cream, crumbled bacon, and scallion slices.
Per serving: Calories: 211; Total fat 10.3g; Sodium 645mg; Total Carbs 1.3g; Fiber 8.3g; Sugars 13.1g; Protein 11.2g

Buttery Mushrooms

Prep time: 10 minutes. | Cooking time: 10 minutes. | Serves: 4

8 ounces cremini mushrooms, halved
2 tablespoons salted butter,
melted
¼ teaspoon salt
¼ teaspoon ground black pepper

1. In a suitable bowl, toss mushrooms with butter, then sprinkle with black pepper and salt. 2. Place into ungreased air fryer basket. Set the temperature to 400°F/204°C and set the timer for almost 10 minutes, shaking the basket halfway through cooking. Mushrooms will be tender when done. Serve warm.
Per serving: Calories: 222; Total fat 14.3g; Sodium 343mg; Total Carbs 4.8g; Fiber 5g; Sugars 9.7g; Protein 12.3g

"Faux-Tato" Hash

Prep time: 10 minutes. | Cooking time: 12 minutes. | Serves: 4

1 pound radishes, ends removed, quartered
¼ medium yellow onion, peeled and diced
½ medium green bell pepper, seeded and chopped
2 tablespoons salted butter, melted
½ teaspoon garlic powder
¼ teaspoon ground black pepper

1. In a suitable bowl, mix radishes, onion, and bell pepper. Toss with butter. 2. Sprinkle garlic powder and black pepper over mixture in bowl, then spoon into ungreased air fryer basket. 3. Set the temperature to 320°F/160°C and set the timer for almost 12 minutes. Shake basket halfway through cooking. Radishes will be tender when done. Serve warm.
Per serving: Calories: 333; Total fat 18.5g; Sodium 576mg; Total Carbs 8.2g; Fiber 5g; Sugars 10g; Protein 8.1g

Savory Zucchini Boats

Prep time: 10 minutes. | Cooking time: 10 minutes. | Serves: 4

1 large zucchini, ends removed, halved lengthwise
6 grape tomatoes, quartered
¼ teaspoon salt
¼ cup feta cheese
1 tablespoon balsamic vinegar
1 tablespoon olive oil

1. Use a spoon to scoop out 2 tablespoons from center of each zucchini half, making just enough space to fill with tomatoes and feta. 2. Place tomatoes evenly in centers of zucchini halves and sprinkle with salt. Place into ungreased air fryer basket. Set the temperature to 350°F/177°C and set the timer for almost 10 minutes. When done, zucchini will be tender. 3. Transfer boats to a serving tray and sprinkle with feta, then drizzle with vinegar and olive oil. Serve warm.
Per serving: Calories: 263; Total fat 10.6g; Sodium 718mg; Total Carbs 3g; Fiber 7.1g; Sugars 9.9g; Protein 4.3g

Bacon-Jalapeño Cheesy "Breadsticks"

Prep time: 10 minutes. | Cooking time: 15 minutes. | Serves: 8

2 cups shredded mozzarella cheese
¼ cup grated parmesan cheese
¼ cup chopped pickled jalapeños
2 large eggs, whisked
4 slices cooked sugar-free bacon, chopped

1. Mix all the recipe ingredients in a suitable bowl. 2. Cut a suitable piece of parchment paper to fit inside air fryer basket. 3. Dampen your hands with a bit of water and press out mixture into a circle to fit on ungreased parchment. You may need to separate into two smaller circles, depending on the size of air fryer. 4. Place parchment with cheese mixture into air fryer basket. Set the temperature to 320°F/160°C and set the timer for almost 15 minutes. Carefully flip when 5 minutes remain on timer. The top will be golden brown when done. Slice into eight sticks. Serve warm.
Per serving: Calories: 161; Total fat 12.7g; Sodium 355mg; Total carbs 7.1g; Fiber 2.4g; Sugars 2.2g; Protein 7.9g

Onion Rings

Prep time: 10 minutes. | Cooking time: 5 minutes. | Serves: 8

1 large egg
¼ cup coconut flour
2 ounces plain pork rinds, finely
crushed
1 large white onion, peeled and sliced into 8 (¼") rings

1. Whisk egg in a suitable bowl. Place coconut flour and pork rinds in two separate suitable bowls. Dip each onion ring into egg, then coat in coconut flour. Dip coated onion ring in egg once more, then press gently into pork rinds to cover all sides. 2. Place rings into ungreased air fryer basket. Set the temperature to 400°F/204°C and set the timer for almost 5 minutes, turning the onion rings halfway through cooking. Onion rings will be golden and crispy when done. Serve warm.
Per serving: Calories: 361; Total fat 10.3g; Sodium 1557mg; Total Carbs 2.2g; Fiber 5.7g; Sugars 3.6g; Protein 16.7g

Dinner Rolls

Prep time: 10 minutes. | Cooking time: 12 minutes. | Serves: 6

1 cup shredded mozzarella cheese
1 ounce cream cheese, broken into small pieces
1 cup blanched finely ground
almond flour
¼ cup ground flaxseed
½ teaspoon baking powder
1 large egg, whisked

1. Place mozzarella, cream cheese, and flour in a suitable microwave-safe bowl. Microwave on high 1 minute. Mix until smooth. 2. Add flaxseed, baking powder, and egg to mixture until fully combined and smooth. Microwave an additional 15 seconds if dough becomes too firm. 3. Separate dough into six equal pieces and roll each into a ball. Place rolls into ungreased air fryer basket. Set the temperature to 320°F/160°C and set the timer for almost 12 minutes, turning rolls halfway through cooking. Allow rolls to cool completely before serving. for almost 5 minutes.
Per serving: Calories: 448; Total fat 8.5g; Sodium 247mg; Total Carbs 7.7g; Fiber 32.5g; Sugars 6g; Protein 27g

A Go-To Bread!

Prep time: 10 minutes. | Cooking time: 10 minutes. | Serves: 6

1 pound radishes, ends removed, quartered
2 tablespoons salted butter, melted
½ teaspoon garlic powder
½ teaspoon dried parsley
¼ teaspoon dried oregano
¼ teaspoon ground black pepper
¼ cup grated parmesan cheese

1. Place radishes into a suitable bowl and drizzle with butter. Sprinkle with garlic powder, parsley, oregano, and pepper, then place into ungreased air fryer basket. Set the temperature to 350°F/177°C and set the timer for almost 10 minutes, shaking the basket three times during cooking. Radishes will be done when tender and golden. 2. Place radishes into a suitable serving dish and sprinkle with parmesan. Serve warm.
Per serving: Calories: 373; Total fat 12g; Sodium 1364mg; Total Carbs 3.3g; Fiber 31.3g; Sugars 6.4g; Protein 19.1g

Flatbread Dippers

Prep time: 10 minutes. | Cooking time: 8 minutes. | Serves: 4

1 cup shredded mozzarella cheese
1 ounce cream cheese, broken into small pieces
½ cup blanched finely ground almond flour

1. Place mozzarella into a suitable microwave-safe bowl. Add cream cheese pieces. Microwave on high 60 seconds, then stir to combine. Add flour and stir until a soft ball of dough forms. 2. Cut dough ball into two equal pieces. Cut a piece of parchment to fit into air fryer basket. Press each dough piece into a 5" round on ungreased parchment. 3. Place parchment with dough into air fryer basket. Set the temperature to 350°F/177°C and set the timer for almost 8 minutes. Carefully flip the flatbread over halfway through cooking. Flatbread will be golden brown when done. 4. Let flatbread cool 5 minutes, then slice each round into six triangles. Serve warm.
Per serving: Calories: 114; Total fat 2.6g; Sodium 242mg; Total Carbs 12.5g; Fiber 1.6g; Sugars 0.8g; Protein 10.5g

Mini Spinach and Sweet Pepper Poppers

Prep time: 10 minutes. | Cooking time: 8 minutes. | Serves: 4

4 ounces cream cheese, softened
1 cup chopped fresh spinach leaves
½ teaspoon garlic powder
8 mini sweet bell peppers, tops removed, seeded, and halved lengthwise

1. In a suitable bowl, mix cream cheese, spinach, and garlic powder. Place 1 tablespoon mixture into each sweet pepper half and press down to smooth. 2. Place poppers into ungreased air fryer basket. Set the temperature to 400°F/204°C and set the timer for almost 8 minutes. Poppers will be done when cheese is browned on top and peppers are tender-crisp. Serve warm.
Per serving: Calories: 162; Total fat 8.7g; Sodium 135mg; Total carbs 19g; Fiber 2.7g; Sugars 1g; Protein 5g

Crispy Green Beans

Prep time: 10 minutes. | Cooking time: 8 minutes. | Serves: 4

2 teaspoons olive oil
½ pound fresh green beans, ends trimmed
¼ teaspoon salt
¼ teaspoon ground black pepper

1. In a suitable bowl, drizzle olive oil over green beans and sprinkle with black pepper and salt.
Place green beans into air fryer basket. 2. Set the temperature to 350°F/177°C and set the timer for almost 8 minutes. Serve.
Per serving: Calories: 277; Total fat 21g; Sodium 925mg; Total Carbs 0.1g; Fiber 4.8g; Sugars 8.1g; Protein 6.7g

Pesto Vegetable Skewers

Prep time: 10 minutes. | Cooking time: 8 minutes. | Serves: 4

1 medium zucchini, trimmed and cut into ½" slices	and cut into 1" squares
½ medium yellow onion, peeled and cut into 1" squares	16 whole cremini mushrooms
1 medium red bell pepper, seeded	⅓ cup basil pesto
	½ teaspoon salt
	¼ teaspoon ground black pepper

1. Divide zucchini slices, onion, and bell pepper into eight even portions. 2. Place on 6" skewers for a total of eight kebabs. 3. Add 2 mushrooms to each skewer and brush kebabs generously with pesto. 4. Sprinkle each kebab with salt and black pepper on all sides, then place into ungreased air fryer basket. Set the temperature to 375°F/191°C and set the timer for almost 8 minutes, turning kebabs halfway through cooking. Vegetables will be browned at the edges and tender-crisp when done. Serve warm.
Per serving: Calories: 60; Total fat 0.3g; Sodium 295mg; Total Carbs 14g; Fiber 2.6g; Sugars 2.3g; Protein 2g

Cauliflower Rice-Stuffed Peppers

Prep time: 10 minutes. | Cooking time: 15 minutes. | Serves: 4

2 cups uncooked cauliflower rice	¼ teaspoon salt
¾ cup drained canned petite diced tomatoes	¼ teaspoon ground black pepper
2 tablespoons olive oil	4 medium green bell peppers, tops removed, seeded
1 cup shredded mozzarella cheese	

1. In a suitable bowl, mix all the recipe ingredients except bell peppers. Scoop mixture evenly into peppers. 2. Place peppers into ungreased air fryer basket. Set the temperature to 350°F/177°C and set the timer for almost 15 minutes. Peppers will be tender and cheese will be melted when done. Serve warm.
Per serving: Calories: 223; Total fat 13.1g; Sodium 591mg; Total Carbs 2.5g; Fiber 4.2g; Sugars 1g; Protein 5.3g

Pan Pizza

Prep time: 10 minutes. | Cooking time: 8 minutes. | Serves: 2

1 cup shredded mozzarella cheese	2 tablespoons chopped black olives
¼ medium red bell pepper, seeded and chopped	2 tablespoons crumbled feta cheese
½ cup chopped fresh spinach leaves	

1. Sprinkle mozzarella into an ungreased 6" round nonstick baking dish in an even layer. Add remaining ingredients on top. 2. Place dish into air fryer basket. Set the temperature to 350°F/177°C. 3. Set the timer for almost 8 minutes. Slice and serve.
Per serving: Calories: 203; Total fat 13.5g; Sodium 990mg; Total Carbs 7.9g; Fiber 4.4g; Sugars 8.9g; Protein 5.9g

Vegetable Burgers

Prep time: 10 minutes. | Cooking time: 12 minutes. | Serves: 4

8 ounces cremini mushrooms	onion
2 large egg yolks	1 clove garlic, peeled and finely minced
½ medium zucchini, trimmed and chopped	½ teaspoon salt
¼ cup peeled and chopped yellow	¼ teaspoon ground black pepper

1. Place all the recipe ingredients into a food processor and pulse twenty times until finely chopped and combined. 2. Separate mixture into four equal sections and press each into a burger shape. Place burgers into ungreased air fryer basket. Set the temperature to 375°F/191°C and set the timer for almost 12 minutes, turning burgers halfway through cooking. Burgers will be browned and firm when done. 3. Place burgers on a suitable plate and let cool 5 minutes before serving.
Per serving: Calories: 241; Total fat 20.1g; Sodium 608mg; Total Carbs 3.4g; Fiber 2.9g; Sugars 8g; Protein 4.5g

Roasted Spaghetti Squash

Prep time: 10 minutes. | Cooking time: 45 minutes. | Serves: 6

1 (4-pound) spaghetti squash, halved and seeded	4 tablespoons salted butter, melted
2 tablespoons coconut oil	1 teaspoon garlic powder

2 teaspoons dried parsley

1. Brush shell of spaghetti squash with coconut oil. Brush inside with butter. Sprinkle inside with garlic powder and parsley. 2. Place squash skin side down into ungreased air fryer basket, working in batches if needed. Set the temperature to 350°F/177°C and set the timer for almost 30 minutes. When the timer beeps, flip squash and cook an additional 15 minutes until fork-tender. 3. Use a fork to remove spaghetti strands from shell and serve warm.
Per serving: Calories: 310; Total fat 25.9g; Sodium 131mg; Total carbs 9.7g; Fiber 5.1g; Sugars 3.4g; Protein 13g

Alfredo Eggplant Stacks

Prep time: 10 minutes. | Cooking time: 12 minutes. | Serves: 6

1 large eggplant, ends trimmed, cut into ¼" slices	1 cup alfredo sauce
1 medium beefsteak tomato, cored and cut into ¼" slices	8 ounces fresh mozzarella cheese, cut into 18 slices
	2 tablespoons fresh parsley leaves

1. Place 6 slices eggplant in bottom of an ungreased 6" round nonstick baking dish. Place 1 slice tomato on top of each eggplant round, followed by 1 tablespoon alfredo and 1 slice mozzarella. Repeat with remaining ingredients. for almost three repetitions. 2. Cover dish with foil sheet and place dish into air fryer basket. Set the temperature to 350°F/177°C and set the timer for almost 12 minutes. Eggplant will be tender when done. 3. Sprinkle parsley evenly over each stack. Serve warm.
Per serving: Calories: 327; Total fat 17.6g; Sodium 654mg; Total Carbs 6.7g; Fiber 3.4g; Sugars 17.8g; Protein 7.8g

Crab Rangoons

Prep time: 15 minutes| Cook time: 25 minutes| Serves: 10

5 teaspoons olive oil, divided	cheese, softened
5 large eggs, divided	1 teaspoon onion powder
1 (6-ounce) can crab meat, drained and finely shredded	½ teaspoon garlic powder
5 tablespoons full-fat cream	¼ teaspoon salt

1. In a pan heat 1 teaspoon oil. In a small bowl, beat one egg. Pour egg into the pan, coating the entire bottom. 2. With the help of spatula, lift the egg edges as it becomes firm. Tilt the pan to allow egg to fill in the gaps along the edge of the pan, creating a thin, solid pancake shape. Cook for a minute, then transfer to a plate. Repeat and make four additional egg pancakes, heating 1 teaspoon oil before cooking each egg. 3. Cut egg pancakes evenly into quarters, making twenty egg triangle shapes. 4. Combine crab, cream cheese, onion powder, garlic powder, and salt in a medium mixing bowl. 5. Dollop equal amounts of the crab mixture (about 1 teaspoon each) in the center of the egg triangles. Fold over and pinch to close. Repeat until the mixture is gone. 6. Spread out half the rangoons, without letting them touch, on the crisper tray in an air fryer basket. Bake for 9 minutes at 400°F/204°C. Repeat with the remaining half until all rangoons are "fried." Serve immediately.
Per Serving: Calories 96; Fat 7g; Sodium 169mg; Carbs 1g; Fiber 0g; Sugar 0g; Protein 7g

Cheesy Broccoli Sticks

Prep time: 10 minutes. | Cooking time: 16 minutes. | Serves: 2

1 (10-ounce) steamer bag broccoli florets, cooked according to package instructions	crisps, finely ground
	½ cup shredded sharp cheddar cheese
1 large egg	½ teaspoon salt
1 ounce parmesan 100% cheese	½ cup ranch dressing

1. Let cooked broccoli cool 5 minutes, then place into a food processor with egg, cheese crisps, cheddar, and salt. Process on low for almost 30 seconds until all the recipe ingredients are combined and begin to stick. 2. Cut a sheet of parchment paper to fit air fryer basket. Take one scoop of mixture, for almost 3 tablespoons, and roll into a 4" stick shape, pressing down gently to flatten the top. Place stick on ungreased parchment into air fryer basket. Repeat with remaining mixture to form eight sticks. 3. Set the temperature to 350°F/177°C and set the timer for almost 16 minutes, turning sticks halfway through cooking. Sticks will be golden brown when done. 4. Serve warm with ranch dressing on the side for dipping.
Per serving: Calories: 282; Total fat 4g; Sodium 684mg; Total Carbs 4.7g; Fiber 5.5g; Sugars 6.9g; Protein 8.9g

Zucchini Fritters

Prep time: 10 minutes. | Cooking time: 12 minutes. | Serves: 4

1½ medium zucchini, trimmed and grated	1 large egg, whisked
½ teaspoon salt	¼ teaspoon garlic powder
	¼ cup grated parmesan cheese

1. Place grated zucchini on a kitchen towel and sprinkle with ¼ teaspoon salt. Wrap in towel and let sit 30 minutes, then wring out as much excess moisture as possible. 2. Place zucchini into a suitable bowl and mix with egg, remaining salt, garlic powder, and parmesan. Cut a piece of parchment to fit air fryer basket. Divide mixture into four mounds, for almost ⅓ cup each, and press out into 4" rounds on ungreased parchment. 3. Place parchment with rounds into air fryer basket. Set the temperature to 400°F/204°C and set the timer for almost 12 minutes, turning fritters halfway through cooking. Fritters will be crispy on the edges and tender but firm in the center when done. Serve warm.
Per serving: Calories: 366; Total fat 15g; Sodium 67mg; Total Carbs 8.9g; Fiber 14g; Sugars 24.4g; Protein 7.5g

Crispy Cabbage Steaks

Prep time: 10 minutes. | Cooking time: 10 minutes. | Serves: 4

1 small head green cabbage, cored and cut into ½"-thick slices	1 clove garlic, peeled and finely minced
¼ teaspoon salt	½ teaspoon dried thyme
¼ teaspoon ground black pepper	½ teaspoon dried parsley
2 tablespoons olive oil	

1. Sprinkle each side of cabbage with black pepper and salt, then place into ungreased air fryer basket, working in batches if needed. 2. Drizzle each side of cabbage with olive oil, then sprinkle with remaining ingredients on both sides. 3. Set the temperature to 350°F/177°C and set the timer for almost 10 minutes, turning "steaks" halfway through cooking. Cabbage will be browned at the edges and tender when done. Serve warm.
Per serving: Calories: 441; Total fat 33.9g; Sodium 759mg; Total Carbs 4.9g; Fiber 2.2g; Sugars 3.6g; Protein 21.4g

Eggplant Parmesan

Prep time: 10 minutes. | Cooking time: 17 minutes. | Serves: 4

1 medium eggplant, ends trimmed, sliced into ½" rounds	1 ounce 100% cheese crisps, finely crushed
¼ teaspoon salt	½ cup low-carb marinara sauce
2 tablespoons coconut oil	½ cup shredded mozzarella cheese
½ cup grated parmesan cheese	

1. Sprinkle eggplant rounds with salt on both sides and wrap in a kitchen towel for almost 30 minutes. Press to remove excess water, then drizzle rounds with coconut oil on both sides. 2. In a suitable bowl, mix parmesan and cheese crisps. Press each eggplant slice into mixture to coat both sides. 3. Place rounds into ungreased air fryer basket. Set the temperature to 350°F/177°C and set the timer for almost 15 minutes, turning rounds halfway through cooking.
When the pot beeps, spoon marinara over rounds and sprinkle with mozzarella. 4. Continue cooking an additional 2 minutes at 350°F/177°C until cheese is melted. Serve warm.
Per serving: Calories: 238; Total fat 10.6g; Sodium 149mg; Total carbs 0.6g; Fiber 0.4g; Sugars 0.2g; Protein 33g

Keto Tater Tots

Prep time: 5 minutes| Cook time: 30 minutes| Serves: 8

1½ pounds riced cauliflower	1½ cups shredded whole milk mozzarella cheese
4 tablespoons avocado oil, divided	2 cloves minced garlic
1 large egg	¾ teaspoon salt, divided

1. In a pan, fry cauliflower rice with 2 tablespoons oil for 5–10 minutes until soft and brown. 2. In a bowl, whisk egg and mix in cheese, garlic, and ½ teaspoon salt. 3. Combine browned cauliflower rice with egg mixture. Stir the mixture well to melt the cheese. 4. Form cauliflower tots using a spoon or melon scoop. 5. In a pan over medium heat, fry tots using the remaining 2 tablespoons of oil. 6. Space tots apart in a single layer, turning every 3–5 minutes until browned on all sides. 7. Repeat until all tots are cooked. Sprinkle with remaining ¼ teaspoon salt and serve hot.
Per Serving: Calories 154; Fat 12g; Carbs 5g; Fiber

2g; Sugar 2g; Protein 7g

Parmesan Cauliflower

Prep time: 10 minutes| Cook time: 35 minutes| Serves: 4

16 ounces cauliflower, cut into bite-sized florets	¼ teaspoon salt
4 tablespoons melted unsalted butter	¼ teaspoon black pepper
2 tablespoons olive oil	1 cup grated Parmesan cheese
	2 teaspoons parsley flakes

1. Preheat the oven to 400°F/204°C. Prepare a baking sheet with parchment paper. 2. Toss cauliflower, melted butter, and olive oil in a large mixing bowl. Add salt and pepper. 3. Place coated cauliflower on the baking sheet. Keep cauliflower in a single layer so it cooks evenly. Bake for 25–30 minutes or until soft. 4. Remove from oven and dust with Parmesan cheese and parsley. Return to oven for 5 minutes to melt the cheese. 5. Remove from the oven and serve warm.
Per Serving: Calories 294; Fat 23g; Sodium 632mg; Carbs 9g; Fiber 2g; Sugar 2g; Protein 9g

Pesto Pasta

Prep time: 5 minutes| Cook time: 15 minutes| Serves: 6

¼ cup pine nuts	½ cup olive oil
4 cloves garlic, peeled and chopped	½ cup grated or shredded Parmesan cheese, divided
1½ cups fresh basil leaves	1 head cauliflower, cut into florets

1. Pulse the pine nuts, garlic, basil, oil, and ¼ cup Parmesan cheese in a small blender until liquefied, about 1–2 minutes. 2. Steam florets until tender, for about 10–15 minutes. Place florets in a medium mixing bowl and gently fold in pesto sauce. 3. Serve warm and sprinkle with remaining Parmesan cheese.
Per Serving: Calories 270; Fat 23g; Sodium 193mg; Carbs 10g; Fiber 3g; Sugar 3g; Protein 6g

Fried Zuck Patties

Prep time: 30 minutes| Cook time: 15 minutes| Serves: 8

1 pound zucchini	mozzarella cheese
1 teaspoon salt	½ cup blanched almond flour
2 large beaten eggs	¼ cup grated Parmesan cheese
2 medium green onions, chopped	¼ cup flaxseed meal
1½ teaspoons lemon pepper	4 tablespoons coconut oil
1 cup shredded whole milk	

1. Grate zucchini and sprinkle with salt. Drain the grated zucchini for 15 minutes or more in a large colander. Turn shreds often to speed up drainage. Squeeze the mixture using a cheesecloth to remove excess moisture. 2. Mix grated zucchini with beaten eggs and green onions in a large bowl. 3. Mix all ingredients except for the oil. Add to zucchini mixture, stirring well. 4. Form "zuck" patties 3" in diameter and ½" thick. 5. In a pan heat oil. Fry patties for 3–5 minutes per side. 6. When "Zuck" patties are thoroughly cooked and firm throughout, place on a paper towel-lined plate to drain and cool.
Per Serving: Calories 199; Fat 16g; Sodium 457mg; Carbs 5g; Fiber 2g; Sugar 2g; Protein 8g

Roasted Broccoli Salad

Prep time: 10 minutes. | Cooking time: 7 minutes. | Serves: 4

2 cups fresh broccoli florets, chopped	⅛ teaspoon ground black pepper
1 tablespoon olive oil	¼ cup lemon juice
¼ teaspoon salt	¼ cup shredded parmesan cheese
	¼ cup sliced roasted almonds

1. In a suitable bowl, toss broccoli and olive oil. Sprinkle with black pepper and salt, then drizzle with 2 tablespoons lemon juice. 2. Place broccoli into ungreased air fryer basket. Set the temperature to 350°F/177°C and set the timer for almost 7 minutes, shaking the basket halfway through cooking. Broccoli will be golden on the edges when done. 3. Place broccoli into a suitable serving bowl and drizzle with remaining lemon juice. Sprinkle with parmesan and almonds. Serve warm.
Per serving: Calories: 190; Total fat 11.5g; Sodium 639mg; Total Carbs 8g; Fiber 1.9g; Sugars 13.5g; Protein 7.5g

Stuffed Portobello Mushrooms

Prep time: 10 minutes. | Cooking time: 8 minutes. | Serves: 4

3 ounces cream cheese, softened
½ medium zucchini, trimmed and chopped
¼ cup seeded and chopped red bell pepper
1½ cups chopped fresh spinach

leaves
4 large Portobello mushrooms, stems removed
2 tablespoons coconut oil, melted
½ teaspoon salt

1. In a suitable bowl, mix cream cheese, zucchini, pepper, and spinach. 2. Drizzle mushrooms with coconut oil and sprinkle with salt. 3. Scoop ¼ zucchini mixture into each mushroom. 4. Place mushrooms into ungreased air fryer basket. Set the temperature to 400°F/204°C and set the timer for almost 8 minutes. Portobellos will be tender and tops will be browned when done. Serve warm.
Per serving: Calories: 200; Total fat 6.3g; Sodium 647mg; Total Carbs 3g; Fiber 7g; Sugars 18.6g; Protein 7g

Cauliflower Pizza Crust

Prep time: 10 minutes. | Cooking time: 7 minutes. | Serves: 2

1 (12-ounce) steamer bag cauliflower, cooked according to package instructions
½ cup shredded sharp cheddar cheese

1 large egg
2 tablespoons blanched finely ground almond flour
1 teaspoon Italian seasoning

1. Let cooked cauliflower cool for almost 10 minutes. Using a kitchen towel, wring out excess moisture from cauliflower and place into food processor. 2. Add cheddar, egg, flour, and Italian seasoning to processor and pulse ten times until cauliflower is smooth and all the recipe ingredients are combined. 3. Cut two pieces of parchment paper to fit air fryer basket. Divide cauliflower mixture into two equal portions and press each into a 6" round on ungreased parchment. 4. Place crusts on parchment into air fryer basket. Set the temperature to 360°F/182°C and set the timer for almost 7 minutes, gently turning crusts halfway through cooking. 5. Store crusts in refrigerator in an airtight container up to 4 days or freeze between sheets of parchment in a sealable storage bag for up to 2 months.
Per serving: Calories: 357; Total fat 8.5g; Sodium 168mg; Total Carbs 4.1g; Fiber 10g; Sugars 54.7g; Protein 6.5g

Roasted Salsa

Prep time: 10 minutes. | Cooking time: 30 minutes. | Serves: 8

2 large San Marzano tomatoes, cored and cut into large chunks
½ medium white onion, peeled and large-diced
½ medium jalapeño, seeded and

large-diced
2 cloves garlic, peeled and diced
½ teaspoon salt
1 tablespoon coconut oil
¼ cup fresh lime juice

1. Place tomatoes, onion, and jalapeño into an ungreased 6" round nonstick baking dish. Add garlic, then sprinkle with salt and drizzle with coconut oil. 2. Place dish into air fryer basket. Set the temperature to 300 degrees F and set the timer for almost 30 minutes. Vegetables will be dark brown around the edges and tender when done. 3. Pour the prepared mixture into a food processor or blender. Add lime juice. Process on low speed 30 seconds until only a few chunks remain. 4. Transfer salsa to a sealable container and refrigerate at least 1 hour. Serve chilled.
Per serving: Calories: 229; Total fat 12.6g; Sodium 875mg; Total Carbs 6.2g; Fiber 4.6g; Sugars 8.9g; Protein 5.4g

Sweet Pepper Nachos

Prep time: 10 minutes. | Cooking time: 5 minutes. | Serves: 2

6 mini sweet peppers, seeded and sliced in half
¾ cup shredded Colby jack cheese

¼ cup sliced pickled jalapeños
½ medium avocado, peeled, pitted, and diced
2 tablespoons sour cream

1. Place peppers into an ungreased 6" round nonstick baking dish. Sprinkle with Colby jack cheese and top with jalapeños. 2. Place dish into air fryer basket. Set the temperature to 350°F/177°C and set the timer for almost 5 minutes. Cheese will be melted and bubbly when done. 3. Remove dish from air fryer and top with avocado. Drizzle with sour cream. Serve warm.
Per serving: Calories: 111; Total fat 5.4g; Sodium 1357mg; Total carbs 8.7g; Fiber 2g; Sugars 3.9g; Protein 9.1g

Lemon Caper Cauliflower Steaks

Prep time: 10 minutes. | Cooking time: 15 minutes. | Serves: 4

1 small head cauliflower, leaves and core removed, cut into 4 (½"-thick) "steaks"
4 tablespoons olive oil
1 medium lemon, zested and

juiced
¼ teaspoon salt
⅛ teaspoon ground black pepper
1 tablespoon salted butter, melted
1 tablespoon capers, rinsed

1. Brush each cauliflower "steak" with ½ tablespoon olive oil on both sides and sprinkle with lemon zest, salt, and pepper on both sides. 2. Place cauliflower into ungreased air fryer basket. Set the temperature to 400°F/204°C and set the timer for almost 15 minutes, turning cauliflower halfway through cooking. Steaks will be golden at the edges and browned when done. 3. Transfer steaks to four medium plates. In a suitable bowl, whisk remaining olive oil, butter, lemon juice, and capers, and pour evenly over steaks. Serve warm.
Per serving: Calories: 240; Total fat 11.8g; Sodium 440mg; Total Carbs 3.9g; Fiber 6.7g; Sugars 8.8g; Protein 2.2g

Crispy Eggplant Rounds

Prep time: 10 minutes. | Cooking time: 10 minutes. | Serves: 4

1 large eggplant, ends trimmed, cut into ½" slices
½ teaspoon salt
2 ounces parmesan 100% cheese

crisps, finely ground
½ teaspoon paprika
¼ teaspoon garlic powder
1 large egg

1. Sprinkle eggplant rounds with salt. 2. Place rounds on a kitchen towel for almost 30 minutes to draw out excess water. 3. Pat rounds dry. 4. In a suitable bowl, mix cheese crisps, paprika, and garlic powder. 5. In a separate suitable bowl, whisk egg. 6. Dip each eggplant slice in egg, then gently press into cheese crisps to coat both sides. 7. Set eggplant rounds into ungreased air fryer basket. 8. Set the temperature to 400°F/204°C and set the timer for 10 minutes. Serve warm.
Per serving: Calories: 400; Total fat 15.2g; Sodium 644mg; Total Carbs 3.6g; Fiber 6.3g; Sugars 2.3g; Protein 42.2g

White Cheddar and Mushroom Soufflés

Prep time: 10 minutes. | Cooking time: 12 minutes. | Serves: 4

3 large eggs, whites and yolks separated
½ cup sharp white cheddar cheese
3 ounces cream cheese, softened

¼ teaspoon cream of tartar
¼ teaspoon salt
¼ teaspoon ground black pepper
½ cup cremini mushrooms, sliced

1. In a suitable bowl, whip egg whites until stiff peaks form. for almost 2 minutes. In a separate suitable bowl, beat cheddar, egg yolks, cream cheese, cream of tartar, salt, and pepper until well-mixed. 2. Fold egg whites into cheese mixture, being careful not to stir. Fold in mushrooms, then pour mixture evenly into four ungreased 4" ramekins. 3. Place ramekins into air fryer basket. Set the temperature to 350°F/177°C and set the timer for almost 12 minutes. Eggs will be browned on the top and firm in the center when done. Serve warm.
Per serving: Calories: 180; Total fat 10.3g; Sodium 672mg; Total Carbs 4.6g; Fiber 6g; Sugars 3.5g; Protein 7.8g

Pesto Spinach Flatbread

Prep time: 10 minutes. | Cooking time: 8 minutes. | Serves: 4

1 cup blanched finely ground almond flour
2 ounces cream cheese
2 cups shredded mozzarella

cheese
1 cup chopped fresh spinach leaves
2 tablespoons basil pesto

1. Place flour, cream cheese, and mozzarella in a suitable microwave-safe bowl and microwave on high 45 seconds, then stir. 2. Fold in spinach and microwave an additional 15 seconds. Stir until a soft dough ball forms. 3. Cut two pieces of parchment paper to fit air fryer basket. Separate dough into two sections and press each out on ungreased parchment to create 6" rounds. 4. Spread 1 tablespoon pesto over each flatbread and place rounds on parchment into ungreased air fryer basket. Set the temperature to 350°F/177°C and set the timer for almost 8 minutes, turning crusts halfway through cooking. Flatbread will be golden when done. Serve.
Per serving: Calories: 338; Total fat 3.6g; Sodium 155mg; Total Carbs 4.7g; Fiber 2.3g; Sugars 47g; Protein 2.4g

Herb Cloud Eggs

Prep time: 10 minutes. | Cooking time: 8 minutes. | Serves: 2

2 large eggs, whites and yolks separated
¼ teaspoon salt
¼ teaspoon dried oregano

2 tablespoons chopped fresh chives
2 teaspoons salted butter, melted

1. In a suitable bowl, whip egg whites until stiff peaks form, for almost 3 minutes. 2. Place egg whites evenly into two ungreased 4" ramekins. 3. Sprinkle evenly with salt, oregano, and chives. 4. Place 1 whole egg yolk in center of each ramekin and drizzle with butter. 5. Place ramekins into air fryer basket. Set the temperature to 350°F/177°C and set the timer for almost 8 minutes. Egg whites will be fluffy and browned when done. Serve warm.

Per serving: Calories: 264; Total fat 10g; Sodium 9mg; Total Carbs 5.4g; Fiber 6.8g; Sugars 3.5g; Protein 8g

Spinach and Artichoke-Stuffed Peppers

Prep time: 10 minutes. | Cooking time: 15 minutes. | Serves: 4

2 ounces cream cheese, softened
½ cup shredded mozzarella cheese
½ cup chopped fresh spinach leaves

¼ cup chopped canned artichoke hearts
2 medium green bell peppers, halved and seeded

1. In a suitable bowl, mix cream cheese, mozzarella, spinach, and artichokes. Spoon ¼ cheese mixture into each pepper half. 2. Place peppers into ungreased air fryer basket. Set the temperature to 320°F/160°C and set the timer for almost 15 minutes. Peppers will be tender and cheese will be bubbling and brown when done. Serve warm.

Per serving: Calories: 197; Total fat 17g; Sodium 426mg; Total Carbs 2.5g; Fiber 3g; Sugars 4.8g; Protein 1.9g

Roasted Brussels Sprouts

Prep time: 10 minutes. | Cooking time: 10 minutes. | Serves: 6

1 pound fresh Brussels sprouts, halved
2 tablespoons coconut oil
½ teaspoon salt

¼ teaspoon ground black pepper
½ teaspoon garlic powder
1 tablespoon salted butter, melted

1. Place Brussels sprouts into a suitable bowl. 2. Drizzle with coconut oil and sprinkle with salt, pepper, and garlic powder. 3. Place Brussels sprouts into ungreased air fryer basket. Set the temperature to 350°F/177°C and set the timer for almost 10 minutes, shaking the basket three times during cooking. Brussels sprouts will be dark golden and tender when done. 4. Place cooked sprouts in a suitable serving dish and drizzle with butter. Serve warm.

Per serving: Calories: 229; Total fat 12.6g; Sodium 875mg; Total Carbs 6.2g; Fiber 4.6g; Sugars 8.9g; Protein 5.4g

Crustless Spinach and Cheese Frittata

Prep time: 10 minutes. | Cooking time: 20 minutes. | Serves: 4

6 large eggs
½ cup heavy whipping cream
1 cup frozen chopped spinach, drained
1 cup shredded sharp cheddar

cheese
¼ cup peeled and diced yellow onion
½ teaspoon salt
¼ teaspoon ground black pepper

1. In a suitable bowl, whisk eggs and cream. Whisk in spinach, cheddar, onion, salt, and pepper. 2. Pour mixture into an ungreased 6" round nonstick baking dish. Place dish into air fryer basket. 3. Set the temperature to 320°F/160°C and set the timer for almost 20 minutes. Eggs will be firm and slightly browned when done. Serve immediately.

Per serving: Calories: 161; Total fat 8.1g; Sodium 692mg; Total Carbs 0.6g; Fiber 5g; Sugars 8.2g; Protein 5.2g

Chocolaty Cheesecake Bars

Prep time: 50 minutes| Cook time: 55 minutes| Serves: 6

Brownie layer
2 ounces bittersweet chocolate, chopped
½ cup butter softened
⅓ cup raw unsweetened cocoa powder
½ cup almond flour
2 large eggs
½ cup sugar substitute

½ teaspoon pure vanilla extract
¼ teaspoon salt
Cheesecake layer
2 large eggs
16 ounces cream cheese, softened
⅓ cup sugar substitute
¼ cup heavy cream
½ teaspoon pure vanilla extract

1. Preheat the oven to 325°F/163°C. 2. Grease an 8x8 baking dish oil. 3. Melt the butter along with chocolate and stir until well combined. 4. Whisk the almond flour, cocoa powder, and salt together in a small bowl. 5. Whisk the eggs along with sugar substitute, and vanilla extract in a large bowl until frothy. Slowly whisk in the melted chocolate mixture. 6. Add in the flour mix and stir until smooth. Pour into the prepared baking dish and bake for 20 minutes. Cool the cake completely. 7. Mix together the cream cheese, eggs, sugar substitute, heavy cream, and vanilla extract with an electric mixer for the cheesecake layer. 8. Reduce the oven heat to 300°F/149°C. Pour the batter over the baked brownies and return to the oven for 40 to 45 minutes or until set. Cool it before serving.
Per Serving: Calories 556; Fat 54g; Sodium 489mg; Carbs 12g; Fiber 3g; Sugar 5g; Protein 13g

Chocolate Pudding

Prep time: 5 minutes| Cook time: 5 minutes| Serves: 4

2 cups coconut milk, canned
¼ cup raw unsweetened cocoa powder
1 tablespoon stevia
2 tablespoons gelatin

4 tablespoons water
½ cup whipping cream
1 ounce chopped bittersweet chocolate (optional for garnish)

1. Heat the coconut milk, cocoa powder, and stevia in a small saucepan. Stir until the cocoa powder and stevia have dissolved. 2. Mix the gelatin with the water and add to the saucepan. Stir until well combined. 3. Pour the mixture into 4 small ramekins or glasses. 4. Place the hot ramekins in the refrigerator to cool for at least 1 hour.
Per Serving: Calories 389; Fat 37g; Sodium 894mg; Carbs 14g; Fiber 5g; Sugar 7g; Protein 8g

Nuts Squares

Prep time: 10 minutes| Cook time: 25 minutes| Serves: 6

1 cup pecans (halved)
3 tablespoons pure Grade B maple syrup
½ cup almond flour
¼ cup flax meal
¼ cup unsweetened, shredded

coconut
¼ cup coconut oil, melted
1 egg, beaten
2 tablespoons sugar substitute
⅓ cup sugar-free chocolate chips

1. Preheat the oven to 350°F/ 177°C. Prepare a baking sheet by lining it with parchment paper. Place the pecans on the baking sheet and bake for 7 minutes, until toasted and fragrant. 2. Allow the pecans to cool when done. Chop the pecans once cooled, reserving a few halves for garnish. 3. Mix the flax meal, almond flour, chopped pecans, and shredded coconut in a large bowl. 4. Stir in the maple syrup, coconut oil, egg, and sugar substitute. Mix well. Add the sugar-free chocolate chips if using. 5. Transfer the dough into a 9-inch by 3-inch loaf pan that has been prepared with nonstick cooking spray. 6. Bake at 350°F/177°C temperature setting for 20 minutes, or until a toothpick inserted comes out clean. 7. Remove from oven and allow to cool. 8. Cut into squares and enjoy!
Per Serving: Calories 233; Fat 21g; Sodium 433mg; Carbs 12g; Fiber 4g; Sugar 4g; Protein 5g

Delicious Chocolate Lava Cake

Prep time: 10 minutes| Cook time: 13 minutes| Serves: 4

½ cup raw unsweetened cocoa powder
¼ cup butter, melted
4 eggs
¼ cup sugar-free and gluten-free

chocolate sauce
½ teaspoon ground cinnamon
½ teaspoon sea salt
1 teaspoon pure vanilla extract
¼ cup raw stevia

1. Pour 1 tablespoon of chocolate sauce into 4 cavities of an ice cube tray and freeze it. 2. Preheat oven to 350°F/177°C. Prepare 4 ramekins by greasing with oil or butter. 3. Whisk together the cocoa powder, stevia, cinnamon, and sea salt in a small bowl. 4. Whisk eggs one by one in a bowl. Add the melted butter and vanilla extract. Stir until well combined. 5. Fill each prepared ramekin halfway with the mixture. 6. Remove the chocolate sauce from the freezer and place one in each of the ramekins. 7. Cover the chocolate with the remaining cake batter. 8. Bake the cake for 13 to 14 minutes or until just set. Transfer from the oven to a wire rack and allow to cool for 5 minutes. 9. Carefully remove the cakes from the ramekins. Enjoy your tasty and healthy chocolate lava cake by cutting into its molten center.
Per Serving: Calories 189; Fat 17g; Sodium 84mg; Carbs 3g; Fiber 3g; Sugar 3g; Protein 8g

Three-Layered Chocolate Cream Cake

Prep time: 30 minutes| Cook time: 60 minutes| Serves: 8

4 ounces unsweetened chocolate
½ cup butter
1½ cups powdered sweetener, divided
3 eggs
½ cup + 8 tablespoons raw unsweetened cocoa powder

1 vanilla pod
Pinch of sea salt
1 cup whipping cream
Coconut whipped cream
1 can coconut milk, refrigerated overnight

1. Preheat the oven to 325°F/163°C. Spray a little cooking oil into a pan smaller than 8 inches. 2. Combine the chocolate and butter in a double boiler and melt them together. Stir in ½ cup of sweetener and stirring over low heat until everything is well combined. Remove from heat and let cool a little bit. 3. Separate the eggs, and beat the whites until stiff peaks form. Add ¼ cup of sweetener little by little. 3. Whisk the yolks together with another ¼ cup of sweetener. Add the chocolate mixture to the yolks and stir well. Mix in ½ cup cocoa, and then scrape the vanilla seeds from the pod and add to the mix along with salt. 5. Fold in egg whites slowly to the chocolate mixture, but do not over mix. 6. Bake it for 1 hour. Let it cool thoroughly, and then remove it from the pan. Let it cool thoroughly, and then remove it from the pan. Cream: 1. To prepare the 3 types of filling, beat the whipping cream for about 6-7 minutes until it gets very thick. Slowly add ½ cup of sweetener. 2. Divide the cream into halves and place one half in a bowl. Divide the remaining cream into halves again, and remember to put in the other 2 separate bowls. You will have 3 bowls, one with ½ of the cream and two with ¼ of the cream. 3. Take a bowl with ¼ cream, add 1 tablespoon of cocoa powder and mix well. This will be the lightest-colored cream. 4. Add ½ the cream to the bowl, and add 3 tablespoons of cocoa powder. Mix until well distributed. This will be the middle-colored cream. 5. Add to the last bowl with ¼ cream. This will be the darkest cream.
Assembling: 1. Slice the cake horizontally into 3 slices using a very sharp knife. 2. Place the bottom part on a serving plate and cover with the middle-colored cream. Repeat with the second cake layer. 3. Top the third cake layer and cover it with the light-colored cream on top, followed by the darkest cream. 4. Cut into 8 slices and enjoy
Per Serving: Calories 304; Fat 27g; Sodium 678mg; Carbs 11g; Fiber 6g; Sugar 2g; Protein 7g

Strawberry Cheesecakes

Prep time: 10 minutes| Cook time: 0 minutes| Serves: 4

Crust
½ cup almond flour
3 tablespoons butter, melted
¼ cup sugar substitute
Filling
6 strawberries
3 tablespoons sugar

8 ounces cream cheese
⅓ cup sour cream
½ teaspoon pure vanilla extract
4 strawberries, quartered (for garnish)
Fresh mint leaves (for garnish)

1. To prepare the crust, place the almond flour, melted butter, and sugar substitute in a medium bowl and mix well to combine. 2. Divide the mixture evenly into 4 small serving bowls or ramekins, lightly pressing with your hands. 3. To prepare the filling, puree the strawberries in a food processor. 4. Add the sugar substitute, vanilla extract, cream cheese, and sour cream. Blend until smooth and creamy. 5. Spoon the mixture over the crust and chill for at least 1 hour.
Per Serving: Calories 489; Fat 47g; Sodium 678mg; Carbs 12g; Fiber 3g; Sugar 6g; Protein 8g

Strawberries Coconut Whip

Prep time: 5 minutes| Cook time: 3 minutes| Serves: 4

2 cans coconut cream, refrigerated
4 cups strawberries

1 ounce chopped unsweetened 70% dark chocolate

1. Scoop the solidified coconut cream into a large bowl and blend with a hand mixer for about 5 minutes until stiff peaks form. Slice the strawberries and arrange them in 4 small serving bowls. 2. Dollop the coconut whipped cream on top of the strawberries. 3. Garnish with chopped dark chocolate and additional berries. 4. Serve and enjoy!
Per Serving: Calories 342; Fat 31g; Sodium 532mg; Carbs 15g; Fiber 5g; Sugar 6g; Protein 15g

Regular Carrot Cake with Cream Cheese Frosting

Prep time: 15 minutes| Cook time: 30 minutes| Serves: 6

Carrot cake
1½ cups carrots, grated finely
¾ cups sugar substitute
¼ cup brown sugar substitute
½ cup coconut oil, melted
2 large eggs
¼ cup flax meal
½ teaspoon baking soda
½ teaspoon ground cinnamon

¼ teaspoon ground nutmeg
¾ cup almond flour
Cream cheese frosting
8 ounces cream cheese, softened
2 tablespoons pure Grade B maple syrup
¼ teaspoon pure vanilla extract
¼ cup toasted walnuts, chopped (optional for garnish)

1. Preheat the oven to 350°F/177°C temperature setting and grease a 9-inch round cake pan with oil. 2. Blend the sugars, coconut oil, and eggs using a hand mixer. 3. Whisk the all dry ingredients together until well combined. Add the dry ingredients slowly and keep blending until no lumps remain. 4. Add in the grated carrots and pour the cake batter into the cake pan. Bake the cake for 30 minutes. 5. Remove from oven and allow to cool. Beat the cream cheese, maple syrup, and vanilla extract until light and fluffy to prepare the frosting. 6. Top the cake with the frosting, sprinkle with toasted walnuts, slice, and serve!
Per Serving: Calories 479; Fat 45g; Sodium 236mg; Carbs 14g; Fiber 5g; Sugar 7g; Protein 11g

Coconut Nut Cookies

Prep time: 10 minutes| Cook time: 15 minutes| Serves: 6

1¼ cups almond flour
½ cup unsweetened, shredded coconut
3 large eggs
6 tablespoons butter, softened

⅓ cup pure Grade B maple syrup
1 teaspoon almond extract
¼ teaspoon ground cinnamon
¼ teaspoon sea salt

1. Preheat the oven to 350°F/177°C. Prepare a metal baking sheet with parchment paper or non-stick spray. 2. Use a hand mixer to blend the maple syrup with the softened butter until smooth and creamy. 3. Add the eggs and mix well. Add the almond flour, almond extract, cinnamon, and salt with the mixer on low, mixing until combined. 4. Stir in the shredded coconut. Drop the spoonful onto the baking sheet. 5. Bake for 12-15 minutes, until golden brown around the edges.
Per Serving: Calories 271; Fat 25g; Sodium 347mg; Carbs 5g; Fiber 3g; Sugar 5g; Protein 7g

Peanut Butter with Jelly Cookies

Prep time: 10 minutes| Cook time: 12 minutes| Serves: 6

⅔ cup creamy peanut butter
⅓ cup sugar-free strawberry preserves
⅓ cup almond flour
1 egg

½ cup sugar substitute
¼ teaspoon pure vanilla extract
¼ teaspoon baking powder
¼ teaspoon sea salt

1. Preheat the oven to 350°F/177°C. Prepare a metal baking sheet by lining it with parchment paper or nonstick spray. 2. Beat the egg with the peanut butter and sugar substitute in a large bowl until smooth and creamy. Add the almond flour along with baking powder, salt, and vanilla extract. Mix well to form a dough. 3. Shape mix into balls and place them on the prepared baking sheet. 4. Make a small well in the middle of each cookie and fill with about 1 teaspoon of the preserves. 5. Bake it for 10-12 mins, until the cookies are golden brown. Cool on a wire rack, and enjoy!
Per Serving: Calories 209; Fat 18g; Sodium 452mg; Carbs 7g; Fiber 2g; Sugar 8g; Protein 9g

Chocolate Truffles

Prep time: 10 minutes| Cook time: 20 minutes| Serves: 6

4 ounces unsweetened dark chocolate
1 tablespoon raw unsweetened cocoa powder
1 tablespoon pure maple syrup

1½ tablespoons butter
⅓ cup heavy cream
¼ teaspoon pure vanilla extract
¼ teaspoon ground cinnamon
Pinch of sea salt

1. Chop the dark chocolate finely. 2. Heat the cream in a saucepan. Mix in the chopped chocolate and butter. Stir until melted and well combined. Mix in the chopped chocolate and butter. Stir until melted and well combined. 3. Remove from heat and stir the vanilla extract, maple syrup, salt, and cinnamon. 4. Place mixture in the fridge for at least 2 hours. 5. Remove the mixture from the fridge once cooled and shape them into small balls using your palms. 6. Roll balls in cocoa powder until coated fully. Store in an airtight container in the fridge.
Per Serving: Calories 160; Fat 11g; Sodium 333mg; Carbs 11g; Fiber 1g; Sugar 2g; Protein 2g

Chocolate Coconut Torts

Prep time: 5 minutes| Cook time: 7 minutes| Serves: 6

4 ounces unsweetened dark chocolate
¼ cup unsweetened, shredded coconut
1 cup coconut flour

1 tablespoon chocolate protein powder
4 tablespoons coconut oil
⅓ cup heavy cream

1. Chop the dark chocolate into small pieces. 2. Heat the cream in a pan over medium-low heat. Add the chocolate and coconut oil and stir until melted and well combined. 3. Stir in the coconut flour and protein powder while removed from heat. Cool the mix for at least 2 hours in fridge. 4. Once cooled, shape into small balls using your palms. 5. Roll balls in the shredded coconut until coated fully.
Per Serving: Calories 326; Fat 27g; Sodium 348mg; Carbs 12g; Fiber 3g; Sugar 6g; Protein 9g

Mini Chocolaty Avocado Tarts

Prep time: 15 minutes| Cook time: 8 minutes| Serves: 4

Tart crust
2 tablespoons almond flour
1 tablespoon maple syrup
1 large egg white
¼ cup flax meal
Middle layer
4 tablespoons creamy peanut butter

2 tablespoons butter
Top layer
1 medium avocado
4 tablespoons raw unsweetened cocoa powder
¼ cup sugar substitute
2 tablespoons heavy cream
½ teaspoon pure vanilla extract

1. Preheat the oven to 350°F/177°C. 2. Mix the almond flour, flax meal, 1 tablespoon of sugar substitute, and egg white in a small bowl. 3. Press the mix into 4 small tart tins. Bake for about 8 minutes, until golden. Remove from oven and allow to cool slightly. 4. Melt the peanut butter with regular butter in a small saucepan over medium-low heat and stir until well combined. Divide evenly between the baked tart shells. Chill for 30 minutes. 5. Mix the avocado, cocoa powder, sugar substitute, heavy cream, and vanilla extract in a blender or food processor. 6. Remove the chilled tarts from the fridge, top with the blended avocado mixture, and return to the refrigerator for at least 1 hour. 7. Serve and enjoy!
Per Serving: Calories 367; Fat 33g; Sodium 357mg; Carbs 5g; Fiber 10g; Sugar 3g; Protein 11g

Nutty Chocolate Milkshake

Prep time: 5 minutes| Cook time: 0 minutes| Serves: 4

2 cups unsweetened coconut, almond, or dairy-free milk of choice
1 banana, sliced and frozen
¼ cup unsweetened coconut flakes
1 cup ice cubes

¼ cup macadamia nuts, chopped
3 tablespoons sugar-free sweetener
2 tablespoons raw unsweetened cocoa powder
Whipped coconut cream (optional for garnish)

1. Mix all the ingredients in blender until smooth and creamy. If desired, divide evenly between 4 "mocktail" glasses and top with whipped coconut cream. 2. Add a cocktail umbrella and toasted coconut for added flair. 3. Enjoy your delicious Choco-nut smoothie!
Per Serving: Calories 199; Fat 17g; Sodium 347mg; Carbs 12g; Fiber 4g; Sugar 8g; Protein 3g

Nutty Chocolate Fudge

Prep time: 10 minutes| Cook time: 5 minutes| Serves: 4

2 tablespoons raw unsweetened cocoa powder
2 tablespoons sugar substitute
3 tablespoons coconut oil
¼ cup chopped walnuts
¼ cup heavy cream
1 teaspoon pure vanilla extract

1. Place the coconut oil in a metal bowl atop a pot of simmering water. Stir until melted. 2. Whisk in the cocoa powder along with sugar substitute. Remove from heat and stir in the walnuts, heavy cream, and vanilla extract. 3. Stir until well combined and pour into chocolate molds or a square tray. 4. Let cool, then transfer to the fridge to harden. 5. Remove from the fridge and enjoy your delicious chocolate walnut fudge.
Per Serving: Calories 168; Fat 18g; Sodium 478mg; Carbs 3g; Fiber 1g; Sugar 2g; Protein 3g

Creamy Coconut Brownies

Prep time: 10 minutes| Cook time: 25 minutes| Serves: 6

¾ cup coconut butter, melted
⅓ cup coconut cream
¼ cup raw unsweetened cocoa powder
¼ cup coconut flour
2 tablespoons butter, melted
½ cup sugar substitute
1 egg
1 teaspoon pure vanilla extract
¼ teaspoon baking soda
Pinch of sea salt

1. Whisk the coconut flour, cocoa powder, sugar substitute, baking soda, and salt together in a large bowl. 2. Whisk the coconut butter, coconut cream, and butter together in a separate bowl until well combined. Whisk in the egg and vanilla extract. 3. Stir in the dry ingredients slowly into the wet ingredients and mix well. 4. Transfer the mixture into a 9-inch by 3-inch loaf pan that has been prepared with nonstick cooking spray. 5. Bake at 350°F/177°C temperature setting for 20 minutes or until a toothpick inserted comes out clean. Cut into squares and enjoy!
Per Serving: Calories 175; Fat 17g; Sodium 541mg; Carbs 5g; Fiber 3g; Sugar 8g; Protein 3g

Blueberry Ice Cream

Prep time: 15 minutes| Cook time: 0 minutes| Serves: 4

¼ cup sour cream
1 cup heavy whipping cream
¼ cup fresh blueberries
1 egg yolk, beaten
2 teaspoons pure vanilla extract

1. Whip the sour cream with a hand mixer until frothy. 2. Whip the heavy cream in a separate bowl until soft peaks form. 3. Fold the sour cream with the whipped cream carefully. Puree the blueberries in a food processor or blender until smooth. 4. Stir the blueberry puree, egg yolk, and vanilla extract into the whipped cream mixture. Mix until just combined. 5. Transfer mixture into a loaf pan and freeze for 2 hours, stirring well every 30 minutes. 6. Scoop into serving bowls and enjoy your fresh blueberry ice cream!
Per Serving: Calories 153; Fat 15g; Sodium 690mg; Carbs 3g; Fiber 0g; Sugar 3g; Protein 2g

Chocolate Macaroons

Prep time: 10 minutes| Cook time: 25 minutes| Serves: 3

1 cup unsweetened shredded coconut
2 ounces dark chocolate (80% cocoa or higher)
2 large egg whites
¼ cup sugar substitute
2 tablespoons coconut oil
1 teaspoon pure vanilla extract
Pinch of sea salt

1. Preheat the oven to 350°F/177°C. Prepare a metal baking sheet by lining it with parchment paper. 2. Spread the shredded coconut evenly onto the baking sheet and place in the oven to toast for 3-5 minutes or until light brown and fragrant. 3. Beat the egg whites with an electric mixer in a large mixing bowl. Add the sugar substitute slowly and continue mixing until stiff peaks form. 4. Stir in the coconut along with vanilla extract, and salt. 5. Prepare a baking sheet with parchment paper. Shape into balls and drop them onto the prepared baking sheet. 6. Bake for 15-18 minutes until golden brown. Cool it on a wire rack. 7. Melt the chocolate with the coconut oil. Stir until well combined. 8. Drizzle the macaroons with the melted chocolate and enjoy!
Per Serving: Calories 143; Fat 12g; Sodium 689mg; Carbs 8g; Fiber 2g; Sugar 6g; Protein 3g

Regular Peanut Butter Cookies

Prep time: 10 minutes| Cook time: 14 to 16 minutes| Serves: 6

½ cup creamy peanut butter
½ cup coconut flour
¼ cup sugar substitute
1 egg
¼ teaspoon pure vanilla extract
Pinch of sea salt

1. Preheat the oven to 350°F/177°C. Prepare a metal baking sheet by lining it with parchment paper or non-stick cooking spray. 2. Using an electric mixer, blend all ingredients until a smooth dough forms. 3. Shape the dough into walnut-size balls and arrange them on the prepared baking sheet. 4. Using a fork, make crisscross marks on top of the balls to form cookies and bake for 14-16 minutes, until golden brown.
Per Serving: Calories 160; Fat 14g; Sodium 421mg; Carbs 5g; Fiber 3g; Sugar 3g; Protein 7g

Chocolate Tart

Prep time: 20 minutes| Cook time: 30 minutes| Serves: 4

Crust
1 cup coconut flour
¼ cup flaxseed meal
3 tablespoons sugar substitute
½ cup butter
4 egg whites
Filling
½ cup raw unsweetened cocoa powder
1 cup heavy cream
2½ teaspoons gelatin powder
¼ cup sugar substitute
1 teaspoon pure vanilla extract
¼ cup pistachios, sliced

For the crust: 1. Preheat the oven to 375°F/191°C. Prepare a tiny tart or pie pan with nonstick cooking spray. Prepare a tiny tart or pie pan with nonstick cooking spray. 2. Combine all the crust in a food processor and pulse until well combined. Press the mix in tart pan and bake it for about 15 minutes. Remove from oven and allow to cool.
To prepare the filling: 1. Combine all stuffing (reserving the pistachios) in a blender or food processor and blend until smooth and creamy. 2. Pour the mixture into the crust, cover with plastic wrap, and refrigerate for at least 2 hours. 3. Sprinkle with the reserved pistachios, and serve!
Per Serving: Calories 490; Fat 46g; Sodium 235mg; Carbs 13g; Fiber 7g; Sugar 8g; Protein 13g

Peanut Butter Bars

Prep time: 10 minutes| Cook time: 5 minutes| Serves: 24

½ cup unsweetened dark chocolate baking chips
½ cup coconut oil
½ cup unsweetened peanut butter
1 teaspoon pure vanilla extract
2 tablespoons sugar substitute
1 teaspoon sea salt

1. Prepare a mini muffin tin with liners. 2. Add the dark chocolate, coconut oil, vanilla extract, sugar substitute, and sea salt to a stockpot and stir until thoroughly melted. 3. Pour 2 teaspoons of the chocolate mix into the base of each lined muffin tin and top with a scoop of peanut butter. Set in the freezer for about 5 minutes to harden. 4. Remove the muffin pan from the freezer and top with another 2 teaspoons of the melted chocolate mixture to thoroughly cover the peanut butter. 5. Set the pan in the freezer and freeze for another 15-20 minutes or until the peanut butter cups are hardened. 6. Store leftovers in the fridge.
Per Serving: Calories 107; Fat 10g; Sodium 714mg; Carbs 4g; Fiber 1g; Sugar 3g; Protein 2g

Strawberry Milkshake

Prep time: 2 minutes| Cook time: 0 minutes| Serves: 2

1 cup crushed ice cubes
½ cup sliced strawberries, divided
¼ cup heavy whipping cream
1 tablespoon full-fat cream cheese, softened
2 cups unsweetened vanilla
almond milk
1 scoop of low-carb vanilla protein powder
1 teaspoon pure vanilla extract
4 (1-gram) packets of sweetener, 0g net carbs

1. In a blender, add ice, then remaining ingredients, holding back 2 strawberry slices, and blend 1–2 minutes until creamy. 2. Divide evenly between two tall glasses. Garnish each glass with 1 strawberry slice. Serve immediately.
Per Serving: Calories 231; Fat 16g; Sodium 287mg; Carbs 8g; Fiber 2g; Sugar 4g; Protein 14g

Buttery Pecan Ice Cream

Prep time: 10 minutes| Cook time: 0 minutes| Serves: 4

½ cup chopped pecans
⅛ teaspoon xanthan gum
2 egg yolks
1 teaspoon pure vanilla extract

¼ cup sugar substitute
2 tablespoons butter
1 cup heavy cream

1. Melt butter over medium heat. Whisk the heavy cream into the butter after it has melted and become slightly brown. 2. Stir in the sugar substitute and mix until dissolved. 3. Add the xanthan gum and whisk until well combined. Transfer to a large metal bowl and allow to cool. 4. Add the egg yolks slowly, one at a time, using a hand mixer. 5. Stir in the pecans and vanilla extract. 6. Place the bowl in the freezer for at least 4 hours, stirring well every hour. 7. Remove from the freezer and scoop into serving bowls. 8. Garnish with additional chopped pecans, if desired, and serve!
Per Serving: Calories 230; Fat 24g; Sodium 421mg; Carbs 2g; Fiber 1g; Sugar 2g; Protein 3g

Minty Chocolate Shake

Prep time: 5 minutes| Cook time: 0 minutes| Serves: 2

1 cup full-fat coconut milk
2 tablespoons unsweetened dark chocolate, chopped
½ cup mint leaves

½ avocado pitted
1 teaspoon pure vanilla extract
1 tablespoon sugar substitute
½ cup ice

1. Add all the ingredients into blender. 2. Blend them until smooth. 3. Enjoy right away.
Per Serving: Calories 247; Fat 21g; Sodium 314mg; Carbs 18g; Fiber 7g; Sugar 8g; Protein 4g

Chocolate Almonds

Prep time: 10 minutes| Cook time: 5 minutes| Serves: 8

¾ cup unsweetened dark chocolate baking chips
1½ cups whole raw almonds

1 teaspoon pure vanilla extract
Pinch of sea salt

1. Prepare a baking sheet by paper lining and add the chocolate chips to a stockpot with the vanilla extract over low heat. Stir the chocolate until melted. 2. Add the almonds to the stockpot with the melted chocolate and stir until the almonds are coated. 3. Place the almonds onto the lined baking sheet. 4. Sprinkle with salt and set in the fridge for at least 30 minutes before serving.
Per Serving: Calories 183; Fat 15g; Sodium 314mg; Carbs 7g; Fiber 4g; Sugar 7g; Protein 4g

Healthy Almond Cookies

Prep time: 10 minutes| Cook time: 10 minutes| Serves: 18

1 cup unsweetened almond butter
½ cup sugar substitute
¼ cup unsweetened dark chocolate baking chips

1 egg
1 teaspoon baking soda
1 teaspoon pure vanilla extract
Pinch of sea salt

1. Preheat the oven to 350°F/191°C temperature setting and prepare a baking sheet by lining it with parchment paper. Add the almond butter, egg, sugar substitute, and vanilla to a large mixing bowl and stir well. 2. Add in the remaining ingredients and stir. 3. Drop the dough by 1-inch rounds onto the baking sheet and bake for 10 minutes or until the edges are brown and lightly crispy.
Per Serving: Calories 137; Fat 10g; Sodium 236mg; Carbs 10g; Fiber 1g; Sugar 3g; Protein 3g

Snicker Bites

Prep time: 10 minutes| Cook time: 0 minutes| Serves: 12

1 cup unsweetened peanut butter
¼ cup sugar substitute
¼ cup unsweetened dark chocolate baking chips
3 tablespoons coconut flour

2 tablespoons unsweetened almond milk
1 teaspoon ground cinnamon
1 teaspoon pure vanilla extract
Pinch of sea salt

1. Prepare a baking sheet with parchment paper. 2. Mix all the ingredients well. Set in the fridge for 30 minutes. 3. Remove from the fridge, roll into 12 bite-sized balls, and place on the lined baking

sheet. Set in the refrigerator for another hour before serving.
Per Serving: Calories 194; Fat 14g; Sodium 259mg; Carbs 12g; Fiber 3g; Sugar 5g; Protein 7g

Delicious Swoop Cream

Prep time: 10 minutes| Cook time: 0 minutes| Serves: 8

1 cup heavy whipping cream
¼ teaspoon liquid sweetener, 0g

net carbs
½ teaspoon pure vanilla extract

1. In a medium bowl of an electric mixer, whip all ingredients on high speed 1–2 minutes until soft peaks form.
Serve cool.
Per Serving: Calories 103; Fat 10g; Sodium 11mg; Carbs 1g; Fiber 0g; Sugar 1g; Protein 1g

Blueberry Smoothie

Prep time: 3 minutes| Cook time: 0 minutes| Serves: 2

1 cup ice cubes
¼ cup blueberries
1 cup spinach
1 cup unsweetened vanilla almond milk
1 scoop berry-flavored low-carb

protein powder
3 tablespoons heavy whipping cream
½ teaspoon pure vanilla extract
4 (1-gram) packets of sweetener, 0g net carbs

1. In a blender, add ice, then the remaining ingredients. 2. Pulse 1–2 minutes until desired consistency is reached. Serve immediately.
Per Serving: Calories 328; Fat 19g; Sodium 360mg; Carbs 12g; Fiber 3g; Sugar 7g; Protein 27g

Caramel Macchiato

Prep time: 3 minutes| Cook time: 3 minutes| Serves: 2

14 ounces brewed macchiato, hot and unsweetened
¼ cup heavy whipping cream
½ teaspoon pure vanilla extract

1 (1-gram) packet sweetener, 0g net carbs
2 tablespoons sugar-free caramel syrup

1. In an emersion blender, add all and pulse 15–30 seconds to blend. Serve immediately in two coffee mugs while still hot.
Per Serving: Calories 125; Fat 11g; Sodium 41mg; Carbs 5g; Fiber 0g; Sugar 1g; Protein 1g

Piña Colada

Prep time: 3 minutes| Cook time: 0 minutes| Serves: 2

1½ cups ice
½ teaspoon sugar-free pineapple drink enhancer
1 cup unsweetened canned coconut milk (12–14% coconut fat)

1 (1½-ounce) shot of unflavored white rum
1 teaspoon 100% lemon juice
4 whole raspberries
2 green leaves from a pineapple crown

1. Add ice and remaining ingredients except for raspberries and pineapple leaves in a blender. 2. Pulse 1–2 minutes until desired consistency is reached, adding water if needed. Divide evenly between two tall glasses. 3. Using a toothpick, pierce two raspberries and one pineapple leaf—balance garnish on the lip of the glass. Repeat for a second glass. Serve immediately.
Per Serving: Calories 199; Fat 15g; Sodium 60mg; Carbs 2g; Fiber 0g; Sugar 0g; Protein 2g

Cayenne Chocolate Pudding

Prep time: 10 minutes| Cook time: 0 minutes| Serves: 2

3 tablespoons unsweetened canned coconut milk
2 medium avocados, peeled and pitted
½ cup ice cubes
2 tablespoons unsweetened 100% cocoa powder

1 teaspoon pure vanilla extract
1 teaspoon ground cinnamon
2 tablespoons sweetener, 0g net carbs
⅛ teaspoon salt
⅛ teaspoon ground cayenne pepper

1. Add all chocolate pudding ingredients to a food processor and pulse until even and creamy, 2–3 minutes, stopping midway from scraping down sides with a rubber spatula. Serve immediately.
Per Serving: Calories 299; Fat 24g; Sodium 159mg; Carbs 18g; Fiber 12g; Sugar 2g; Protein 4g

Sweet Iced Tea

Prep time: 5 minutes| Cook time: 0 minutes| Serves: 4

4 cups unsweetened brewed herbal tea, chilled
4 cups sugar-free lemonade, chilled

3 (1-gram) packets of sweetener, 0g net carbs
8 thin slices of lemon

1. Add all tea ingredients in a pitcher and stir to combine until sweetener is dissolved. Divide evenly among four tall glasses and serve immediately while still chilled.
Per Serving: Calories 6; Fat 0g; Sodium 34mg; Carbs 2g; Fiber 0g; Sugar 0g; Protein 0g

Fast Fudge

Prep time: 15 minutes| Cook time: 10 minutes| Serves: 20

2 cups unsweetened 100% cocoa powder
¾ cup unsalted butter, softened
1 cup water

⅔ cup whole milk
1 cup sweetener, 0g net carbs
1 teaspoon pure vanilla extract
¼ teaspoon salt

1. Grease a 9" × 9" baking dish. 2. Add cocoa powder and butter in the top pan of a double boiler and stir to combine. 3. Boil water over medium-high heat for a double boiler. Reduce heat to low and cover with the top pan. Stir cocoa mixture constantly while slowly adding milk, sweetener, vanilla, and salt until fudge is thoroughly blended and creamy, approximately 10 minutes. Fudge will become increasingly more and challenging to stir. 4. Transfer fudge to prepared baking dish. Using a spatula, evenly press fudge into all corners of the container. Cover and refrigerate. 5. Serve cold. Cut into serving-sized squares right before serving.
Per Serving: Calories 90; Fat 8g; Sodium 35mg; Carbs 10g; Fiber 3g; Sugar 1g; Protein 2g

Salty Pecan Bark

Prep time: 25 minutes| Cook time: 1 minutes| Serves: 6

1 cup sugar-free chocolate chips
1 tablespoon coconut oil

1 cup pecan halves
⅛ teaspoon salt

1. Prepare a baking sheet with parchment paper. 2. In a microwave-safe bowl, add chocolate chips with oil and microwave on high 30 seconds. Stir and microwave again 30 seconds. 3. Stir in pecans until coated. 4. Spread the mixture in even layer on the prepared baking sheet. Sprinkle with salt. 5. Freeze at least 20 minutes to harden. 6. Break into 1"–2" pieces and serve—store leftovers in a medium resealable container.
Per Serving: Calories 276; Fat 24g; Sodium 48mg; Carbs 21g; Fiber 11g; Sugar 1g; Protein 4g

Chocolate Chip Cookies

Prep time: 10 minutes| Cook time: 20 minutes| Serves: 8

1 ¼ cups superfine blanched almond flour
3 ½ tablespoons full-fat cream cheese, softened
¼ cup unsalted butter, softened

¼ cup sweetener, 0g net carbs
½ teaspoon pure vanilla extract
¼ cup whole macadamia nuts
2 tablespoons sugar-free chocolate chips

1. Preheat the oven to 350°F/177°C. Prepare a baking sheet with parchment paper. 2. Combine all the ingredients well except nuts and chocolate chips. Stir until thoroughly mixed and a dough forms. 3. Fold in nuts and chocolate chips until evenly incorporated. 4. Scoop out dough in 1" balls and pat down to no more than ¼" thickness. Place on parchment paper with at least ½" between cookies. 5. Bake for 20 minutes until cookies start to brown. 6. Transfer to a plate and serve warm.
Per Serving: Calories 231; Fat 21g; Sodium 24mg; Carbs 9g; Fiber 3g; Sugar 1g; Protein 5g

Strawberries Ice Cream

Prep time: 5 minutes| Cook time: 0 minutes| Serves: 2

¾ cup frozen sliced unsweetened strawberries
¾ cup heavy whipping cream, icy

6 (1-gram) packets of sweetener, 0g carbs

1. Add all ingredients and pulse 30–60 seconds until smooth and thick in a food processor. 2. Divide between two chilled bowls and serve

immediately.
Per Serving: Calories 327; Fat 31g; Sodium 34mg; Carbs 8g; Fiber 1g; Sugar 5g; Protein 2g

Sweet Bacon Cupcakes

Prep time: 10 minutes| Cook time: 20 minutes| Serves: 20

Cupcakes
½ cup unsalted butter, softened
1 cup full-fat cream cheese, softened
1 cup sweetener, 0g net carbs
1 teaspoon pure vanilla extract
2 tablespoons sugar-free pancake syrup
4 large eggs
1 tablespoon baking powder
½ teaspoon salt
2 ½ cups superfine blanched

almond flour
Maple frosting
1 cup unsalted butter, softened
1½ cups confectioners'-style sweetener, 0g net carbs
3 tablespoons heavy whipping cream
3 tablespoons sugar-free pancake syrup, divided
¼ cup cooked bacon bits
½ cup pecan halves

1. Preheat the oven to 375°F/191°C. Line twenty cups of two muffin tins with twenty cupcake liners. 2. In the medium bowl of an electric mixer, combine butter, cream cheese, sweetener, vanilla, syrup, and eggs. Beat the mix on high speed until smooth. Add baking powder and salt. Beat again, scraping sides of bowl often. Add almond flour and beat until thoroughly combined. 3. Divide batter equally among prepared muffin cups. Bake for 20 minutes until a toothpick inserted into the center of a cupcake comes out clean. Let cool for 3 minutes. 4. Remove cupcakes from tins to a cooling rack. 5. In a small bowl, mix butter, confectioners'-style sweetener, cream, and 2 teaspoons syrup and beat 2–3 minutes until thoroughly combined. 6. Pipe maple frosting onto cupcakes, leaving liners on. Evenly sprinkle bacon bits and pecans on cupcakes. Drizzle with remaining syrup.
Per Serving: Calories 299; Fat 28g; Sodium 232mg; Carbs 15g; Fiber 2g; Sugar 1g; Protein 6g

Avocado Brownies

Prep time: 5 minutes| Cook time: 25 minutes| Serves: 12

2 medium avocados, peeled, pitted, and mashed
2 large eggs, beaten
⅓ cup unsweetened cocoa powder, 100%
⅓ cup superfine blanched almond flour

¾ cup brown sugar substitute, 0g net carbs
1 teaspoon pure vanilla extract
1 teaspoon baking powder
¼ teaspoon salt
½ cup sugar-free chocolate chips

1. Preheat the oven to 350°F/177°C. Grease a 9" × 9" baking dish. 2. Blend all ingredients except chocolate chips. Blend for 2–3 minutes until creamy, often scraping batter from the sides. 3. Fold in chocolate chips and pour them into the prepared baking dish. Bake it for 25 minutes. 4. Slice into twelve servings. Serve warm.
Per Serving: Calories 109; Fat 9g; Sodium 103mg; Carbs 22g; Fiber 5g; Sugar 14g; Protein 3g

Brownie

Prep time: 1 minutes| Cook time: 1 minutes| Serves: 2

1 large egg
1 tablespoon unsweetened 100% cocoa powder
1 tablespoon sweetener

1 tablespoon Carbquik baking mix
⅛ teaspoon pure vanilla extract
⅛ teaspoon salt

1. In a well-greased coffee mug, beat the egg with a fork. 2. Add remaining ingredients and stir thoroughly to combine. 3. Microwave on high covered 45 seconds. Enjoy warm right from the mug.
Per Serving: Calories 100; Fat 6g; Sodium 401mg; Carbs 7g; Fiber 5g; Sugar 0g; Protein 8g

Vanilla Frosting

Prep time: 2 minutes| Cook time: 0 minutes| Serves: 8

3 tablespoons full-fat cream cheese, softened
1½ tablespoon heavy whipping

cream
2 tablespoons sweetener
¼ teaspoon pure vanilla extract

1. Blend all ingredients until smooth. If desired, use an electric hand mixer to smooth out any lumps. 2. Cover and refrigerate until ready to serve. Eat within four days.
Per Serving: Calories 23; Fat 2g; Sodium 20mg; Carbs 3g; Fiber 0g; Sugar 0g; Protein 0g

Hibiscus Tea

Prep time: 10 minutes| Cook time: 0 minutes| Serves: 4

6 cups unsweetened brewed hibiscus tea
¾ cup unsweetened canned coconut milk, Premium 12–14% coconut fat

6 (1-gram) packets of sweetener, 0g net carbs
2 teaspoons pure vanilla extract
1½ cups ice cubes
¼ cup fresh mint leaves

1. Add tea, coconut milk, sweetener, and vanilla to a pitcher and stir to combine until sweetener is dissolved. 2. Divide evenly among four tall glasses over ice. Top with mint leaves and serve.
Per Serving: Calories 66; Fat 6g; Sodium 26mg; Carbs 2g; Fiber 0g; Sugar 0g; Protein 1g

Berries and Cream Syrup

Prep time: 10 minutes. | Cooking time: 4 minutes. | Serves: 8

1 cup fresh strawberries
1 cup fresh blackberries
½ cup fresh blueberries
2 tablespoons lemon juice

1 tablespoon water
2 tablespoons heavy cream
¼ teaspoon xanthan gum
1 cup water

1. Place all berries, lemon juice, and water into 7-cup glass bowl. 2. Insert steam rack in Instant Pot and place bowl on top. 3. Add 1 cup water to pot. Turn the pot's lid to close. Hit the manual button and adjust time for almost 4 minutes. 4. When the pot beeps, quick-release the pressure. Pour berries and juice into a food processor or blender. 5. Pulse until smooth. Use fine-mesh strainer to remove seeds and fruit skin from mixture. 6. Whisk in heavy cream and xanthan gum. Keep in sealed container or mason jar in fridge.
Per serving: Calories: 389; Total fat 12.7g; Sodium 685mg; Total Carbs 0.9g; Fiber 3.5g; Sugars 6.5g; Protein 47.2g

Candied Pecans

Prep time: 10 minutes. | Cooking time: 3 hours. | Serves: 8

2 egg whites
2 cups whole pecans
½ cup powdered erythritol
3 tablespoons melted butter

3 teaspoons cinnamon
1 teaspoon vanilla extract
1 tablespoon water

1. Whisk egg whites and add remaining ingredients to a bowl. Place in Instant Pot and hit the slow cook button. You may use a clear slow cooker lid. 2. Place nut mixture into Instant Pot and stir every 45 minutes for almost 3 hours until pecans are softened. If they begin sticking to pot, add 1 tablespoon of water when stirring.
Per serving: Calories: 314; Total fat 13.3g; Sodium 194mg; Total Carbs 4.9g; Fiber 6.8g; Sugars 16g; Protein 26g

Crustless Berry Cheesecake

Prep time: 10 minutes. | Cooking time: 40 minutes. | Serves: 12

16 ounces' cream cheese, softened
1 cup powdered erythritol
¼ cup sour cream
2 teaspoons vanilla extract

2 eggs
2 cups water
¼ cup blackberries and strawberries for topping

1. In suitable bowl, beat cream cheese and erythritol until lump-free. 2. Add sour cream, vanilla, and eggs and gently fold until well-mixed. 3. Pour batter into 7-inch springform pan. 4. Gently tap pan on counter to remove air bubbles and level batter. 5. Cover top of pan with tinfoil. Pour water into Instant Pot and place steam rack in pot. 6. Carefully lower pan into pot. Hit the cake button and hit the adjust button to set heat to more. Set time for almost 40 minutes. 7. When the pot beeps, natural release the pressure. 8. Carefully lift pan from Instant Pot and allow to cool completely before refrigerating. 9. Place strawberries and blackberries on top of cheesecake and serve.
Per serving: Calories: 271; Total fat 22.9g; Sodium 30mg; Total Carbs 7.1g; Fiber 2.6g; Sugars 9.6g; Protein 3g

Slow Cooker Mint Hot Chocolate

Prep time: 10 minutes. | Cooking time: 60 minutes. | Serves: 4

4 cups unsweetened almond milk
½ cup heavy cream
3 tablespoons unsweetened cocoa powder

½ cup powdered erythritol
¼ cup low-carb chocolate chips
1 teaspoon vanilla extract
½ teaspoon mint extract

1. Place all the recipe ingredients into Instant Pot, place slow cooker lid on pot, and hit the slow cook button. Hit the adjust button to set heat to low and set time for almost 1 hour. 2. Stir occasionally to help chocolate chips melt and incorporate. Serve warm. Whip it!
Per serving: Calories: 345; Total fat 24.3g; Sodium 36mg; Total Carbs 4.9g; Fiber 6.8g; Sugars 23.8g; Protein 3.7g

Almond Butter Fat Bomb

Prep time: 10 minutes. | Cooking time: 3 minutes. | Serves: 6

¼ cup coconut oil
¼ cup no-sugar-added almond butter

2 tablespoons cacao powder
¼ cup powdered erythritol

1. Hit the sauté button on the Instant Pot and add coconut oil to preheat. Let coconut oil melt completely and hit the cancel button. 2. Stir in remaining ingredients. Mixture will be liquid. 3. Pour into 6 silicone molds and place into freezer for almost 30 minutes until set. Store in fridge.
Per serving: Calories: 122; Total fat 10.7g; Sodium 40mg; Total carbs 8.8g; Fiber 1.2g; Sugars 6.6g; Protein 0.8g

Blackberry Crunch

Prep time: 10 minutes. | Cooking time: 5 minutes. | Serves: 4

10 blackberries
½ teaspoon vanilla extract
2 tablespoons powdered erythritol
⅛ teaspoon xanthan gum
1 tablespoon butter

¼ cup chopped pecans
3 teaspoons almond flour
½ teaspoon cinnamon
2 teaspoons powdered erythritol
1 cup water

1. Place blackberries, vanilla, erythritol, and xanthan gum in 4-inch ramekin. Stir gently to coat blackberries. 2. In a suitable bowl, mix remaining ingredients. Sprinkle over blackberries and cover with foil. Hit the manual button and set time for almost 4 minutes. When the pot beeps, quick-release the pressure. Serve warm. Feel free to add scoop of whipped cream on top.
Per serving: Calories: 226; Total fat: 15g; saturated fat: 4g; cholesterol: 31mg; carbohydrates: 20g; Fiber: 3g; Protein: 6g

Peanut Butter Cheesecake Bites

Prep time: 10 minutes. | Cooking time: 15 minutes. | Serves: 8

16 ounces cream cheese, softened
1 cup powdered erythritol
½ cup peanut flour
¼ cup sour cream
2 teaspoons vanilla extract

2 eggs
2 cups water
¼ cup low-carb chocolate chips
1 tablespoon coconut oil

1. In suitable bowl, beat cream cheese and erythritol until smooth. Gently fold in peanut flour, sour cream, and vanilla. Fold in eggs slowly until well-mixed. 2. Pour batter into four 4-inch springform pans or silicone cupcake molds. Cover with foil. Pour water into Instant Pot and place steam rack in pot. 3. Carefully lower pan into the pot. Hit the cake button and hit the adjust button to set heat to more. Set time for almost 15 minutes. When the pot beeps, allow a full natural release. Carefully lift cups from Instant Pot and allow to cool completely before refrigerating. 4. In suitable bowl, microwave chocolate chips and coconut oil for almost 30 seconds and whisk until smooth. Drizzle over cheesecakes. Chill in fridge.
Per serving: Calories 284; Total Fat 23g; Sodium 14mg; Total Carbs 7.5g; Fiber 11.1g; Sugars 4g; Protein 6.1g

Pecan Clusters

Prep time: 10 minutes. | Cooking time: 5 minutes. | Serves: 8

3 tablespoons butter
¼ cup heavy cream
1 teaspoon vanilla extract

1 cup chopped pecans
¼ cup low-carb chocolate chips

1. Hit the sauté button on the Instant Pot and add butter to Instant Pot. Allow butter to melt and begin to turn golden brown. Once it begins to brown, immediately add heavy cream. Hit the cancel button. 2. Add vanilla and chopped pecans to Instant Pot. Allow to cool for almost 10 minutes, stirring occasionally. Spoon mixture onto parchment-lined baking sheet to form eight clusters, and scatter chocolate chips over clusters. Place in fridge to cool.
Per serving: Calories 127; Total Fat 3.5g; Sodium 54mg; Total Carbs 0.6g; Fiber 1g; Sugars 19.7g; Protein 3.9g

Classic Fudge

Prep time: 10 minutes. | Cooking time: 3 minutes. | Serves: 10

1 cup low-carb chocolate chips	¼ teaspoon cinnamon
8 ounces cream cheese	1 teaspoon vanilla extract
¼ cup erythritol	1 cup water

1. Place chocolate chips, cream cheese, erythritol, cinnamon, and vanilla into 7-cup glass bowl. Cover with foil. Place on steam rack inside Instant Pot. Pour water in bottom of pot. 2. Turn the pot's lid to close. Hit the manual button and adjust time for almost 3 minutes. When the pot beeps, allow a natural release. When pressure indicator drops, remove bowl carefully and stir ingredients until smooth. 3. Pour mixture into 8' × 8' parchment-lined pan and chill for almost 2 hours. Slice.
Per serving: Calories 150; Total Fat 3.2g; Sodium 9mg; Total Carbs 1.1g; Fiber 3g; Sugars 24.4g; Protein 1.6g

Lemon Poppy Seed Cake

Prep time: 10 minutes. | Cooking time: 25 minutes. | Serves: 6

1 cup almond flour	¼ cup heavy cream
2 eggs	⅛ cup sour cream
½ cup erythritol	½ teaspoon baking powder
2 teaspoons vanilla extract	1 cup water
1 teaspoon lemon extract	¼ cup powdered erythritol, for
1 tablespoon poppy seeds	garnish
4 tablespoons melted butter	

1. In suitable bowl, mix almond flour, eggs, erythritol, vanilla, lemon, and poppy seeds. 2. Add butter, heavy cream, sour cream, and baking powder. 3. Pour into 7-inch round cake pan. Cover with foil. 4. Pour water into Instant Pot and place steam rack in bottom. Place baking pan on steam rack and Turn the pot's lid to close. Hit the cake button and hit the adjust button to set heat to less. Set time for almost 25 minutes. 5. When the pot beeps, allow a 15-minute natural release, then quick-release the remaining pressure. Let cool completely. Sprinkle with powdered erythritol for serving.
Per serving: Calories 177; Total Fat 9.5g; Sodium 20mg; Total Carbs 1.4g; Fiber 0.1g; Sugars 16.8g; Protein 5.9g

Brownies

Prep time: 10 minutes. | Cooking time: 25 minutes. | Serves: 6

1 cup low-carb chocolate chips	½ teaspoon baking soda
1 tablespoon coconut oil	4 tablespoons melted butter
1 ounce cream cheese, warmed	¾ cup powdered erythritol
¼ cup heavy cream	1 teaspoon gelatin
1 cup almond flour	½ cup cocoa powder
2 eggs	1 cup water

1. In suitable bowl, melt chocolate chips and coconut oil in microwave in 10-second increments until melted and smooth. Keep it aside. 2. In suitable bowl, mix cream cheese, heavy cream, almond flour, eggs, baking soda, butter, erythritol, gelatin, and cocoa powder. Fold in melted chocolate. 3. Pour mixture into 7-inch round cake pan and cover with foil. Pour water into Instant Pot and place steam rack in bottom of pot. Place pan on steam rack and turn the pot's lid to close. Hit the manual button and adjust time for almost 25 minutes. When the pot beeps, allow a natural release. Serve warm.
Per serving: Calories 179; Total Fat 11.9g; Sodium 30mg; Total Carbs 1.9g; Fiber 4.3g; Sugars 23.5g; Protein 7.9g

Cinnammon Chocolate Pudding

Prep time: 10 minutes. | Cooking time: 15 minutes. | Serves: 4

2 cups unsweetened vanilla almond milk	⅛ teaspoon cinnamon
½ cup heavy cream	2 tablespoons cocoa powder
2 egg yolks	¾ teaspoon guar gum
1 teaspoon vanilla extract	¼ cup low-carb chocolate chips

1. Hit the sauté button on the Instant Pot and hit the adjust button to set heat to less. Pour half of almond milk into Instant Pot. Pour in heavy cream. Bring to gentle boil. 2. In suitable bowl, whisk yolks, vanilla, cinnamon, cocoa powder, and guar gum. Slowly whisk into milk mixture and continue quickly whisking until smooth. Hit the cancel button. 3. Add chocolate chips to pot and whisk very quickly until melted. Pour mixture into a suitable bowl and refrigerate for almost 2 hours.

Per serving: Calories: 106; Total fat 7.7g; Sodium 7mg; Total carbs 9.9g; Fiber 2.6g; Sugars 8.2g; Protein 1.4g

Chocolate Cheesecake

Prep time: 10 minutes. | Cooking time: 50 minutes. | Serves: 12

2 cups pecans	2 teaspoons vanilla extract
2 tablespoons butter	2 cups low-carb chocolate chips
16 ounces cream cheese, softened	1 tablespoon coconut oil
1 cup powdered erythritol	2 eggs
¼ cup sour cream	2 cups water
2 tablespoons cocoa powder	

1. At 400°F/204°C, preheat your oven. Place pecans and butter into food processor. Pulse until dough-like consistency. Press into bottom of 7-inch springform pan. Bake for almost 10 minutes then keep it aside to cool. 2. While crust bakes, mix cream cheese, erythritol, sour cream, cocoa powder, and vanilla in suitable bowl using a rubber spatula. Keep it aside. 3. In suitable bowl, mix chocolate chips and coconut oil. Microwave in 20-second increments until chocolate begins to melt and then stir until smooth. Gently fold chocolate mixture into cheesecake mixture. 4. Add eggs and gently fold in, careful not to overmix. Pour mixture over cooled pecan crust. Cover with foil. 5. Pour water into Instant Pot and place steam rack on bottom. Place cheesecake on steam rack and turn the pot's lid to close. Hit the manual button and adjust time for almost 40 minutes. When the pot beeps, allow a natural release. Carefully remove and let cool completely. Serve chilled.
Per serving: Calories: 374; Total fat 27.9g; Sodium 3mg; Total Carbs 5.1g; Fiber 3.8g; Sugars 26.1g; Protein 1.3g

Chocolate Mug Cake

Prep time: 10 minutes. | Cooking time: 20 minutes. | Serves: 1

1 cup water	2 tablespoons erythritol
¼ cup almond flour	½ teaspoon vanilla extract
2 tablespoons coconut flour	1 tablespoon butter
1 egg	2 teaspoons cocoa powder

1. Pour water into Instant Pot. In suitable bowl, mix remaining ingredients. Pour into 4-inch ramekin or oven-safe mug. Cover with foil. 2. Place steam rack into pot and place mug onto steam rack. Turn the pot's lid to close. Hit the manual button and adjust time for almost 20 minutes. When the pot beeps, allow a natural release. Serve warm.
Per serving: Calories: 444; Total fat 31.2g; Sodium 75mg; Total Carbs 4.4g; Fiber 6g; Sugars 31.7g; Protein 4.4g

Vanilla Tea Cake

Prep time: 10 minutes. | Cooking time: 25 minutes. | Serves: 8

1 cup almond flour	4 tablespoons melted butter
2 eggs	¼ cup heavy cream
½ cup erythritol	½ teaspoon baking powder
2 teaspoons vanilla extract	1 cup water

1. In suitable bowl, mix all the recipe ingredients except water. Pour into 7-inch round cake pan. Cover with foil. 2. Pour water into Instant Pot and place steam rack in bottom. Place baking pan on steam rack and turn the pot's lid to close. Hit the cake button and hit the adjust button to set heat to less. Set time for almost 25 minutes. 3. When the pot beeps, allow a 15-minute natural release, then quick-release the remaining pressure. Let cool completely.
Per serving: Calories: 207; Total fat 6g; Sodium 32mg; Total Carbs 9.5g; Fiber 3.9g; Sugars 31.1g; Protein 2.2g

Slow Cooker Peanut Butter Fudge

Prep time: 10 minutes. | Cooking time: 2 hours. | Serves: 12

1 cup low-carb chocolate chips	¼ cup no-sugar-added peanut
8 ounces cream cheese	butter
¼ cup erythritol	1 teaspoon vanilla extract

1. Place all the recipe ingredients into Instant Pot and cover with slow cooker lid. 2. Allow to cook on low for almost 1 hour and stir. Smooth mixture and allow to cook additional 30 minutes. Pour mixture into 8' × 8' parchment-lined pan and chill for almost 2 hours. Slice.
Per serving: Calories 213; Total Fat 12.1g; Sodium 60mg; Total Carbs 6.5g; Fiber 4.4g; Sugars 18g; Protein 2.4g

Espresso Cream

Prep time: 10 minutes. | Cooking time: 9 minutes. | Serves: 4

1 cup heavy cream	¼ cup low-carb chocolate chips
½ teaspoon espresso powder	½ cup powdered erythritol
½ teaspoon vanilla extract	3 egg yolks
2 teaspoons unsweetened cocoa powder	1 cup water

1. Hit the sauté button on the Instant Pot and add heavy cream, espresso powder, vanilla, and cocoa powder. 2. Bring mixture to boil and add chocolate chips. 3. Hit the cancel button. Stir quickly until chocolate chips are completely melted. 4. In suitable bowl, whisk erythritol and egg yolks. 5. Fold mixture into Instant Pot chocolate mix. Ladle into four (4-inch) ramekins. 6. Rinse inner pot and replace. Pour in 1 cup of water and place steam rack on bottom of pot. 7. Cover ramekins with foil and carefully place on top of steam rack. Turn the pot's lid to close. 8. Hit the manual button and adjust time for almost 9 minutes. Allow a full natural release. 9. When the pressure indicator drops, carefully remove ramekins and allow to completely cool, then refrigerate. Serve chilled with whipped topping.
Per serving: Calories: 179; Total fat 14.3g; Sodium 493mg; Total Carbs 2.3g; Fiber 2.4g; Sugars 8.7g; Protein 0.9g

Walnut Crust Pumpkin Cheesecake

Prep time: 10 minutes. | Cooking time: 50 minutes. | Serves: 6

2 cups walnuts	⅔ cup pumpkin purée
3 tablespoons melted butter	2 teaspoons pumpkin spice
1 teaspoon cinnamon	1 teaspoon vanilla extract
16 ounces cream cheese, softened	2 eggs
1 cup powdered erythritol	1 cup water
⅓ cup heavy cream	

1. At 350°F/177°C, preheat your oven. Add walnuts, butter, and cinnamon to food processor. Pulse until ball forms. Scrape down sides as necessary. Dough should hold in ball. 2. Press into greased 7-inch springform pan. Bake for almost 10 minutes or until it begins to brown. Remove and keep it aside. While crust is baking, make cheesecake filling. 3. In suitable bowl, stir cream cheese until completely smooth. Using rubber spatula, mix in erythritol, heavy cream, pumpkin purée, pumpkin spice, and vanilla. 4. In suitable bowl, whisk eggs. Slowly add them into suitable bowl, folding gently until just combined. 5. Pour mixture into crust and cover with foil. Pour water into Instant Pot and place steam rack on bottom. Place pan onto steam rack and Turn the pot's lid to close. Hit the cake button and hit the adjust button to set heat to more. Set timer for almost 40 minutes. 6. When the pot beeps, allow a full natural release. When pressure indicator drops, carefully remove pan and place on counter. Remove foil. Let cool for additional hour and then refrigerate. Serve chilled.
Per serving: Calories: 192; Total fat 6.6g; Sodium 5mg; Total Carbs 0.7g; Fiber 4.2g; Sugars 16.3g; Protein 3.8g

Personal Pumpkin Pie

Prep time: 10 minutes. | Cooking time: 40 minutes. | Serves: 6

Crust	pumpkin purée
1½ cups superfine blanched almond flour	¼ cup heavy whipping cream
½ cup unsalted butter, softened	3 tablespoons 0g net carbs sweetener
½ cup 0g net carbs sweetener	1 large egg
¼ teaspoon salt	1 teaspoon pumpkin pie spice
Filling	¼ teaspoon salt
¾ cup canned 100% pure	¼ teaspoon pure vanilla extract

1. At 425°F/218°C, preheat your oven. Lightly spray a twelve-hole muffin pan with nonstick cooking spray. 2. In a suitable bowl, mix all the recipe ingredients for the crust. Press equal amounts of crust mixture into twelve muffin cups. Use your thumbs to create a bird's-nest shape. Bake 9–10 minutes until edges start browning. 3. Remove from oven and decrease oven temperature to 350°F/177°C. 4. Next, make the filling. In a suitable mixing bowl, use a mixer to blend all filling ingredients. 5. Use an ice cream scoop to transfer equal amounts of filling into the prepared crusts. 6. Bake for 27–30 minutes. Check doneness by pushing a toothpick into the center of a "pie." It's done if the toothpick comes out dry. 7. Remove from your oven and let cool. Serve warm.
Per serving: Calories: 100; Total fat 7.2g; Sodium 113mg; Total carbs 8.3g; Fiber 1.3g; Sugars 5.4g; Protein 2.3g

Chaffle Cannoli

Prep time: 10 minutes. | Cooking time: 5 minutes. | Serves: 6

Chaffles	Cannoli topping
2 tablespoons unsalted butter, softened	1½ tablespoons sugar-free chocolate chips
2 large eggs, beaten	1½ tablespoons 4% milkfat cottage cheese
1 tablespoon 0g net carbs sweetener	1 tablespoon full-fat cream cheese, softened
3 tablespoons superfine blanched almond flour	1½ tablespoons 0g net carbs sweetener
¼ teaspoon baking powder	½ teaspoon pure vanilla extract
½ teaspoon pure vanilla extract	

1. Spray a waffle maker with nonstick cooking spray and preheat. 2. Make the chaffles. In a suitable bowl, mix all chaffle ingredients and whisk until creamy. 3. Evenly distribute batter into two waffle molds and cook for 4 minutes. 4. Remove chaffles and transfer to two serving plates. 5. Next, make the cannoli topping. In a suitable microwave-safe bowl, heat 1 tablespoon chocolate chips 30–60 seconds, stopping to stir halfway through. Stir until creamy and chocolate is fully melted. 6. In a second suitable bowl, mix all remaining cannoli topping ingredients except remaining chocolate chips and stir. Add melted chocolate and stir until mixture is creamy. 7. Create a sling with each chaffle by folding the opposite corners. 8. Stuff each chaffle with equal amounts of cannoli topping and pin the chaffle ends with toothpicks. Sprinkle remaining chocolate chips onto the exposed cannoli topping. 9. Transfer to the refrigerator to chill at least 30 minutes. Serve cold.
Per serving: Calories: 179; Total fat 14.3g; Sodium 493mg; Total Carbs 2.3g; Fiber 2.4g; Sugars 8.7g; Protein 0.9g

Best Attempt Rice Pudding

Prep time: 10 minutes. | Cooking time: 0 minutes. | Serves: 6

¼ cup frozen riced cauliflower	1 teaspoon heavy whipping cream
1 teaspoon whole white chia seeds	2 (1-g) packets 0g net carbs sweetener
1 tablespoon unsweetened vanilla almond milk	⅛ teaspoon ground cinnamon

1. In a suitable microwave-safe glass bowl, microwave cauliflower 30 seconds. 2. Add all remaining ingredients and stir. Keep it aside 5 minutes until chia softens. Serve immediately.
Per serving: Calories: 113; Total fat 1.9g; Sodium 68mg; Total Carbs 4.6g; Fiber 3.5; Sugars 16.3g; Protein 2.4g

Pumpkin Spice Latte

Prep time: 10 minutes. | Cooking time: 0 minutes. | Serves: 2

2 cups unsweetened coffee	2 teaspoons pure vanilla extract
½ cup heavy whipping cream	2 tablespoons unsalted butter, melted
½ cup canned 100% pure pumpkin purée	3 tablespoons 0g net carbs sweetener
1 teaspoon pumpkin pie spice	

1. To your high-speed blender, add all the recipe ingredients and pulse until thoroughly mixed. 2. Evenly pour mixture into two oversized microwave-safe coffee mugs. 3. Microwave each 45 seconds. Serve warm.
Per serving: Calories 127; Total Fat 3.5g; Sodium 54mg; Total Carbs 0.6g; Fiber 1g; Sugars 19.7g; Protein 3.9g

Stunt Double Chocolate Malt

Prep time: 10 minutes. | Cooking time: 0 minutes. | Serves: 1

1 cup cold coffee	¼ cup canned unsweetened, 12%–14% fat coconut milk
1 cup ice	1 tablespoon 100% cocoa powder
4 (1-g) packets 0g net carbs sweetener	½ scoop low-carb chocolate protein powder
1 small avocado, peeled, pitted, and mashed	½ teaspoon pure vanilla extract

1. Put all the recipe ingredients in your high-speed blender. Pulse 30–60 seconds until desired consistency is reached, pausing to scrape the sides of the blender halfway through. 2. Pour malt into an extra-tall glass and enjoy immediately.
Per serving: Calories 284; Total Fat 23g; Sodium 14mg; Total Carbs 7.5g; Fiber 11.1g; Sugars 4g; Protein 6.1g

Mo Milk

Prep time: 10 minutes. | Cooking time: 0 minutes. | Serves: 8

2 cups unsalted, unroasted almonds
6 cups water, and more

¼ teaspoon salt
1 tablespoon pure vanilla extract

1. Add almonds to a suitable bowl and cover with water. Cover with plastic wrap and soak overnight in the refrigerator. 2. Drain and rinse almonds and add them to your high-speed blender along with 6 cups water and remaining ingredients. Blend on high 1–3 minutes until puréed. Stop and scrape the sides of the blender with a spatula as needed. 3. Cover a suitable pitcher with a four-ply layer of cheesecloth. Strain mixture through cheesecloth into the pitcher and discard pulp. If milk in the pitcher still contains almond residue, repeat straining process. Store in the refrigerator until ready to serve. Serve chilled. Enjoy refrigerated within 4 days.
Per serving: Calories 271; Total Fat 11g; Sodium 8mg; Total Carbs 6.7g; Fiber 3.2g; Sugars 32.8g; Protein 4.2g

Sneaky Strawberry Smoothie

Prep time: 10 minutes. | Cooking time: 0 minutes. | Serves: 2

¾ cup ice
½ cup canned unsweetened, 12%–14% fat coconut milk
¾ cup water
½ scoop low-carb vanilla protein powder

½ cup frozen strawberries
¼ teaspoon pure vanilla extract
4 (1-g) packets 0g net carbs sweetener
2 tablespoons unsweetened canned dairy whipped topping

1. In your high-speed blender, pulse all the recipe ingredients except whipped topping on high until desired consistency is achieved. 2. Pour into a tall glass and top with whipped topping. Serve immediately.
Per serving: Calories: 200; Total fat 15.7g; Sodium 31mg; Total Carbs 12.5g; Fiber 2.6g; Sugars 7.3g; Protein 4.9g

Chocolate Chip Fat Bomb

Prep time: 10 minutes. | Cooking time: 2 minutes. | Serves: 12

½ cup coconut oil
½ cup no-sugar-added peanut butter

2 ounces cream cheese, warmed
¼ cup powdered erythritol
¼ cup low-carb chocolate chips

1. Hit the sauté button on the Instant Pot and add coconut oil to preheat. 2. Allow oil to melt and hit the cancel button. 3. Stir in peanut butter, cream cheese, and erythritol. 4. Pour mixture into silicone baking cups or 12-cup muffin tin and sprinkle chocolate chips into each. Place in freezer until firm then keep in fridge.
Per serving: Calories: 113; Total fat 28g; Sodium 139mg; Total Carbs 4.3g; Fiber 2.7g; Sugars 19.2g; Protein 1.5g

Chocolate Mousse

Prep time: 10 minutes. | Cooking time: 5 minutes. | Serves: 4

1 cup heavy whipping cream
½ teaspoon gelatin
1 tablespoon erythritol

1 teaspoon vanilla extract
1 cup chocolate pudding

1. In suitable bowl, place heavy cream and gelatin. Microwave for almost 10 seconds and whisk until gelatin is dissolved. 2. Add erythritol and vanilla. Whisk until soft peaks form. 3. Gently fold in chocolate pudding. Serve chilled.
Per serving: Calories: 170; Total fat 9.8g; Sodium 49mg; Total Carbs 7.4g; Fiber 1.5g; Sugars 15.5g; Protein 3.2g

Strawberry Dessert

Prep time: 10 minutes. | Cooking time: 0 minutes. | Serves: 4

1 cup sliced frozen strawberries
5 (1-g) packets 0g net carbs sweetener
1 cup full-fat, plain, Greek-style

yogurt
2 teaspoons pure vanilla extract
1 tablespoon sugar-free chocolate chips

1. Add all the recipe ingredients except chocolate chips to your high-speed blender. Pulse blender 30 seconds until mixture is creamy. 2. Divide into two dessert bowls and put in the freezer for almost 30 minutes. 3. Top each serving with equal amounts of chocolate chips. Serve immediately.
Per serving: Calories: 444; Total fat 31.2g; Sodium 75mg; Total

Carbs 4.4g; Fiber 6g; Sugars 31.7g; Protein 4.4g

Chilly Cheesecake Bars

Prep time: 10 minutes. | Cooking time: 50 minutes. | Serves: 8

1 cup superfine blanched almond flour
7 tablespoons unsalted butter, melted
8 tablespoons 0g net carbs sweetener

14 ounces full-fat cream cheese, softened
1 large egg, beaten
2 teaspoons pure vanilla extract
1 teaspoon 100% lemon juice
½ cup sugar-free chocolate chips

1. Preheat oven to 370°F/188°C. Grease a 9" × 5" loaf pan. 2. In a suitable bowl, mix flour, butter, and 2 tablespoons sweetener. 3. Transfer to a loaf pan and press evenly into bottom. Bake for 5 minutes. Remove from oven. 4. In a suitable mixing bowl, add remaining ingredients except chocolate chips. Use a mixer to combine, stopping to scrape the sides of the bowl and the beaters. Fold in chocolate chips. 5. Transfer the prepared mixture to the loaf pan, pouring over the crust, and bake covered for 40–45 minutes until firm. 6. Remove from your oven and transfer to the refrigerator. Let chill 30 minutes. Cut into eight bars. Serve cold.
Per serving: Calories: 207; Total fat 6g; Sodium 32mg; Total Carbs 9.5g; Fiber 3.9g; Sugars 31.1g; Protein 2.2g

Double Chocolate Ahoy Cookies

Prep time: 10 minutes. | Cooking time: 17 minutes. | Serves: 6

6 tablespoons unsalted butter, melted
1 large egg
1 teaspoon pure vanilla extract
9 tablespoons 0g net carbs sweetener

2 cups superfine blanched almond flour
1 teaspoon baking powder
⅛ teaspoon salt
½ cup sugar-free chocolate chips
½ tablespoon 100% cocoa powder

1. At 370°F/188°C, preheat your oven. Layer a suitable baking sheet with parchment paper. 2. In a suitable mixing bowl, mix butter, egg, vanilla, and ½ cup (8 tablespoons) sweetener and beat with a mixer 1–2 minutes until smooth. 3. Slowly beat in flour, baking powder, and salt until well blended and a batter forms. Fold in chocolate chips. 4. In a suitable bowl, mix cocoa powder and remaining 1 tablespoon sweetener. Scoop out 1" balls of dough and roll them in the cocoa mixture until completely covered. 5. Place balls spread out on the prepared baking sheet. Using your thumb, press down slightly on each ball to create a traditional cookie shape (cookies will not rise much). 6. Bake for 15–17 minutes until cookies are firm and starting to brown. Serve warm.
Per serving: Calories 177; Total Fat 9.5g; Sodium 20mg; Total Carbs 1.4g; Fiber 0.1g; Sugars 16.8g; Protein 5.9g

Christmas Dessert Salad

Prep time: 10 minutes. | Cooking time: 0 minutes. | Serves: 4

2 cups boiling water
1 (0.3-ounce) box sugar-free strawberry gelatin mix
2 cups cold water
1 (0.3-ounce) box sugar-free lime

gelatin mix
1 cup full-fat sour cream
1 cup unsweetened canned dairy whipped topping
2 tablespoons crushed pretzels

1. In a suitable heat-safe bowl, carefully stir 1 cup boiling water and strawberry gelatin until gelatin is dissolved. 2. Add 1 cup cold water and stir to combine. 3. Pour ¼ cup strawberry gelatin mix into each of eight parfait cups. Clean the bowl. 4. Cover these cups with plastic wrap and refrigerate 4 hours until firm. 5. In the same bowl, stir to mix remaining 1 cup boiling water and lime gelatin mix. Stir until gelatin is dissolved. Stir in remaining 1 cup cold water. 6. Cover it with plastic wrap and refrigerate 4 hours until firm. 7. Top each cup of set strawberry gelatin with 2 tablespoons sour cream. 8. Stir set lime gelatin while still in the suitable bowl until it's a uniform consistency of approximately ½" chunks. Add ¼ cup lime gelatin to each parfait cup. 9. Top each parfait cup with 2 tablespoons whipped topping. Finally, sprinkle even amounts of crushed pretzels on top of each cup. Serve immediately while still chilled.
Per serving: Calories 150; Total Fat 3.2g; Sodium 9mg; Total Carbs 1.1g; Fiber 3g; Sugars 24.4g; Protein 1.6g

Chapter 9 Sauces, Staples, Broths, and Dressings

Avocado-Herb Butter

Prep time: 25 minutes plus 4 hours to chill| Cook time: 0 minutes| Yields: 2 cups

¼ cup butter, at room temperature
1 avocado, peeled, pitted, and quartered
Juice of ½ lemon
2 teaspoons chopped cilantro
1 teaspoon chopped fresh basil
1 teaspoon minced garlic
Sea salt
Freshly ground black pepper

1. Place the butter, avocado, lemon juice, cilantro, basil, and garlic in a food processor and process until smooth. 2. Season the butter with salt and pepper. Shape it into a log on the parchment paper. Place the parchment butter log in the refrigerator until it is firm, about 4 hours. Slice and serve with fish or chicken. Store unused butter wrapped tightly for up to 1 week.
Per Serving (1 tablespoon): Calories 22; Fat 2g; Sodium 245mg; Carbs 1g; Fiber 0g; Sugar 0g; Protein 0g

Cinnamon Butter

Prep time: 15 minutes| Cook time: 1 hours| Serves: 16

1 cup butter, at room temperature
10 drops of, or another liquid sugar substitute
1 teaspoon pure vanilla extract
1 teaspoon ground cinnamon
¼ teaspoon salt

Mix the butter, stevia, vanilla, cinnamon, and salt in a medium bowl
Per Serving: Calories 103; Fat 12g; Sodium 247mg; Carbs 0g; Fiber 0g; Sugar 0g; Protein 0g

Horseradish Butter

Prep time: 7 minutes| Cook time: 0 minutes| Serves: 24

1 cup butter, softened
½ cup coconut oil
1 teaspoon prepared horseradish
1 garlic clove
1 tablespoon fresh chopped basil
1 tablespoon fresh chopped oregano
½ teaspoon freshly ground black pepper
¼ teaspoon sea salt

1. In a blender, pulse the butter, coconut oil, horseradish, garlic, basil, oregano, pepper, and salt until well blended. 2. Scoop the butter mixture onto a double layer of plastic wrap. 3. Fold the wrap over the butter mixture, creating a long tube. Roll in the wrap and twist the ends. Refrigerate or freeze the butter cylinder until it is substantial. Cut off a slice of butter to top vegetables, fish, or steak. Store the butter for up to 1 month.
Per Serving: Calories 108; Fat 12g; Sodium 112mg; Carbs 0g; Fiber 0g; Sugar 0g; Protein 0g

Ghee

Prep time: 2 minutes| Cook time: 6 hours| Yields: 2 cups

1 pound unsalted butter, diced

1. Place the butter in the slow cooker. 2. Cook on low with the lid open for 6 hours. Pour the melted butter through a fine-mesh cheesecloth into a bowl. 3. Cool the ghee for 30 minutes and pour it into a jar. Refrigerate for up to 2 weeks.
Per Serving: Calories 100; Fat 11g; Sodium 25mg; Carbs 0g; Fiber 0g; Sugar 0g; Protein 0g

Strawberry Butter

Prep time: 25 minutes| Cook time: 0 minutes| Yields: 3 cups

2 cups shredded unsweetened coconut
1 tablespoon coconut oil
¾ cup fresh strawberries
½ tablespoon freshly squeezed lemon juice
1 teaspoon alcohol-free pure vanilla extract

1. Puree the coconut in a food processor until it is buttery and smooth for about 15 minutes. 2. Add the coconut oil, strawberries, lemon juice, and vanilla to the coconut butter and process until very smooth. 3. Remove strawberry seeds by passing it from the fine sieve. 4. Store the strawberry butter in an airtight container in the refrigerator for up to 2 weeks. Serve chicken or fish with a spoon of this butter on top.

Per Serving: Calories 23; Fat 2g; Sodium 12mg; Carbs 1g; Fiber 0g; Sugar 0g; Protein 0g

Beef Bone Broth

Prep time: 15 minutes| Cook time: 4 hours 40 minutes| Serves: 2

1 pound beef bones
1 tablespoon apple cider vinegar
1 teaspoon sea salt
4 quarts water

1. Preheat the oven to 400°F/204°C. Spread the beef bones on a rimmed baking sheet. 2. Roast uncovered for 40 minutes or until browned. Transfer the bones to a large pot. Pour the oil from the roasting pan and use a fat separator to discard the fat. 3. Transfer the remaining bits to the pot. Add the salt, vinegar, and water to the pot and bring a gentle simmer. 4. Cook partially covered for 4 hours, skimming fat off the surface as it rises.
Per Serving: Calories 45; Fat 1g; Sodium 0mg; Carbs 0g; Fiber 0g; Sugar 0g; Protein 9g

Chicken Bone Broth

Prep time: 5 minutes| Cook time: 4 hours| Serves: 2 quarts

1 pound chicken bones, preferably roasted
1 tablespoon apple cider vinegar
1 teaspoon sea salt
4 quarts of cold water

1. Place the chicken bones, vinegar, and salt in a large pot. Cover with the water and bring to a simmer over medium heat. 2. Reduce the heat to simmer for about 4 hours, or until reduced to about 2 quarts. 3. Allow the stock to cool thoroughly before refrigerating.
Per Serving: Calories 45; Fat 1g; Sodium 35mg; Carbs 0g; Fiber 0g; Sugar 0g; Protein 9g

Italian Seasoning

Prep time: 5 minutes| Cook time: 0 minutes| Serves: 12

2 tablespoons dried basil
2 tablespoons dried oregano
2 tablespoons dried rosemary
2 tablespoons garlic powder
2 tablespoons dried thyme
2 teaspoons red pepper flakes

1. Combine all the spices. Store the spices in a sealed container at room temperature for up to 6 months.
Per Serving (1 tablespoon): Calories 11; Fat 0g; Sodium 35mg; Carbs 2g; Fiber 1g; Sugar 0g; Protein 0g

Ranch Seasoning

Prep time: 5 minutes| Cook time: 0 minutes| Serves: 10

6 tablespoons dried dill
1 tablespoon pink Himalayan salt
1 tablespoon freshly ground black
pepper
1 tablespoon onion powder
1 tablespoon garlic powder

1. Combine all the spices. Store the spices in a sealed container at room temperature for up to 6 months.
Per Serving: Calories 12; Fat 0g; Sodium 61mg; Carbs 3g; Fiber 1g; Sugar 1g; Protein 1g

Buttermilk Ranch Dressing

Prep time: 10 minutes| Cook time: 0 minutes| Yields: 1½ cups

½ cup heavy (whipping) cream
1 teaspoon apple cider vinegar
½ cup mayonnaise
¼ cup sour cream
1 tablespoon freshly squeezed lemon juice
2 tablespoons chopped fresh parsley
2 tablespoons chopped fresh chives
½ teaspoon minced garlic
¼ teaspoon ground cayenne pepper
Sea salt
Freshly ground black pepper

1. Stir the heavy cream and vinegar in a small bowl, and set aside for 10 minutes. 2. In a bowl, whisk the mayonnaise with sour cream, lemon juice, parsley, chives, garlic, cayenne pepper, and the reserved cream mixture until blended. 3. Season with salt and pepper.
Per Serving: Calories 74; Fat 6g; Sodium 24mg; Carbs 3g; Fiber 0g; Sugar 0g; Protein 2g

Lemon-Garlic Dressing

Prep time: 10 minutes| Cook time: 0 minutes| Yields: 1 cup

½ cup sour cream
¼ cup extra-virgin olive oil
1 tablespoon Dijon mustard
¼ cup freshly squeezed lemon juice
2 teaspoons minced garlic

2 teaspoons chopped fresh basil
2 teaspoons chopped fresh parsley
2 teaspoons chopped fresh thyme
Sea salt
Freshly ground black pepper

1. Whisk the sour cream, olive oil, Dijon mustard, lemon juice, garlic, basil, parsley, and thyme in a medium bowl until well blended. Season the dressing with salt and pepper. Refrigerate it for up to 1 week.
Per Serving (2 tablespoons): Calories 98; Fat 10g; Sodium 32mg; Carbs 1g; Fiber 0g; Sugar 0g; Protein 1g

Beef Stock

Prep time: 15 minutes| Cook time: 12 hours| Serves: 8 to 10

2 to 3 pounds of beef bones (beef marrow, knuckle bones, ribs, and any other bones)
8 black peppercorns
5 thyme sprigs
3 garlic cloves, peeled and crushed
2 bay leaves

1 carrot, washed and chopped into 2-inch pieces
1 celery stalk, chopped into big chunks
½ onion, peeled and quartered
1-gallon water
1 teaspoon extra-virgin olive oil

1. Preheat the oven to 350°F/177°C. Place the beef bones in a deep baking pan and roast them in the oven for about 30 minutes. 2. Place the bones to a large pot and add the peppercorns, thyme, garlic, bay leaves, carrot, celery, and onion. 3. Add the water, covering the bones thoroughly, ultimately bring to a boil over high heat, then lower the heat to simmers. Check the stock every hour for the first 3 hours, and skim off any foam from on the top. Simmer for 12 hours in total, and then remove the pot from the heat. Cool the stock for about 30 minutes. 4. Remove any large bones with tongs and strain the stock through a fine-mesh sieve. Discard the leftover vegetables and bones. 5. Pour the stock into containers with tight-fitting lids and cool thoroughly before refrigerating.
Per Serving: Calories 65; Fat 5g; Sodium 25mg; Carbs 1g; Fiber 0g; Sugar 0g; Protein 4g

Grapefruit-Tarragon Dressing

Prep time: 5 minutes| Cook time: 0 minutes| Serves: 4 to 6

½ cup avocado oil mayonnaise
2 tablespoons Dijon mustard
1 teaspoon dried tarragon
Zest and juice of ½ grapefruit (about 2 tablespoons juice)

½ teaspoon salt
¼ teaspoon freshly ground black pepper
1 to 2 tablespoons water (optional)

1. In a large mason jar or glass measuring cup, shake the mayonnaise, Dijon, tarragon, grapefruit zest and juice, salt, and pepper until smooth and creamy. If a thinner dressing is preferred, thin it out with water.
Per Serving: Calories 86; Fat 7g; Sodium 124mg; Carbs 6g; Fiber 0g; Sugar 0g; Protein 1g

Harissa Oil

Prep time: 15 minutes| Cook time: 5 minutes| Serves: 1 cup

4 to 6 medium-hot dried chiles
2 to 4 hot dried chiles de árbol
2 tablespoons coriander seeds
1 tablespoon cumin seeds
1 teaspoon caraway seeds
4 large garlic cloves, chopped

2 tablespoons tomato paste
2 teaspoons smoked paprika
1 teaspoon salt
1 cup extra-virgin olive oil, divided

1. Remove the stems and tops from the dried chiles and discard any loose seeds. In a bowl place chilies and cover with boiling water. Allow to steep for 30 minutes or until softened. 2. Remove from the water, drain off any excess liquid, and roughly chop, discarding any seeds and membranes. 3. In a large dry pan, toast the coriander, cumin, and caraway seeds over medium-high heat until very fragrant. 4. In a blender, add the chopped chiles, garlic, tomato paste, paprika, and salt and pulse until thick paste forms. 5. With the food processor running, stream in ¾ cup olive oil until well combined. 6. Transfer to a large glass jar and stir in the remaining ¼ cup of olive oil.
Per Serving: Calories 266; Fat 26g; Sodium 341mg; Carbs 6g; Fiber 1g; Sugar 0g; Protein 2g

Chimichurri

Prep time: 5 minutes| Cook time: 5 minutes| Serves: 8

1 cup fresh cilantro
2 cups fresh parsley
¼ cup red wine vinegar
3 garlic cloves, halved

½ teaspoon ground cumin
½ teaspoon red pepper flakes
¼ teaspoon pink Himalayan salt
¼ cup extra-virgin olive oil

1. Place the cilantro, parsley, vinegar, garlic, cumin, red pepper flakes, and salt in a blender or food processor. 2. Blend until the ingredients break down, about 20 seconds. Slowly pour in the oil blend until the oil is fully incorporated.
Per Serving: Calories 66; Fat 6g; Sodium 144mg; Carbs 2g; Fiber 1g; Sugar 2g; Protein 1g

Traditional Caesar Dressing

Prep time: 10 minutes plus 10 minutes to cool| Cook time: 5 minutes| Yields: 1½ cups

2 teaspoons minced garlic
4 large egg yolks
¼ cup wine vinegar
½ teaspoon dry mustard
Dash Worcestershire sauce

1 cup extra-virgin olive oil
¼ cup freshly squeezed lemon juice
Sea salt
Freshly ground black pepper

1. In a pan, add the garlic with egg yolks, vinegar, mustard, and Worcestershire sauce and whisk on low heat until bubbly and thicken about 5 minutes. 2. Remove from the heat and let it stand for about 10 minutes to cool. Transfer the yolk mixture to a bowl and whisk in the olive oil in a thin stream. 3. Whisk the lemon juice in a sauce and season the dressing with salt and pepper.
Per Serving (2 tablespoons): Calories 180; Fat 20g; Sodium 121mg; Carbs 1g; Fiber 0g; Sugar 0g; Protein 1g

Basic Marinara

Prep time: 10 minutes. | Cooking time: 65 minutes. | Serves: 4

2 tablespoons plus ¼ cup olive oil, extra-virgin
2 tablespoons unsalted butter
½ small onion, finely minced
2 ribs celery, finely minced
¼ cup minced carrot (about 1 small carrot)
4 cloves garlic, minced

1 teaspoon salt
¼ teaspoon black pepper
1 (32-ounce) can crushed tomatoes, with juices
2 tablespoons balsamic vinegar
1 teaspoon dried oregano
1 teaspoon dried rosemary
½ to 1 teaspoon red pepper flakes

1. Preheat 2 tablespoons oil and melt the butter in a suitable saucepan over medium heat. 2. Add the onion, celery, and carrot and sauté until just starting to get tender, for almost 5 minutes. Add the garlic, salt, and pepper and sauté for an additional 30 seconds. 3. Whisk in the tomatoes and their juices, vinegar, remaining ¼ cup of olive oil, oregano, rosemary, and red pepper. 4. Cook to a simmer, cover, reduce heat to low, and simmer for almost 30 to 60 minutes to allow the flavors to blend. Serve warm. The sauce will keep, tightly covered in the refrigerator, for up to 1 week. Cooled sauce can be frozen for up to 3 months.
Per serving: Calories: 11; Total fat 0.1g; Sodium 37mg; Total carbs 1.9g; Fiber 0.1g; Sugars 1.4g; Protein 0.5g

Cashew Hummus

Prep time: 10 minutes. | Cooking time: 0 minutes. | Serves: 8

1 cup raw cashews
2 small cloves garlic, peeled
3 tablespoons tahini
1 tablespoon lemon juice

1 teaspoon salt
½ teaspoon smoked paprika
¼ cup olive oil, extra-virgin

1. Place the cashews in a suitable bowl and cover with cold water. Cover the bowl and soak in the refrigerator overnight or up to 24 hours. 2. Drain the water from the cashews and place them in the bowl of a food processor. Add the garlic and tahini and process until smooth but thick. Add the lemon juice, salt, and paprika and pulse until well combined. 3. With the processor running, stream in the olive oil and process until very smooth and silky but not runny. Serve with raw veggies for dipping, such as celery, cucumber, bell pepper, or broccoli. Leftover hummus can be stored in a sealed container in the refrigerator for up to 4 days.
Per serving: Calories: 59; Total fat 4.3g; Sodium 0mg; Total carbs 5.8g; Fiber 0g; Sugars 5.8g; Protein 0g

Ranch Dressing

Prep time: 10 minutes| Cook time: 60 minutes| Serves: 16

1 cup mayonnaise
1 cup sour cream
¼ cup buttermilk
1 tablespoon onion powder
1 tablespoon dried parsley

2 teaspoons garlic powder
½ teaspoon salt
½ teaspoon dried dill
½ teaspoon mustard powder
¼ teaspoon celery salt

1. Mix the mayonnaise, sour cream, buttermilk, onion powder, parsley, garlic powder, salt, dill, mustard powder, and celery salt in a large bowl. 2. Whisk well to incorporate.
Per Serving: Calories 93; Fat 8g; Sodium 211mg; Carbs 5g; Fiber 0g; Sugar 2g; Protein 1g

Keto Peanut Butter Cups

Prep time: 10 minutes. | Cooking time: 1 minute. | Serves: 16

½ cup cacao butter or coconut oil
¼ cup unsweetened cocoa powder
2 to 4 teaspoons sweetener, sugar-free

½ teaspoon cinnamon
½ teaspoon salt
½ cup unsweetened creamy peanut butter or almond butter

1. Layer a mini muffin tin with 16 liners. 2. Place the cacao butter and cocoa powder into a microwave-safe bowl and microwave on high for almost 30 to 45 seconds or until melted. Stir until creamy. 3. Whisk in the sweetener (if using), cinnamon (if using), and salt. Spoon half of the chocolate mixture into the 16 cups, spreading to cover the bottom of the liner. Reserve the other half of the chocolate mixture. Place this pan in the freezer for almost 10 minutes to set. 4. In a suitable, microwave-safe bowl, microwave the nut butter for almost 30 seconds, until soft, then spread on top of the chocolate in the cups. Freeze for almost 10 minutes. 5. Microwave the cacao butter mixture for an additional 30 seconds, just to soften it. Dollop the remaining chocolate on top of the nut butter. 6. Return this pan to the freezer and freeze until solid. for almost 2 hours. Once frozen, peanut butter cups can be transferred to a zip-top bag and stored in the refrigerator for up to 2 weeks or the freezer for up to 3 months.
Per serving: Calories: 149; Total fat 16.2g; Sodium 116mg; Total carbs 2.2g; Fiber 0.8g; Sugars 0.6g; Protein 1.6g

Mustard Shallot Vinaigrette

Prep time: 10 minutes| Cook time: 0 minutes| Serves: 8

½ cup olive oil
½ cup apple cider vinegar
3 tablespoons Dijon mustard
1 shallot, minced

½ teaspoon salt
¼ teaspoon freshly ground black pepper

1. Add the olive oil, cider vinegar, mustard, shallot, salt, and pepper in a blender or food processor. Pulse for about 1 minute until combined.
Per Serving: Calories 117; Fat 13g; Sodium 222mg; Carbs 1g; Fiber 0g; Sugar 0g; Protein 0g

Herbed Balsamic Dressing

Prep time: 4minutes| Cook time: 0 minutes| Serves: 8

1 cup extra-virgin olive oil
¼ cup balsamic vinegar
2 tablespoons chopped fresh oregano

1 teaspoon chopped fresh basil
1 teaspoon minced garlic
Sea salt
Freshly ground black pepper

1. Whisk the olive oil with vinegar in a bowl until emulsified, about 3 minutes. Whisk in the oregano, basil, and garlic until well combined, about 1 minute. 2. Season the dressing with salt and pepper.
Per Serving: Calories 83; Fat 9g; Sodium 35mg; Carbs 0g; Fiber 0g; Sugar 0g; Protein 0g

Herbed Infused Olive Oil

Prep time: 5 minutes| Cook time: 45 minutes| Serves: 8

1 cup extra-virgin olive oil
4 large garlic cloves, smashed

4 (4- to 5-inch) sprigs of rosemary

1. Heat the olive oil, garlic, and rosemary sprigs in a medium pan over low heat. Cook until fragrant and garlic is very tender, for 30 to 45 minutes, stirring occasionally. 2. Remove the rosemary and garlic with a slotted spoon and pour the oil into a glass container. 3. Allow

cooling thoroughly before covering.
Per Serving: Calories 241; Fat 27g; Sodium 11mg; Carbs 1g; Fiber 0g; Sugar 0g; Protein 0g

Ginger with Lime Dressing

Prep time: 5 minutes| Cook time: 0 minutes| Serves: 8

1 cup extra-virgin olive oil
Juice of 3 limes
2 inches fresh ginger, peeled
1 teaspoon ground cumin

⅓ teaspoon ground cardamom
1 drop of liquid stevia
Sea salt

1. Blend the oil, lime juice, ginger, cumin, cardamom, stevia, and salt in a high-powered blender. Refrigerate the dressing in a covered container for up to 1 week.
Per Serving: Calories 245; Fat 27g; Sodium 321mg; Carbs 0g; Fiber 0g; Sugar 0g; Protein 0g

Garlic and Herb Marinade

Prep time: 15 minutes| Cook time: 0 minutes| Serves: 8

½ cup olive oil
Juice and zest of ½ lemon
Juice and zest of ½ lime
1½ teaspoons minced garlic

2 teaspoons chopped fresh basil
2 teaspoons chopped fresh thyme
1 teaspoon chopped fresh oregano
¼ teaspoon sea salt

1. Whisk the olive oil, lemon and lime juices and zests, garlic, basil, thyme, oregano, and salt in a medium bowl until well combined.
Per Serving: Calories 122; Fat 14g; Sodium 111mg; Carbs 1g; Fiber 0g; Sugar 0g; Protein 0g

Lemon-Tahini Dressing

Prep time: 5 minutes| Cook time: 0 minutes| Serves: 8 to 10

½ cup tahini
¼ cup lemon juice
¼ cup extra-virgin olive oil

1 garlic clove, finely minced or ½ teaspoon of garlic powder
2 teaspoons salt

1. In a jar with a lid, mix tahini, lemon juice, olive oil, garlic, and salt. Cover and shake well until combined and creamy. Refrigerate for up to 2 weeks.
Per Serving: Calories 121; Fat 12g; Sodium 211mg; Carbs 3g; Fiber 1g; Sugar 1g; Protein 2g

Any-Herb Pesto

Prep time: 10 minutes. | Cooking time: 0 minutes. | Serves: 8

4 cups packed baby arugula leaves
1 cup packed basil leaves
1 cup walnuts, chopped
½ cup shredded parmesan cheese

2 small garlic cloves, peeled and smashed
½ teaspoon salt
¾ cup olive oil

1. In a food processor, pulse the arugula, basil, walnuts, cheese, and garlic until very finely chopped. Add the salt. With the processor running, stream in the olive oil until well blended and smooth. 2. Transfer the prepared mixture to a glass container and store, tightly covered in the refrigerator, for up to 2 weeks.
Per serving: Calories: 102; Total fat 8.5g; Sodium 54mg; Total carbs 6g; Fiber 2.1g; Sugars 2.9g; Protein 2.4g

Bacon Jam

Prep time: 10 minutes. | Cooking time: 4 hrs. | Serves: 12

3 tablespoons bacon fat, melted and divided
1 pound cooked bacon, chopped into ½-inch pieces
1 sweet onion, diced

½ cup apple cider vinegar
¼ cup granulated erythritol
1 tablespoon minced garlic
1 cup brewed decaffeinated coffee

1. Lightly grease the insert of the slow cooker with 1 tablespoon of the bacon fat. 2. Add the remaining 2 tablespoons of the bacon fat, bacon, onion, apple cider vinegar, erythritol, garlic, and coffee to the insert. Stir to combine. 3. Cook uncovered for almost 3 to 4 hours on high, until the liquid has thickened and reduced. 4. Cool completely. Store the bacon jam in the refrigerator in a sealed container for up to 3 weeks.
Per serving: Calories: 179; Total fat 14.3g; Sodium 493mg; Total Carbs 2.3g; Fiber 2.4g; Sugars 8.7g; Protein 0.9g

Coconut-Curry Simmer Sauce

Prep time: 10 minutes. | Cooking time: 5 minutes. | Serves: 12

1 (14½-ounce) can full-fat coconut milk	1 tablespoon soy sauce
Zest and juice of 1 lime	1 teaspoon ground ginger
2 tablespoons curry powder	1 teaspoon garlic powder
	½ to 1 teaspoon cayenne pepper

1. Whisk all the recipe ingredients in a suitable saucepan over medium-high heat and bring just below a boil. Remove from heat and allow to cool to room temperature. The sauce will keep, tightly covered in the refrigerator, for up to 1 week.
Per serving: Calories: 100; Total fat 7.2g; Sodium 113mg; Total carbs 8.3g; Fiber 1.3g; Sugars 5.4g; Protein 2.3g

Red Wine Vinaigrette

Prep time: 10 minutes. | Cooking time: 0 minutes. | Serves: 8

½ cup olive oil	as rosemary, basil, thyme, or oregano
½ cup red wine vinegar	
1 tablespoon Dijon or stone-ground mustard	½ teaspoon salt
½ to 1 teaspoon dried herbs such	¼ teaspoon black pepper

1. In a suitable bowl or canning jar, mix all the recipe ingredients and whisk or shake until well combined. The dressing will keep, tightly covered in the refrigerator, for up to 2 weeks. Be sure to bring it to room temperature and shake well before serving, as the oil and vinegar will naturally separate.
Per serving: Calories: 204; Total fat 2.5g; Sodium 35mg; Total Carbs 6.4g; Fiber 1g; Sugars 37.3g; Protein 1g

Easiest Creamy Caesar Dressing

Prep time: 10 minutes. | Cooking time: 0 minutes. | Serves: 8

1 cup mayonnaise	1 teaspoon anchovy paste
2 small garlic cloves, pressed with a garlic press (or 1 teaspoon garlic powder)	1 teaspoon Worcestershire sauce
	½ cup freshly grated parmesan cheese
2 tablespoons freshly squeezed lemon juice, from 1 lemon	¼ teaspoon salt
2 teaspoons Dijon mustard	¼ teaspoon black pepper

1. In a canning jar or suitable bowl, mix the mayonnaise, garlic, lemon juice, mustard, anchovy paste, and Worcestershire and whisk well. 2. Add the cheese, salt, and pepper and whisk until well combined and smooth. The dressing will keep, tightly covered in the refrigerator, for up to 1 week. Shake or whisk again before serving.
Per serving: Calories: 192; Total fat 6.6g; Sodium 5mg; Total Carbs 0.7g; Fiber 4.2g; Sugars 16.3g; Protein 3.8g

Basil Dressing

Prep time: 10 minutes| Cook time: 0 minutes| Serves: 1 cup

1 avocado, peeled and pitted	lime juice
¼ cup sour cream	1 teaspoon minced garlic
¼ cup extra-virgin olive oil	Sea salt
¼ cup chopped fresh basil	Freshly ground black pepper
1 tablespoon freshly squeezed	

1. Place the avocado, sour cream, olive oil, basil, lime juice, and garlic in a food processor and pulse until smooth. Season the dressing with salt and pepper.
Per Serving: Calories 173; Fat 17g; Sodium 321mg; Carbs 1g; Fiber 0g; Sugar 0g; Protein 5g

Tangy Citrus-Poppyseed Dressing

Prep time: 10 minutes. | Cooking time: 0 minutes. | Serves: 8

½ cup mayonnaise	sugar-free
2 tablespoons buttermilk	1 teaspoon dried tarragon
2 tablespoons sour cream	½ teaspoon salt
Zest and juice of 1 small orange	¼ teaspoon black pepper
2 teaspoons sweetener of choice,	1 tablespoon poppy seeds

1. In a canning jar or suitable bowl, mix the mayonnaise, buttermilk, sour cream, orange zest and juice, sweetener (if using), tarragon, salt, and pepper and whisk well. 2. Add the poppy seeds and shake or whisk until well combined and smooth. The dressing will keep

covered tightly in the refrigerator for up to 1 week. Shake or whisk again before serving.
Per serving: Calories: 242; Total fat 17g; Sodium 17mg; Total Carbs 8.8g; Fiber 2.9g; Sugars 14g; Protein 5.4g

Marinara Sauce

Prep time: 10 minutes. | Cooking time: 8 hours. | Serves: 12

3 tablespoons olive oil, extra-virgin	2 teaspoons minced garlic
2 (28-ounce) cans crushed tomatoes	½ teaspoon salt
	1 tablespoon chopped fresh basil
½ sweet onion, finely chopped	1 tablespoon chopped fresh oregano

1. Lightly grease the insert of the slow cooker with 1 tablespoon of the olive oil. 2. Add the remaining 2 tablespoons of the olive oil, tomatoes, onion, garlic, and salt to the insert, stirring to combine. 3. Cover and cook on low for almost 7 to 8 hours. 4. Remove the cover and stir in the basil and oregano. 5. Store the cooled sauce in a sealed container in the refrigerator for up to 1 week.
Per serving: Calories: 166; Total fat 19g; Sodium 2mg; Total carbs 0.5g; Fiber 0.1g; Sugars 0.1g; Protein 0.2g

Bolognese Sauce

Prep time: 10 minutes. | Cooking time: 7 to 8 hours. | Serves: 10

3 tablespoons olive oil, extra-virgin	1 tablespoon minced garlic
1 pound ground pork	2 celery stalks, chopped
½ pound ground beef	1 carrot, chopped
½ pound bacon, chopped	2 (28-ounce) cans diced tomatoes
1 sweet onion, chopped	½ cup coconut milk
	¼ cup apple cider vinegar

1. Lightly grease the insert of the slow cooker with 1 tablespoon of the olive oil. 2. In a suitable skillet over medium-high heat, heat the remaining 2 tablespoons of the olive oil. Add the pork, beef, and bacon, and sauté until cooked through. for almost 7 minutes. 3. Stir in the onion and garlic and sauté for an additional 2 minutes. 4. Transfer the meat mixture to the insert and add the celery, carrot, tomatoes, coconut milk, and apple cider vinegar. 5. Cover and cook on low for almost 7 to 8 hours. 6. Serve, or cool completely, and store in the refrigerator in a sealed container for up to 4 days or in the freezer for almost 1 month.
Per serving: Calories: 31; Total fat 0.5g; Sodium 2mg; Total carbs 7.5g; Fiber 2.1g; Sugars 4.2g; Protein 0.7g

Bone and Veggies Broth

Prep time: 10 minutes. | Cooking time: 24 hrs. | Serves: 8

1 tablespoon olive oil, extra-virgin	1 carrot, chopped
2 chicken carcasses, separated into pieces	½ sweet onion, cut into eighths
	2 tablespoons apple cider vinegar
2 garlic cloves, crushed	2 bay leaves
1 celery stalk, chopped	½ teaspoon black peppercorns
	Water

1. Lightly grease the insert of the slow cooker with the olive oil. 2. Place the chicken bones, garlic, celery, carrot, onion, apple cider vinegar, bay leaves, and peppercorns in the insert. Add water until the liquid reaches about 1½ inches from the top of the insert. 3. Cover and cook on low for almost 24 hours. 4. Strain the broth through a fine-mesh cheesecloth and throw away the solids. 5. Store the broth in sealed containers in the refrigerator for up to 5 days or in the freezer for up to 1 month.
Per serving: Calories: 34; Total fat 3g; Sodium 8mg; Total carbs 1.5g; Fiber 0.5g; Sugars 0g; Protein 1g

Golden Caramelized Onions

Prep time: 10 minutes. | Cooking time: 10 hours. | Serves: 12

6 sweet onions, sliced	½ teaspoon salt
¼ cup olive oil, extra-virgin	

1. In a suitable bowl, toss the onions, oil, and salt. Transfer the prepared mixture to the insert of the slow cooker. 2. Cover and cook on low for almost 9 to 10 hours. 3. Serve, or store after cooling in a sealed container in the refrigerator for up to 5 days.
Per serving: Calories: 67; Total fat 6.1g; Sodium 149mg; Total carbs 2.5g; Fiber 1.3g; Sugars 0.4g; Protein 1.9g

Spinach-Cheese Spread

Prep time: 10 minutes. | Cooking time: 6 hrs. | Serves: 8

1 tablespoon olive oil, extra-virgin
8 ounces cream cheese
1 cup sour cream
½ cup shredded cheddar cheese
½ cup shredded mozzarella
cheese
½ cup parmesan cheese
½ sweet onion, finely chopped
2 teaspoons minced garlic
12 ounces chopped spinach

1. Grease an 8-by-4-inch loaf pan with the olive oil. 2. In a suitable bowl, stir the cream cheese, sour cream, cheddar, mozzarella, parmesan, onion, garlic, and spinach until well mixed. 3. Transfer the prepared mixture to the loaf pan and place this pan in the insert of the slow cooker. Cover and cook on low for almost 5 to 6 hours. Serve warm.

Per serving: Calories: 40; Total fat 3.1g; Sodium 81mg; Total carbs 2.7g; Fiber 0.5g; Sugars 1.5g; Protein 1g

Carolina Barbecue Sauce

Prep time: 10 minutes. | Cooking time: 3 hours. | Serves: 2 cups

3 tablespoons olive oil, extra-virgin
2 (6 ounces) cans tomato paste
½ cup apple cider vinegar
½ cup water
¼ cup granulated erythritol
1 tablespoon smoked paprika
1 teaspoon garlic powder
1 teaspoon onion powder
½ teaspoon chili powder
¼ teaspoon salt

1. Grease the insert of the slow cooker with 1 tablespoon olive oil. 2. In a suitable bowl, beat the tomato paste, remaining olive oil, vinegar, water, erythritol, paprika, garlic powder, onion powder, chili powder, and salt until blended. 3. Pour the prepared mixture into a slow cooker insert. 4. Cover and cook on low for almost 3 hours. 5. After cooling, store the sauce in a container in the refrigerator for up to 2 weeks.

Per serving: Calories: 33; Total fat 3.5g; Sodium 62mg; Total carbs 0.6g; Fiber 0.2g; Sugars 0.1g; Protein 0.2g

Roasted Garlic

Prep time: 10 minutes. | Cooking time: 8 hours. | Serves: 12

6 heads garlic
¼ cup olive oil
Salt, for seasoning

1. Lay a suitable sheet of foil sheet on your counter. 2. Cut the top off the heads of garlic, exposing the cloves. 3. Place the garlic, cut side up, on the foil and drizzle them with the olive oil. 4. Lightly season the garlic with salt. 5. Loosely fold the foil around the garlic to form a packet. 6. Place the packet in the insert of the slow cooker. 7. Cover and cook on low for almost 8 hours. 8. Let the garlic cool for almost 10 minutes and then squeeze the cloves out of the papery skins. 9. Store the garlic in a sealed container in the refrigerator for up to 1 week.

Per serving: Calories: 47; Total fat 1.7g; Sodium 5mg; Total carbs 8.5g; Fiber 0.5g; Sugars 6.7g; Protein 0.3g

Herbed Vegetable Broth

Prep time: 10 minutes. | Cooking time: 8 hours. | Serves: 8

1 tablespoon olive oil, extra-virgin
4 garlic cloves, crushed
2 celery stalks with greens, chopped
1 sweet onion, quartered
1 carrot, chopped
½ cup chopped parsley
4 thyme sprigs
2 bay leaves
½ teaspoon black peppercorns
½ teaspoon salt
8 cups water

1. Lightly grease the insert of the slow cooker with the olive oil. 2. Place the garlic, celery, onion, carrot, parsley, thyme, bay leaves, peppercorns, and salt in the insert. Add the water. 3. Cover and cook on low for almost 8 hours. 4. Strain the broth through a fine-mesh cheesecloth and throw away the solids. 5. Store the broth in sealed containers in the refrigerator for up to 5 days or in the freezer for up to 1 month.

Per serving: Calories: 41; Total fat 2.1g; Sodium 35mg; Total carbs 5.1g; Fiber 0.1g; Sugars 4g; Protein 0.4g

Crab Sauce

Prep time: 10 minutes. | Cooking time: 6 hrs. | Serves: 24

8 ounces cream cheese
8 ounces goat cheese
1 cup sour cream
½ cup grated asiago cheese
1 sweet onion, finely chopped
1 tablespoon granulated erythritol
2 teaspoons minced garlic
12 ounces crabmeat, flaked
1 scallion, white and green parts, chopped

1. In a suitable bowl, stir the cream cheese, goat cheese, sour cream, asiago cheese, onion, erythritol, garlic, crabmeat, and scallion until well mixed. 2. Transfer the prepared mixture to an 8-by-4-inch loaf pan and place this pan in the insert of the slow cooker. 3. Cover and cook on low for almost 5 to 6 hours. Serve warm.

Per serving: Calories: 93; Total fat 7.1g; Sodium 632mg; Total carbs 7.9g; Fiber 1.9g; Sugars 3.7g; Protein 0.8g

Herbed Beef Bone Broth

Prep time: 10 minutes. | Cooking time: 24 hours. | Serves: 8

1 tablespoon olive oil, extra-virgin
2 pounds beef bones with marrow
2 celery stalks with greens, chopped
1 carrot, chopped
1 sweet onion, quartered
4 garlic cloves, crushed
2 tablespoons apple cider vinegar
½ teaspoon whole black peppercorns
½ teaspoon salt
2 bay leaves
5 parsley sprigs
4 thyme sprigs
Water

1. Lightly grease the insert of the slow cooker with the olive oil. 2. Place the beef bones, celery, carrot, onion, garlic, apple cider vinegar, peppercorns, salt, bay leaves, parsley, and thyme in the insert. Add water until the liquid reaches about 1½ inches from the top. 3. Cover and cook on low for almost 24 hours. 4. Strain the broth through a fine-mesh cheesecloth and throw away the solids. 5. Store the broth in sealed containers in the refrigerator for up to 5 days or in the freezer for up to 1 month.

Per serving: Calories: 78; Total fat 8.5g; Sodium 42mg; Total carbs 1.1g; Fiber 0.6g; Sugars 0.1g; Protein 0.4g

Herbed Chicken Stock

Prep time: 15 minutes| Cook time: 12 hours plus 30 minutes to cool| Serves: 8 cups

2 chicken carcasses
6 black peppercorns
4 thyme sprigs
3 bay leaves
2 celery stalks, cut into quarters
1 carrot, washed and chopped roughly
1 sweet onion, peeled and quartered
1 gallon of cold water

1. Place the chicken carcasses in a large stockpot with peppercorns, thyme, bay leaves, celery, carrot, and onion. Add the water, covering them thoroughly, and bring it to a boil over high heat. 2. Lower heat to simmer, stirring every few hours, for 12 hours. When done let the stock cool for 30 minutes. Remove any large bones with tongs and then strain the stock through a fine-mesh sieve. Discard the solid bits. 3. Pour the stock into containers with tight-fitting lids and cool thoroughly. Refrigerate for up to 5 days, or freeze for 3 months.

Per Serving: Calories 73; Fat 5g; Sodium 41mg; Carbs 2g; Fiber 0g; Sugar 0g; Protein 5g

Enchilada Sauce

Prep time: 10 minutes. | Cooking time: 7 to 8 hours. | Serves: 8

¼ cup olive oil, extra-virgin
2 cups puréed tomatoes
1 cup water
1 sweet onion, chopped
2 jalapeño peppers, chopped
2 teaspoons minced garlic
2 tablespoons chili powder
1 teaspoon ground coriander

1. Lightly grease the insert of the slow cooker with 1 tablespoon of the olive oil. 2. Place the remaining 3 tablespoons of the olive oil, tomatoes, water, onion, jalapeño peppers, garlic, chili powder, and coriander in the insert. 3. Cover and cook on low 7 to 8 hours. 4. Serve over poultry or meat. After cooling, store the sauce in a sealed container in the refrigerator for up to 1 week.

Per serving: Calories: 114; Total fat 0.4g; Sodium 2mg; Total Carbs 9.6g; Fiber 3.7g; Sugars 23.7g; Protein 1.2g

Conclusion

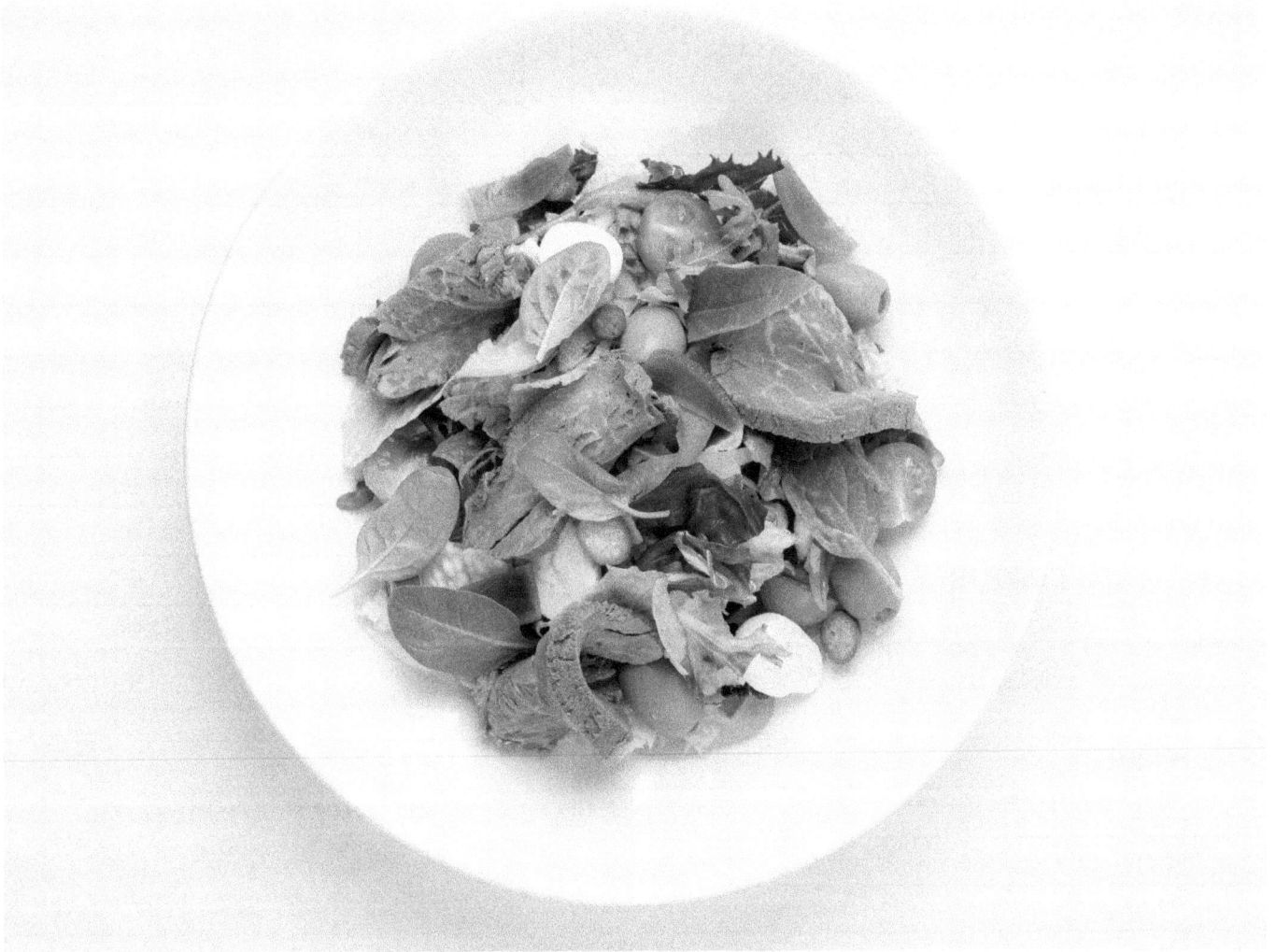

So, what do you think? Is the ketogenic diet worth a try? It was my pleasure to write such a comprehensive text on the low-carb, high-fat approach. And it will be more exciting to see my readers using this dietary regime to cope with their health problems. Since I have said it before, the more keto success stories I hear, the more I feel proud to be a part of this keto family. So why don't you join in and become an active member of this worldwide community, spread the word and share your experience with others as well? You can recommend this book to your friends and family as well to help them get started with the basics of the ketogenic diet. If you have health enthusiasts around you, then you can always try gifting them this ketogenic diet book and make them live the healthy and active life they ever dreamed of.

Appendix 1 Measurement Conversion Chart

VOLUME EQUIVALENTS (LIQUID)

US STANDARD	US STANDARD (OUNCES)	METRIC (APPROXIMATE)
2 tablespoons	1 fl.oz	30 mL
¼ cup	2 fl.oz	60 mL
½ cup	4 fl.oz	120 mL
1 cup	8 fl.oz	240 mL
1½ cup	12 fl.oz	355 mL
2 cups or 1 pint	16 fl.oz	475 mL
4 cups or 1 quart	32 fl.oz	1 L
1 gallon	128 fl.oz	4 L

TEMPERATURES EQUIVALENTS

FAHRENHEIT(F)	CELSIUS(C) (APPROXIMATE)
225 °F	107 °C
250 °F	120 °C
275 °F	135 °C
300 °F	150 °C
325 °F	160 °C
350 °F	180 °C
375 °F	190 °C
400 °F	205 °C
425 °F	220 °C
450 °F	235 °C
475 °F	245 °C
500 °F	260 °C

VOLUME EQUIVALENTS (DRY)

US STANDARD	METRIC (APPROXIMATE)
⅛ teaspoon	0.5 mL
¼ teaspoon	1 mL
½ teaspoon	2 mL
¾ teaspoon	4 mL
1 teaspoon	5 mL
1 tablespoon	15 mL
¼ cup	59 mL
½ cup	118 mL
¾ cup	177 mL
1 cup	235 mL
2 cups	475 mL
3 cups	700 mL
4 cups	1 L

WEIGHT EQUIVALENTS

US STANDARD	METRIC (APPROXINATE)
1 ounce	28 g
2 ounces	57 g
5 ounces	142 g
10 ounces	284 g
15 ounces	425 g
16 ounces (1 pound)	455 g
1.5 pounds	680 g
2 pounds	907 g

Appendix 2 Recipes Index

Lightning Source UK Ltd.
Milton Keynes UK
UKHW032241060223
416580UK00007B/707

9 781801 218306